Immunology of Human Papillomaviruses

Immunology of Human Papillomaviruses

Edited by

Margaret A. Stanley
Department of Pathology
University of Cambridge
Cambridge, United Kingdom

Plenum Press ● New York and London

Library of Congress Cataloging-in-Publication Data

Immunology of human papillomaviruses / edited by Margaret A. Stanley.
      p.   cm.
   Includes bibliographical references and index.
   ISBN 0-306-44714-2
   1. Papillomavirus diseases--Immunological aspects--Congresses.
I. Stanley, Margaret A. II. International Workshop on HPV
Immunology (2nd : 1993 : Cambridge, England)
   [DNLM: 1. Papillomavirus, Human--immunology--congresses.
2. Papovaviridae Infections--immunology--congresses. 3. Tumor Virus
Infections--immunology--congresses. QW 165.5.P2 I33 1994]
QR201.P26I56 1994
616'.0194--dc20
DNLM/DLC
for Library of Congress   94-10556
                                                     CIP

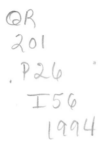
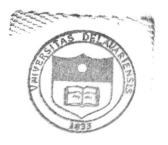

Proceedings of the Second International Workshop on HPV Immunology, held July 5–7, 1993, in
Cambridge, United Kingdom

ISBN 0-306-44714-2

©1994 Plenum Press, New York
A Division of Plenum Publishing Corporation
233 Spring Street, New York, N.Y. 10013

PREFACE

This volume represents a series of papers presented at the Second International Workshop on HPV Immunology held at the University of Cambridge July 5-7 1993. This Workshop and its predecessor held in Amsterdam in May 1992 were two of the major activities of the European Concerted Action "Immunology of Human Papillomavirus and Vaccine Development". The Concerted Action (CA) was supported by grants from the Commission of the European Communities (EC), the French Association for Cancer Research (ARC) and the European Association for Medical Research (EAMR). Twenty-two laboratories throughout Europe and Scandinavia were members of the CA, the objectives of which were to develop collaborations, implement scientific exchanges and co-operate in a collective effort to develop vaccination strategies for HPV.

HPV's are ubiquitous pathogens and evidence which has been accumulated over the past decade leaves little doubt that infection with certain HPV types (the so called "oncogenic HPV's" 16, 18 and their relatives) is the major risk factor in the development of cancer of the uterine cervix in women. Since an infectious agent, a virus, is implicated as the main aetiologic factor in this disease, the possibility is raised that if one could prevent HPV infection or treat established infections this would be an effective anti-cancer strategy against what is the commonest cancer in women worldwide. The development and implementation of such strategies requires an understanding of the host immune response to HPV, - the mechanisms underlying virus clearance (or the failure of these) and the establishment of protective immunity. Meeting these objectives for papillomaviruses is more difficult than for most other viral pathogens. Papillomaviruses are strictly intraepithelial pathogens: they are slow growing and establish chronic persistent lesions of skin and internal mucosae. Viral gene expression is confined to keratinocytes and is linked inextricably to the differentiation programme of the epithelium. Vegetative viral growth and virus assembly occur only in terminally differentiating cells far removed from systemic immune defences.

These facets of papillomavirus biology and the consequences for the host response were addressed in presentations at the Workshop. The meeting format was one of keynote talks from internationally recognised authorities, oral presentations and posters. The sessions covered HPV gene expression, T cell responses, epitope recognition, MHC expression, serology and vaccine development. The chapters in this book are representative of the plenary and poster sessions although not all the presentations are included. Contributions to the volume were made voluntarily in order to encourage presentation of unpublished data and to implement widespread participation.

The meeting was highly successful due to the participation of those who attended and their truly international backgrounds. More than 150 people from Europe, USA, South America, South Africa, China, India, South East Asia and Australasia attended. Particularly important were the keynote speakers David Lane, Peter Parham, Klas Kärre, Herman Waldmann, Lutz Gissmann, Kes Melief and Alan Rickinson who reviewed viral and cellular immunological topics of related importance thus broadening and informing the discussions for HPV.

Particular thanks and acknowledgement must be given to: the Scientific Committee of Peter Beverley, Arséne Burny, Lutz Gissmann, Mark Krul, Kes Melief, Gim Meneguzzi, Bodil Norrild and Peter Stern for the content and balance of the programme: to Hans Stauss, Peter Beverley and Peter Stern of the local organising committee for their hard work: to Philip Stanley of CRTT Ltd for the smooth conference organisation and administration and to Ann Aves for indefatigable secretarial support.

The Workshop and the publication of these Proceedings were generously supported by the EC, ARC and EAMR. I am grateful also to Cantab Pharmaceuticals Research plc; British Biotechnology Ltd; The Wellcome Foundation; Roche Products Ltd and Murex Diagnostics Ltd for their sponsorship of the Workshop.

Margaret Stanley

Department of Pathology
University of Cambridge

CONTENTS

HPV GENE EXPRESSION

HUMORAL RESPONSES TO HPV

CELL MEDIATED IMMUNITY TO HPV

ANIMAL MODELS AND THERAPEUTIC STRATEGIES

THE ANTIBODY RESPONSE AGAINST P53 IN CANCER PATIENTS

Greg Matlashewski

Institute of Parasitology and the McGill Cancer Centre
McGill University
21,111 Lakeshore Road
Ste Anne De Bellevue
Montreal
Quebec
Canada H9X 3V9

INTRODUCTION

The most common genetic alteration described to date associated with human tumour cells are those associated the p53 gene (reviewed in [1,2] and [3]). Frequently, the genetic alterations include missense mutations within the most conserved regions of the protein coding sequence giving rise to the synthesis of a mutant p53 protein. The wild type p53 is thought to act in a policeman role to stop the proliferation of, or mediate apoptosis, in cells which have sustained damage to their genome (reviewed in [3] and [4]). Replication should not occur in cells which have sustained genetic mutations to ensure that the genotypic and phenotypic integrity of the cell will be maintained. This can be considered as a safeguard against either defective cells, or worse, transformed cells. In this manner, the p53 gene product acts as a defence measure against the development of tumours and alterations in this gene can therefore be considered as a significant step toward tumorigenesis.

The idea that p53 is associated with this damage control role comes largely from the observations that high levels of p53 can be induced by DNA damaging agents and that the induced p53 inhibits cell proliferation at the late G1 phase of the cell cycle, possibly allowing for repair of damaged DNA before entry into S phase.[5,6]. This hypothesis is further supported by the important observation that mice with deleted p53 genes develop normally, are immunologically competent and are fertile[7]. However, these p53 null mice developed a variety of tumours at a very early age. This observation revealed that p53 acts as a tumour inhibitor and is not involved in biochemical pathways needed for essential cellular activity. Finally, cells derived from such p53 null mice are unable to undergo DNA damage induced apoptosis [8,9]. Taken together, abrogation of the p53 pathway appears to contribute to the propagation of cells with genetic lesions which is the basis for tumour development.

Efforts are underway to define the biological activity of p53. Wild-type p53 has been shown to be capable of regulating the transcription of various cellular genes. For example, genes which contain a TATA box in their promoters are repressed by wild-type but not mutant p53 [10,11]. The shut-down of this broad class of genes by increasing the level of wild type p53 could be important for the p53-mediated G1 arrest following DNA damage. Interestingly, p53 is also capable of binding to specific DNA sequences resulting in the stimulation of gene expression [12,13]. These target genes may include those responsible for growth arrest and/or DNA repair.

Mutant p53 by itself is capable of immortalising primary cells and together with the activated *ras* oncogene, can fully transform primary cells (reviewed in [1,2] and [3]). It is presently unclear whether the mutant p53 acts as a dominant oncogene in this manner through complexing and inactivation the wild-type p53 or whether there is a gain of function associated with the mutant p53 molecules. In *in vitro* transformation assays it has also been demonstrated that the wild-type p53 could impair the ability of mutant p53 or viral and cellular oncogenes to cooperate with the activated *ras* oncogene to transform primary cells [14, 15]. This, together with the observation that p53 is a common target in many tumours, led to the assertion that wild-type p53 is an anti-oncogene or tumour suppressor gene. It has also been revealed that the human mutant p53 proteins which cooperate with activated *ras* have a longer cellular half-life than the wild-type p53 protein[16]. This is consistent with the knowledge that the p53 protein levels are generally higher in transformed cells than in normal cells [17]. One reason why different mutant p53s may have a longer half-life is because they are conformationally different from the wild-type p53 proteins. There is also evidence that different mutant p53 proteins may share a similar conformation which is distinct from the wild-type conformation [18]. It is therefore possible that the ubiquitin-dependent protease system which is involved in p53 degradation [19] is more active on wild-type p53 than mutant p53.

DETECTION OF ANTI-P53 ANTIBODIES IN SERA FROM CANCER PATIENTS

It is clear from the above observations that mutant p53 molecules play a role in tumourigenesis. With the current understanding that mutant p53 molecules are often present in higher levels in cancer cells than in normal cells, and that the mutant p53 molecules are conformationally different from wild-type p53, then a logical question would be whether the mutant p53 becomes antigenic in cancer patients. This issue was addressed over ten years ago before it was actually realised that the p53 gene was frequently mutated in cancer cells. In 1982, it was known that p53 levels were higher in many transformed cells than in normal cells and that SV40 transformed cells with high levels of p53 elicited anti-p53 antibodies in tumour bearing mice[20]. Based on this knowledge, Crawford *et al.*[21] looked for anti-p53 antibodies in sera from cancer patients. In this original study, anti-p53 antibodies were detected in sera from patients with primary and secondary breast carcinoma. Fourteen out of 155 sera tested positive for anti-p53 antibodies and no positivities were identified in 164 control sera from women without cancer. This observation gave support to the notion that there was a change in the amount or type of p53 in breast tumours *in vivo*. Subsequent studies at the molecular genetic level confirmed this notion.

In a subsequent study, the presence of anti-p53 antibodies and the levels of p53 protein in the tumour cells was compared in a population of sera from patients with breast and colorectal cancers[22]. In this study, sera containing anti-p53 antibodies were present in 12% of patients with colorectal cancer and 11% of patients with breast cancer. An unexpected result was that about half of the patients with anti-p53 antibodies had undetectable levels of p53 protein in their tumours. Therefore, in these individuals, although the tumours tested were p53 negative, they had at some stage been exposed to immunogenic p53. It is possible that the p53 was unstable in the tumour tissue or that the part of the tumour which was assayed was atypical. Alternatively, the anti-p53 response may have come from another tumour which was undetected or which had regressed. In a more recent study, which examined the anti-p53 antibody response in lung cancer patients, all patients with anti-p53 antibodies (5 of 5) had detectable levels of p53 protein in their tumour derived cells[23]. It however remains to be established whether the level of p53 in the tumours is a critical factor for the development of the anti-p53 response. It was also established in these studies[22,23] that some patients with high p53 levels in their tumour do not produce an anti-p53 antibody response.

It has now been established that an anti-p53 response can occur in patients with a variety of cancers. These include breast[21,22,24-26], colon[22], childhood lymphoma[27], lung[23], and ovary[26]. This list will likely expand as future studies are conducted in this area.

WHICH REGION OF P53 IS ANTIGENIC?

One of the major questions arising from these original studies was whether the immune response was directed against a single epitope on p53 or whether many epitopes were recognised by the anti-p53 sera. This issue was first addressed once a human p53 cDNA was cloned [28]. It was then possible to demonstrate that the amino terminal region containing amino acids 32 through 160 and the carboxy terminal amino acids 306 through 393 of p53 when expressed in *E. coli* were reactive with anti-p53 antibodies from breast cancer patients [29]. This revealed that there were multiple antigenic sites on the p53 molecule. It was later confirmed that the carboxy and amino termini of the p53 protein were the immunodominant regions and that the central mutational hot spot region of the p53 molecule was poorly antigenic [25]. Evidence was also presented that there was a higher proportion of anti-p53 positive sera among breast cancer patients with histological grade 3 tumours than in patients with grade 1 and 2 [25]. This provided the first indication that the circulating anti-p53 antibodies may be associated with a poor prognosis (high histological grade). Clearly, this aspect of the anti-p53 antibody response must be further explored.

WHY DOES P53 BECOME ANTIGENIC?

The percentage of cancer patients with anti-p53 antibodies is lower than the percentage which have tumours with altered p53 protein levels. The reason for this discrepancy is not known. Moreover, the molecular basis for p53 immunogenicity remains to be established. The antibody response could result from the loss of tolerance due to the high levels of p53 in some tumours and the release of p53 into the circulation through tumour necrosis. Alternatively, p53 could be recognised as foreign due to conformational changes associated with mutations within the p53 gene. However, since the antibody response appears to be directed to regions of the p53 molecule which are not mutated [25], this would favour the loss of tolerance due to increased levels of p53 in tumour cells. It has also been postulated that mutant p53's complexing with heat shock protein 70 (HSP70) may be responsible for the anti-p53 response [24]. Wild-type p53 does not complex with HSP70. This is an interesting prospect given that HPS70 is believed to be involved in protein translocation across intracellular membranes and in antigen presentation. Therefore, p53 association with HPS70 could present p53 to the immune system in the tumour cell itself in the absence of tumour necrosis. There is also evidence to suggest that an anti-p53 response occurs in patients with tumours containing missense mutations but not slice/stop or frame shift mutations in the p53 gene [23]. This may be due to the low levels of p53 related proteins resulting from these more drastic mutations. Finally the anti-p53 response could arise from a combination of the above factors. Further experiments comparing the antibody response to parameters including tumour type and grade, p53 levels, p53 mutant half-lives, and tumour necrosis are needed to resolve the issue concerning why only a subset of cancer patients with altered p53 produce anti-p53 antibodies.

ARE MUTANT P53 MOLECULES MORE ANTIGENIC THAN WILD-TYPE P53?

It has been reported that anti-p53 sera from lung cancer patients [23] and from breast cancer patients [24,25,26] could react against wild-type and mutant p53 proteins. This clearly demonstrated that the anti-p53 response was not specific to mutant p53. This was consistent with the observation that the mutational hot spot region of p53 is poorly antigenic [25]. However, the possibility existed that although the antibody response was not mutant p53 specific, the mutant p53 molecules may be more antigenic than the wild-type p53 molecule and this may be seen with antibodies reacting against conformational epitopes. To test this possibility, equal amounts of mutant and wild-type p53 molecules were synthesised in a non-denatured form using an *in vitro* transcription translation coupled system and the products were subjected to immunoprecipitation and Western blot analysis with anti-p53 sera [26]. In this manner, it was demonstrated that the anti-p53 sera from patients with a variety of cancers recognised both mutant and wild-type conformational and denaturation resistant epitopes. It was also demonstrated by dilution and immunoprecipitation analysis that the anti-p53 sera recognised mutant and wild-type p53 equally well, confirming that mutant p53 was not more antigenic than the wild-type p53.

SUMMARY AND CONCLUSIONS

p53 is currently the most intensely studied molecule associated with human cancer. Loss of wild-type p53 activity with the concomitant presence of mutant p53 is a hallmark of many tumour cells and this represents the most common molecular alteration in cancer identified to date. Progress has been rapid in identifying the structural alterations in mutant p53 and the biological consequences associated with these changes. An understanding of the p53 biochemistry may yield new strategies for the development of novel treatments of cancer. Furthermore, the identification of altered p53 in tumour cells may have implications for the prognosis of some tumours.

The analysis of the anti-p53 response may serve as an additional parameter to characterise the structure and/or biology of p53. Future studies are required to explore this possibility and to determine whether the anti-p53 response may also prove to be a useful diagnostic or prognostic indicator of tumours.

ACKNOWLEDGEMENTS

Supported by grants form the National Cancer Institute of Canada and the Natural Sciences and Engineering Research Council of Canada (NSERC). Research at the Institute of Parasitology is partially funded by NSERC and FCAR of Quebec. G.M. holds an MRC Scientist award.

REFERENCES

1. M. Hollstein, D. Sidransky, B. Vogelstein and C. Harris, p53 mutations in human cancer, *Science*, 253:49 (1991).

2. A. Levine, J. Momand and C. Finlay, The p53 tumour suppressor gene, *Nature*, 351: 453 (1991).

3. B Vogelstein and K. Kinzler, p53 function and disfunction, *Cell*, 70: 523 (1992).

4. D. Lane, A death in the life of p53, *Nature*, 362: 786 (1993).

5. M. Kastan, O. Onyekwere, D. Sidransky, B. Vogelstein and R. Craig, Participation of p53 protein in the cellular response to DNA damage, *Cancer Res.*, 51: 6304 (1991).

6. S. Kuerbitz, B. Plukett, W. Walsh and M. Kastan, Wild-type p53 is a cell cycle checkpoint determinant following irradiation, *Proc Natl Acad Sci., USA*, 89: 7491(1992).

7. L. Donehower, M. Harvey, B. Slagle, M. McArthur, C. Montgomery, J. Butel and B. Allan, Mice deficient for p53 are developmentally normal but susceptible to spontaneous tumours, *Nature*, 356:215 (1992).

8. S. Low, E. Schmitt, S. Smith, B. Osborne and T. Jacks, p53 is required for radiation induced apoptosis in mouse thymocytes, *Nature*, 362:847 (1993).

9. A. Clarke, C. Purdie, D. Harrison, R. Morris, C. Bird, M. Hooper and A. Wyllie, Thymocyte apoptosis by p53-dependent and independent pathways, *Nature*, 362:849 (1993).

10. E. Seto, A. Usheva, G. Zambetti, J. Momand, N. Horikosh, R. Weinmann, A. Levine and T. Shenk, Wildtype p53 binds to the TATA-binding protein and represses transcription, *Proc Natl Acad Sci., USA.*, 89:12028 (1992).

11. D. Mack, J. Vartikar, J. Pipas and L. Lamins, Specific repression of TATA-mediated but not initiator-mediated transcription by wildtype p53, *Nature,* 363:281 (1993).

12. S. Kern, J. Pietenpol, S. Thiagalingam, A. Seymour, K. Kinzler and B. Vogelstein, Onocogenic forms or p53 inhibit p53-regulated gene expression, *Science,* 256:827(1992).

13. G. Farmer, J. Bargonetti, H. Zhu, P. Freidman, R. Prywes and C. Prives, Wild-type p53 activates transcription in vitro, *Nature,* 358:83 (1992).

14. C. Finlay, P. Hinds and A. Levine, The p53 proto-oncogene can act as a suppressor of transformation, *Cell,* 57:1083 (1989).

15. D. Eliyahu, D. Michalovitz, S. Eliyahu, O. Pinhasi-Kimhi and M. Oren, Wild-type p53 can inhibit oncogene-mediated focus formation, *Proc Natl Acad Sci., USA,* 86:8763 (1989).

16. P. Hinds, C. Finlay, R. Quartin, S. Baker, E. Fearon, B. Vogelstein and A. Levine, Mutant p53 cDNA clones from human colon carcinomas cooperate with ras in transforming primary rat cells: A comparison of the hot spot mutant phenotypes, *Cell Growth and Diff.*, 1:571 (1990).

17. S. Benchimol, D. Pim and L. Crawford, Radioimmunoassay of the cellular protein p53 in mouse and human cell lines, *EMBO J.,* 1:1055 (1982).

18. J. Gannon, R. Greaves, R. Iggo and D. Lane, Activating mutations in p53 produce a common conformational effect. A monoclonal antibody specific for the mutant form, *EMBO J.,* 9:1595(1990).

19. M. Scheffner, B. Werness, J. Huibregtse, A. Levine and P. Howley, The E6 oncoprotein encoded by human papillomavirus types 16 and 18 promotes the degradation of p53, *Cell,* 63:1129 (1990).

20. D. Lane and L. Crawford, T antigen is bound to a host protein in SV40-transformed cells, *Nature*, 278:261- (1979).

21. L. Crawford, D. Pim and R. Bulbrook, Detection of antibodies against the cellular protein p53 in sera from patients with breast cancer, *Int J Cancer,* 30:403 (1982).

22. L. Crawford, D. Pim and P. Lamb, The cellular protein p53 in human tumours, *Mol Biol Med.,* 2:261(1984).

23. S. Winter, J. Minna, B. Johnson, T. Takashi, A. Gazdar and D. Carbone, Development of antibodies against p53 in lung cancer patients appears to be dependent on the type of p53 mutation, *Cancer Res.*, 52: 4168 (1992).

24. A. Davidoff, D. Iglehart and J. Marks, Immune response to p53 is dependent upon p53/HSP70 complexes in breast cancers, *Proc Natl Acad Sci USA*, 89:3439 (1992).

25. B. Schlichtholz, Y. Legros, D. Gillet, C. Gaillard, M. Marty, D. Lane, F. Calvo and T. Soussi, The immune response to p53 in breast cancer patients is directed against immunodominant epitopes unrelated to the mutational hot spot, *Cancer Res.*, 52:6380 (1992).

26. S. Labrecque, N. Naor, D. Thomas and G. Matlashewski, Analysis of the anti-p53 antibody response in cancer patients, *Cancer Res.*, 53:3468 (1993).

27. C. Caron de Fromentel, L. May, H. Mouriesse, J. Lemerie, K. Chandrasekaran and P. May, Presence of circulating antibodies against cellular protein p53 in a notable proportion of children with B-cell lymphoma, *Int J Cancer*, 39:185 (1987).

28. G. Matlashewski, P. Lamb, D. Pim, J. Peacock, L. Crawford and S. Benchimol, Isolation and characterization of a human p53 cDNA clone: Expression of the human p53 gene, *EMBO J.*, 3:3257 (1984).

29. G. Matlashewski, L. Banks, D. Pim and L. Crawford, Analysis of human p53 proteins and mRNA levels in normal and transformed cells, *Eur J Biochem.*, 154:665 (1986).

ENHANCED PRODUCTION OF WILD-TYPE P53 INHIBITS GROWTH AND DIFFERENTIATION OF NORMAL FORESKIN EPITHELIAL CELLS BUT NOT CELL LINES CONTAINING HUMAN PAPILLOMAVIRUS DNA

Craig D. Woodworth, Hong Wang, Luis M. Alvarez-Salas, and Joseph A. DiPaolo

Laboratory of Biology
National Cancer Institute
Bethesda
MD 20892
USA

INTRODUCTION

Normal human epithelial cells cultured from foreskin or cervical epithelia can be immortalized by a subset of HPV DNAs associated with a high risk of cervical cancer (Pirisi *et al.*, 1987; Woodworth *et al.*, 1989). The HPV-immortalized cell lines exhibit aberrant growth and differentiation when maintained as organotypic cultures (McCance *et al.*, 1988) or *in vivo* (Woodworth *et al.*, 1990). It is hypothesized that HPV oncoproteins E6 and E7 contribute to immortalization through their ability to bind the products of the tumor suppressor genes p53 and Rb, respectively (Munger *et al.*, 1992).

Recent studies have shown that the association between the HPV E6 and p53 proteins results in rapid degradation of p53 via an ubiquitin-mediated pathway (Scheffner *et al.*, 1990). The ability of HPVs to degrade the p53 protein and concomitantly alter epithelial growth and differentiation suggested that the two events may be related and raised two important questions. First, would overexpression of p53 enhance differentiation in normal keratinocytes; and second, would upregulation of p53 reverse aberrant growth and differentiation in HPV-immortalized cell lines. To test these hypotheses, high-titer recombinant retroviruses were constructed encoding wild-type p53 in sense and antisense orientation. These viruses were used to infect normal or HPV-immortalized keratinocytes, and the cells were maintained in organotypic culture (Asselineau *et al.*, 1986) to assess the effects of p53 overexpression on normal squamous differentiation.

RESULTS AND DISCUSSION

Effects on Normal Cells

Secondary cultures of normal foreskin keratinocytes were infected with recombinant retroviruses encoding sense or antisense wild-type p53 (Woodworth *et al.*, 1993). Southern analysis showed that the infected cells contained an average of 1 to 2 copies of the retroviral p53 cDNA per cell and that the transduced gene was intact and unrearranged (data not shown). Western blot analyses of cultures infected with sense constructs demonstrated a 3- to 4-fold upregulation in steady-state levels of p53 protein relative to uninfected cells or cells infected with viruses containing vector-only sequences (Figure 1). Cells infected with antisense p53 constructs had decreased expression. Thus, the retroviruses were valid tools for introducing and overexpressing sense or antisense p53 cDNAs in keratinocytes.

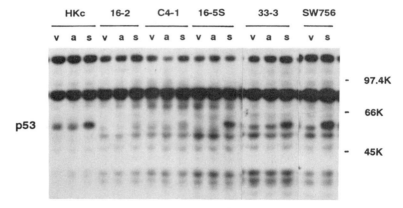

Figure 1. Western analysis of p53 protein levels in normal keratinocytes (HKc), 3 HPV-immortalized cell lines (16-2, 16-5S, 33-3) and two carcinoma-derived cell lines (C4-1, SW756). Cells were infected with retroviruses encoding sense(s), antisense (a) p53 or only vector sequences (v), and cell lysates were analyzed for p53 using the mouse monoclonal antibody to human p53 (PAb1801).

Monolayer cultures of keratinocytes infected with wild-type p53 grew slowly, and the individual cells became flattened (Figure 2A). However, no evidence of cell death or apoptosis was detected. This was in contrast to cells that received either antisense p53, vector sequences alone, or uninfected cultures. All of these cultures contained small round cells which continued to proliferate rapidly (Figure 2B).

To examine whether altered p53 expression influenced differentiation, retrovirus-infected cells were maintained in organotypic culture to promote stratification and keratinization (Asselineau *et al.*, 1986). Upregulation of p53 delayed or inhibited expression of keratin 10 and profilaggrin, two markers of squamous differentiation. Production of these two proteins was confined to the upper 1 to 2 layers of stratified cells (Figure 3). This was in contrast to the stratified epithelia formed by keratinocytes with only endogenous p53 (i.e., those infected with vector-only viruses). Keratin 10 and profilaggrin were expressed abundantly in the majority of superficial cell layers in these cultures. In fact, there was an inverse correlation between p53 and differentiation. In normal cultures endogenous p53 was detected only in the proliferating layer of basal cells and was absent in cells undergoing terminal differentiation (Figure 3). In cultures infected

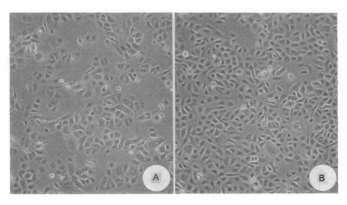

Figure 2. Morphology of keratinocytes infected with retroviruses encoding sense p53 (A) or vector-only sequences (B).

with retroviruses encoding wild-type p53, the protein was expressed in all epithelial layers, and there was a corresponding decrease in production of profilaggrin and keratin 10. Taken together these results suggest that downregulation of p53 during normal differentiation might be necessary to allow complete expression of squamous genes such as keratin 10 and profilaggrin.

Effects on Cell Lines Containing HPV

Three HPV-immortalized cell lines and two cervical carcinoma-derived cell lines containing HPV were infected with retroviruses encoding either sense p53 or vector sequences alone. Western analysis of cultures infected with vector-only viruses

11

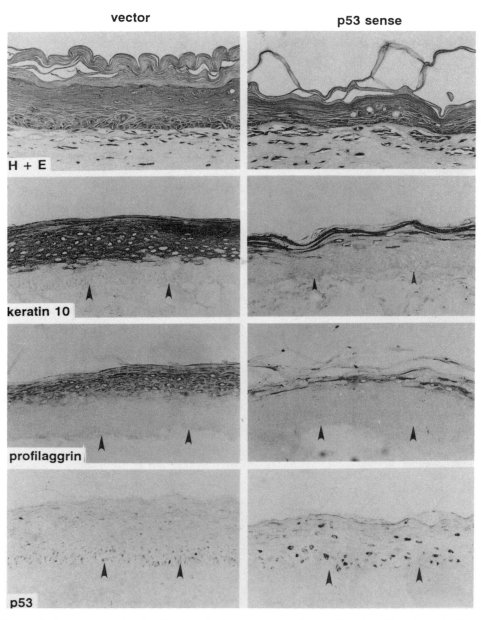

Figure 3. Immunoperoxidase localization of epidermal proteins (keratin 10 and profilaggrin) and p53 in organotypic cultures of retrovirus-infected keratinocytes. Secondary cultures of normal cells were infected with retroviruses encoding vector-only (left panel) or wild-type p53 (right panel). Sections at top were stained with hematoxylin and eosin (H+E).

demonstrated that individual cell lines expressed variable and often decreased levels of endogenous p53 protein (Figure 1). These results are in agreement with findings by other laboratories (Scheffner *et al.*, 1991; Hubbert *et al.*, 1992) and are consistent with the proposed function of the E6 protein in degradation of endogenous p53. Infection of each cell line with retroviruses encoding wild-type p53 in sense orientation resulted in increased steady-state levels of the p53 protein. The magnitude of increase was variable in different cell lines (Figure 1). All of the cell lines containing HPV grew rapidly after infection with retroviruses, and increased cell flattening or apoptosis was not detected in these cultures. No differences in growth rate were observed between cell lines with or without the exogenous retroviral p53 (Figure 4).

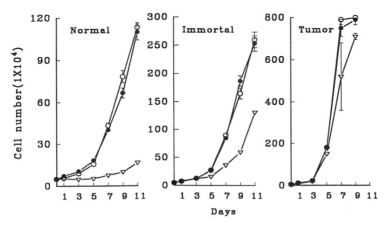

Figure 4. Regulation of cell growth by sense (▽) and antisense (○) p53 retroviruses or viruses encoding vector-only sequences (●). Infected cells were plated at low density and cell number was determined every two days.

To determine whether expression of the retroviral p53 would reverse aberrant epithelial differentiation in HPV-containing cell lines, cells were infected with sense p53 retroviruses and maintained in organotypic cultures. Cell lines containing HPV formed thick dysplastic epithelia regardless of whether they were infected with p53-containing retrovirus or not (data not shown). Thus, upregulation of steady-state levels of the p53 protein did not reverse aberrant differentiation in any of the immortal or carcinoma-derived cell lines.

Increased expression of the wild-type p53 protein inhibits growth of normal epithelial cells as well as many tumor-derived cell lines (Eliyahu *et al.*, 1989; Vogelstein *et al.*, 1992). Recently, it has been proposed that inactivation of p53 function by DNA tumor virus oncoproteins represents a critical and necessary step for transformation of cells (Levine *et al.*, 1991). Results presented here confirm that the majority of HPV-containing cells have decreased steady-state levels of endogenous p53 protein relative to normal keratinocytes. However, upregulation of steady-state levels of p53 in retrovirus-infected cells did not reverse aberrant growth or differentiation characteristic of HPV-containing cell lines. These results suggest that downregulation of total cellular p53 by E6-mediated binding and degradation is not necessarily required to maintain the immortal phenotype of these cell lines. It is expected that high-titer retroviruses encoding sense and antisense p53 cDNAs will prove useful in assessing the normal function of the p53 protein in different cell types.

REFERENCES

Asselineau, D., Bernard, B.A., Bailly, C., Darmon, M., and Pruniéras, M., 1986, Human epidermis reconstructed by culture--is it normal?, *J. Invest. Dermatol.* 86:181.

Eliyahu, D., Michalovitz, D., Eliyahu S., Pinhasi-Kimhi, O., and Oren, M., 1989, Wild type p53 can inhibit oncogene-mediated focus formation, *Proc. Natl. Acad. Sci.* (USA) 86:8763.

Hubbert, N.L., Sedman, S.A., and Schiller, J.T., 1992, Human papillomavirus type 16 E6 increases the degradation rate of p53 in human keratinocytes, *J. Virol.* 66:6237.

Levine, A.J., Momand, J., and Finlay, C.A., 1991, The p53 tumor suppressor gene, *Nature* (Lond.) 352:453.

McCance, D.J., Kopan, R., Fuchs, E., and Laimins, L.A., 1988, Human papillomavirus type 16 alters human epithelial cell differentiation *in vitro*, *Proc. Natl. Acad. Sci.* (USA) 85:7169.

Munger, K., Scheffner, M., Huibregtse, J.M., Howley, P.M., 1992, Interactions of HPV E6 and E7 oncoproteins with tumor suppressor gene products, *Cancer Surv.* 12:197.

Pirisi, L., Yasumoto, S., Feller, M., Doniger, J., and DiPaolo, J.A., 1987, Transformation of human fibroblasts and keratinocytes with human papillomavirus type 16 DNA, *J. Virol.* 61:1061.

Scheffner, M., Munger, K., Byrne, J.C., and Howley, P.M., 1991, The state of the p53 and retinoblastoma genes in human cervical carcinoma cell lines, *Proc. Natl. Acad. Sci.* (USA) 88:5523.

Scheffner, M., Werness, B.A., Huibregtse, J.M., Levine, A.J., and Howley, P.M., 1990, The E6 oncoprotein encoded by human papillomavirus types 16 and 18 promotes the degradation of p53, *Cell* 63:1129.

Vogelstein, B. and Kinzler, K.S., 1992, p53 function and dysfunction, *Cell* 70:523.

Vousden, K.H., 1990, Human papillomavirus oncoproteins, *Semin. Cancer Biol.* 1:415.

Woodworth, C.D., Doniger, J., and DiPaolo, J.A., 1989, Immortalization of human foreskin keratinocytes by various human papillomavirus DNAs corresponds to their association with cervical cancer, *J. Virol.* 63:159.

Woodworth, C.D., Waggoner, S., Barnes, W., Stoler, W.H., and DiPaolo, J.A., 1990, Human cervical and foreskin epithelial cells immortalized by human papillomavirus DNAs exhibit dysplastic differentiation *in vivo*, *Cancer Res.* 50:3709.

Woodworth C.D., Wang, H., Simpson, S., Alvarez-Salas, L.M., and Notario, V. 1993, Overexpression of wild-type p53 alters growth and differentiation of normal human keratinocytes but not human papillomavirus-expressing cell lines, *Cell Growth Diff.* 4:367.

DETECTION OF HUMAN PAPILLOMAVIRUS, EPSTEIN BARR VIRUS AND ELEVATED OR MUTANT P53 EXPRESSION IN SQUAMOUS CELL CARCINOMA OF THE HEAD AND NECK

Ilona Lewensohn-Fuchs[1], Eva Munck-Wikland[2], Zsofia Berke[1,3,4], Gorm Pallesen[5] Annika Linde[6], Klas. G. Wiman[4] and Tina Dalianis[1,3,4]

[1]Dept. of Clinical Virology, F69, [3]Dept. of Clinical Immunology, F79,
Huddinge Hospital
141 86 Huddinge
Sweden
[2]Dept. of Otorhinolaryngology
Karolinska Hospital
104 01 Stockholm
[4]Dept. of Tumour Biology, Karolinska Institute, Box 60400, 104 01
Stockholm
[5]Laboratory of Immunopathology, University Institute of Pathology,
Aarhus Kommunehospital, DK-8000 Aarhus C
Denmark.
[6]Dept. of Virology
National Bacteriological Laboratory and Karolinska Institute
105 21 Stockholm

INTRODUCTION

Human malignancies arising from the head and neck region represent a significant cause of morbidity and mortality world-wide. Tobacco and alcohol are regarded to be the most important risk factors, whereas diet and smokeless tobacco are considered to be of major importance in high endemic areas (for review see Vokes *et al.*, 1993). Increasing evidence suggests that viruses, e.g. Epstein Barr virus (EBV) and human papillomavirus (HPV), as well as mutation of tumour suppressor genes possibly caused by exogenous carcinogens, can contribute to the development of head and neck cancer (for review see Vokes *et al.*, 1993).

Immunology of Human Papillomaviruses
Edited by M.A. Stanley, Plenum Press, New York, 1994

Information on the genetic basis of a possible multistep carcinogenesis in head and neck tumours is accumulating. Mutations of p53 have been described in 50-67% of these tumours (for review see Vokes *et al.*, 1993). Based on the data mentioned above we have accumulated fresh frozen tumour tissue material from 34 Swedish patients with squamous-cell carcinoma of the head, neck and esophagus as well as from 4 controls. In total forty-one biopsies were analysed for the presence of HPV and EBV and presence of mutant or elevated p53. The patients were followed up for a minimum of 8 months, in an attempt to study the presence of these parameters and prognosis.

MATERIAL and METHODS

Study population and specimens and DNA extraction

Forty-one biopsies were collected from 34 patients with head, neck and esophageal cancer, two patients with laryngeal papillomas, and two patients that were undergoing tonsillectomy. The biopsies were divided into two, one was frozen at -70°C without any additives for PCR and p53 ELISA, the other was embedded in paraffin for histopathology and p53 immunohistochemistry.

HPV detection with general primers by PCR and HPV typing by PCR

A nested primer two step PCR according to Evander *et al.*, 1992 was used with the general primer pairs My11/My09 and GP5/GP6. HLA DQ primers were used as controls (Erlich *et al., 1989*). Positive HPV samples were tested by using 2.5 ml of the original DNA extract material for the presence of HPV types 6,16,18, 31 or 33 as described by Evander *et al.*, 1992.

EBV PCR, EBV immunohistochemistry and in situ hybridisation

A nested PCR was performed; including 0.15 mmol/l of primers derived from EBNA-1, EB-3 (bp109332-109351) and EB-4 (bp109609-109628) in 50 ml buffer of 10 mM Tris HCl pH 8.3, 50 mM KCl, 0.1% gelatine, 2.5 mM $MgCl_2$, and 125 mM of each dNTP and 1 unit Taq DNA polymerase and overlaid with mineral oil . 2.5 ml of the amplified product was transferred from the first to the second reaction mixture, which included 0.30 mmol/l of primers EB-1 (bp 109353-109372) and EB-2 (bp109542-109561) was performed. The first round consisting of 20 cycles of 1 min. at 95°C, 1 min at 55°C and 1 min. and the second round 30 cycles of 1 min at 95°C, 1 min at 60°C and 1 min. at 72°C were performed.

Immunostaining was performed using a monoclonal antibody to the immediate-early (BZLF1) protein as described by Sandvej *et al.*, 1992.

In situ hybridisation was performed with BHLF oligonucleotides available with the methodology (DAKO). BHLF deoxy-oligonucleotides are complementary to two abundant immediate early mRNAs encoded proteins (Kieff, E and Liebowitz, D.1990). EBER-1 expression was detected using single stranded digenin labelled riboprobes complementary (anti-sense probe) or anti-complementary (sense, negative control probe) to EBER-1 RNA transcripts.

Mutant p53 measured with an ELISA assay and p53 immunohistochemical staining.

The p53 ELISA assay commercially available from Oncogene Science is based on the mutant specific antibody PAb 240 (Gannon *et al.*, 1990).

Paraffin-embedded biopsies were sectioned, attached to glass slides and stained for p53 with the CM-1 antibody (Novocastra, Newcastle upon Tyne, UK) according to Pignatelli *et al., 1992.*

RESULTS AND DISCUSSION

Detection of HPV

Forty-one biopsies, listed in Table 1, were analysed for the presence of HPV with the nested general primer system and in parallel positively tested for PCR feasibility with HLA DQ-primers (data not shown). Two of the tonsil cancers and one laryngeal cancer as well as one of the laryngeal papillomas were found to be HPV positive with general and specific primers as shown in Table 1. Thus 3 (9%) of the malignancies were HPV positive a frequency comparable to that described by others. HPV type 16 was observed in two tumours of the tonsil in analogy with findings also by others. In the third HPV positive tumour, a laryngeal cancer, HPV type 31 was detected, which to our knowledge has only been detected once before among head and neck cancers. None of the tongue, hypopharyngeal or oesophageal cancers were HPV positive with this method and no HPV was found in the mucous membranes from the two patients that had undergone tonsillectomy for non-neoplastic reasons (Table 1).

Detection of EBV

All forty-one biopsies were analysed with PCR for the presence of EBV. EBV was detected in several locations, but not in any of the hypopharyngeal cancers, or in the mucosa from the two negative controls (Table 1). Of these 11 EBV PCR positive biopsies, 10 were also analysed for BHLF1 and EBER with an *in situ* hybridisation technique, and for BZLF1 with immunohistochemistry in order to detect EBV within the cancer tissues and were found to be negative.

These observations indicate, that the EBV detected by PCR is derived from

Table 1. Summary of primary site, localisation, TNM1 stage, EBV and HPV status analysed by PCR, and p53 status analysed by ELISA and immunostaining.

LOCALISATION	EBV-PCR status	HPV-PCR status	p53 ELISA-status[1]	p53 Immuno-staining.
Oesophagus	-	-	-	Few positive
Oesophagus	-	-	-	+
Oesophagus	-	-	-	N.D.[2]
Oesophagus	-	-	-	-
Oesophagus	-	-	-	-
Oesophagus	+	-	-	-
Oesophagus	+	-	+	+
Oesophagus	-	-	-	+
Oesophagus	-	-	-	-
Hypopharynx	-	-	-	-
Hypopharynx	-	-	+	-
Hypopharynx	-	-	-	+
Hypopharynx*	-	-	-	·+
Hypopharynx (op.)*	-	-	+	+
Hypopharynx (rec.)*	-	-	-	+
Larynx	-	-	+	Few postitive
Larynx	-	-	+	+
Larynx	-	-	-	-
Larynx¤	+	+/31	-	-
Larynx (laryngectomi)¤	+	-	-	-
Larynx	-	-	-	Few positive
Larynx	-	-	-	ND
Tongue	-	-	-	+
Tongue	+	-	+	ND
Tongue	-	-	-	-
Tongue	-	-	-	-
Tongue	-	-	+/-	Few positive
Tongue	+	-	+/-	-
Tonsil	-	+/16	+	Few positive
Tonsil	+	+/16	+/-	Few positive
Tonsil	-	-	-	Few positive
Tonsil	-	-	+/-	Few positive
Gingiva	+	-	+/-	+
Epipharynx	+	-	-	Few positive
Buccae	+	-	-	+
Floor of mouth	-	-	-	-
Laryngeal papilloma	-	-	-	Few positive
Laryngeal papilloma	+	+	-	-
Tonsil	-	-	-	-
Tonsil	-	-	-	-
Floor of the mouth	-	-	-	Few positive

[1] - = OD<0.125, +/- = OD=0.125-0.250, + = OD>0.250

[2] ND = not done,

*or ¤, tumours belonging to the same patients.

contaminating peripheral blood cells, and illustrates the importance of using alternative methodology to PCR for the detection of EBV.

Detection of elevated and/or mutant p53

All 41 biopsy samples were tested for mutated p53 with an ELISA assay. A total of 12/35 (34%) of the cancer biopsies were regarded as positive for mutant p53 with this assay. None of the non-malignant specimens were positive (Table 1). Of the 41 biopsies 38 were tested with immunohistochemistry for the presence of mutated p53 using the CM-1 antibody. Table 1 shows that 21/32 (63%) of the tested cancer biopsies and 2 non-malignant specimens were positive for elevated p53. The other samples were p53 negative. The different methods were not always in concordance (Table 1), which can be explained by that the ELISA technique detects p53 mutations exclusively, while the immunostaining assay detects presence of mutated p53 as well as elevated levels of wild type p53. In addition, the ELISA technique may not detect mutant p53 that is expressed only in a subfraction of the tumour cells.

No mutant p53 was detected in the HPV type 31 positive laryngeal cancer in concordance with previous studies, in contrast the findings in our two tonsil cancers, where HPV type 16 was present and mutant or elevated of p53 was indicated. Sequencing the p53 gene and investigation of whether or not the E6 gene is expressed in these tumours will be of great interest. The finding that two non-malignant lesions displayed positive p53 immunostaining deserves special attention. Both these lesions could be potentially malignant. The p53 positive, HPV negative laryngeal papilloma with a growth pattern resembling cancer, is of particular interest, since it has been shown that squamous cell carcinomas can develop, although rarely from papillomas. The second benign p53 positive lesion, could be a potential second primary tumour, which is commonly encountered in head and neck cancer patients. Taken together, this information suggests that the presence of elevated levels of p53 may be a response to DNA damage, which may result in an increased cancer incidence. It is of interest to sequence the p53 gene in these two specimens.

Follow up with regard to HPV PCR, EBV PCR and p53 status

The follow up period for all patients ranged from 8 months up to 7 years. There are no statistically significant differences with regard to HPV PCR, EBV PCR, or p53 status with regard to prognosis as yet. All patients with HPV positive cancers are still alive.

REFERENCES

Erlich, H.A., and Bugawan, T.L., 1989, HLA class II gene polymorphism; DNA typing, evolution and relationship to disease sucseptibility in PCR Technology; *Principles and Applications for DNA amplification* **Ch 16** pp. 193, Stockholm, New York .

Evander, M., Edlund, K., Boden, E., Gustavsson, Å., Jonsson, M., Karlsson, R., Rylander, E., and Wadell., G., 1992, Comparison of a one-step and a two step polymerase chain reaction with degenerate general primers in a population-based study of human papillomavirus infection in young Swedish women. *J. Clinical Microbiol.* **30,**987.

Gannon, J.V., Greaves, R., Iggo, R, and Lane D.P., 1990, Activating mutations in p53 produce a common conformational effect . A monoclonal antibody specific for the mutant form. *EMBO J.* **9**, 1595.

Kieff, E., and Liebowitz, D., 1990 Epstein-Barr virus and its replication. Editor, Fields, B.N., In Fields Virology 2nd ed. New York: Raven Press, pp 1889.

Pignatelli, M., Stamp, G.W, Kafri, G., Lane, D., and Bodmer, W.F., 1992, Over-expression of p53 nuclear oncoprotein in colorectal adenomas. *Int. J. Cancer.,* **50**, 683.

Sandvej, K., Kreancs, L., Hamilton-Dutoit, S.J., Rindum, J.L., Pindborg, J.J., and Pallesen, G., 1992, Epstein-Barr virus latent and replicative expression in oral hairy leuplakia. *Histopathology,* **20**, 387.

Vokes E.E., Weichselbaum, R.R, Lippman, S.M,and Hong., K.W., 1993, Head and neck cancer, (rev) *N.Engl. J. Med.* 184.

ELEVATED LEVELS OF THE P53 TUMOUR SUPPRESSOR PROTEIN IN THE BASAL LAYER OF RECURRENT LARYNGEAL PAPILLOMAS

[1]Louise J. Clark, [2]Kenneth MacKenzie and [1]E. Kenneth Parkinson

[1]The Beatson Institute for Cancer Research
Garscube Estate
Switchback Road
Bearsden
Glasgow G61 1BD
UK
[2]Department of Otolaryngology
Glasgow Royal Infirmary
Castle Street
Glasgow G4 0SF
UK

INTRODUCTION

A viral aetiology for recurrent respiratory papillomatosis (RRP) has long since been postulated and the human papilloma virus (HPV) types 6,11,16 and 18 have been detected reproducibly in laryngeal papillomas and squamous cell carcinomas of the head and neck (SCCs of the H & N). Whilst the underlying mechanism(s) for the abnormal proliferation of respiratory epithelial cells leading to the formation of papillomas is unknown, it is known that the above HPV types, transform keratinocytes in culture with potencies which correlate with their ability to inactivate the p53 tumour suppressor protein. The E6 proteins of HPVs 16 and 18 complex and degrade the p53 protein[1,2], whereas HPV6 and 11 E6 proteins have been reported to only weakly bind p53 without degradation[2].

Immunology of Human Papillomaviruses
Edited by M.A. Stanley, Plenum Press, New York, 1994

Normally the p53 protein turns over rapidly and is undetectable by conventional immunocytochemistry. However, certain inactive mutant forms of the p53 protein, found in SCCs of the H & N, are stable and detectable by immunocytochemistry and a similar situation may exist in keratinocytes infected with HPV 6 or 11.

We wished to investigate whether recurrent laryngeal papillomas, which contain the HPVs 6 or 11, expressed elevated levels of p53 protein, with the aim of determining whether inactivation of this tumour suppressor protein is implicated in the formation of the papillomas.

MATERIALS AND METHODS

Six patients with recurrent laryngeal papillomatosis were studied. All received laser therapy but no immunotherapy and five were non-smokers. The biopsies were taken before laser treatment and snap frozen in liquid nitrogen. Normal oral mucosa and squamous cell carcinomas from different subjects were used as controls. The immunocytochemistry, PCR and direct sequencing are described elsewhere[3] and the HPV status was confirmed using PCR with specific primers[4].

RESULTS

PCR showed the presence of either HPV 6 or HPV 11 in the recurrent laryngeal papillomas. No evidence of the HPVs 16, 18 or 33 was found (data not shown).

It could be clearly be seen from immunohistochemical staining that whilst the normal control section of human epidermis remained unstained after reaction with the p1801 p53 monoclonal antibody both laryngeal papillomas and carcinomas displayed positive nuclear staining. As described by others the p53 staining in the carcinomas was most intense in the parts of the tumour that were adjacent to the mesenchyme, but was not restricted to the basal epithelial cells. In contrast, the p53 staining in the laryngeal papillomas, was almost exclusively restricted to the basal epithelial cells and was present in all six patients. The adjacent normal epithelium did not stain, nor did normal oral mucosa from disease-free patients (data not shown). Specimens treated without antibody also did not stain.

Direct sequencing, following PCR, of exons 5, 6, 7, 8 and 9 of the p53 gene revealed no mutations. Over 99% of mutations in SCCs of the H & N occur in these regions from our work[3] and others.

Staining of multiple papillomas in the same patient is consistent with a large field change and also with the presence of HPV type 6 or 11. The possible mechanisms of p53 stabilisation and possible inactivation are discussed below, but the results do suggest that the modification of the p53 tumour suppressor protein may be commonly involved in the development of recurrent laryngeal papillomas.

DISCUSSION

We have shown a consistent and widespread elevation in the levels of normal p53 tumour suppressor protein in the basal layer of the multiple recurrent papillomas of six patients, which contain either HPV 6 or 11. The reproducible detection of HPV 6 or 11 in recurrent papilloma patients and its low frequency in solitary papillomas might point to the possibility of immunological defects in these patients and this is currently under investigation.

Elevated p53 levels appear to be specific to recurrent papillomas harbouring HPV6/11 since they have not been reported in studies of solitary papillomas and other hyperplastic lesions[5].

HPV 6 and 11 E6 proteins have been shown experimentally to bind the p53 protein but, unlike HPV 16 and 18 E6 proteins, they do not subsequently degrade it. Therefore it is possible that stabilisation of p53 in recurrent papillomas occurs as a consequence of its interaction with the HPV 6/11 E6 proteins.

However, there is another possible reason for the observed high levels of p53 in recurrent papillomas. The adenovirus 5 E1A protein, which shares homology with the HPV E7 proteins, has recently been shown to induce apoptosis when introduced into cells and appears to mediate this effect by stabilising the p53 protein[6]. Full transformation is only accomplished when p53 is bound and inactivated by the adenovirus 5 E1B protein. Whilst elevation of p53 protein levels by HPV E7 remains to be experimentally demonstrated, it is possible that the HPV 6/11 E7 proteins might elevate p53 protein levels, since the E6 proteins of these viruses do not degrade p53[1,2]. If the HPV 6/11 E7 proteins were to elevate p53 levels and induce apoptosis, this might also explain the incompleteness of the transformed phenotype of the laryngeal papilloma keratinocytes.

ACKNOWLEDGMENTS

This work is supported by grants from the Cancer Research Campaign and L.J. Clark is in receipt of an MRC training fellowship.

REFERENCES

1. M. Scheffner, B.A. Werness, J.M. Humbregtse, A.J. Levine and P.M. Howley, The E6 oncoprotein encoded by human papillomavirus types 16 and 18 promotes the degradation of p53, *Cell* 63:1129 (1990).

2. T. Crook, J.A. Tidy and K.H. Vousden, Degradation of p53 can be targeted by HPV sequences distinct from those required for p53 binding and trans-activation, *Cell* 67:547 (1991).

3. J.E. Burns, M.C. Baird, L.J. Clark, P. Burns, K. Edington, C. Chapman, R. Mitchell, G. Robertson, D. Soutar and E.K. Parkinson, Gene mutations and elevated protein levels in human squamous cell carcinomas and their cell lines, *Br J Cancer* 67:1274 (1993).

4. M.J. Arends, Y.K. Donaldson, E. Duvall, A.H. Wyllie and C. Bird, HPV in full thickness cervical biopsies: high prevalence in CIN 2 and CIN 3 detected by a sensitive PCR method, *J Pathol.* 165:301 (1991).

5. G.R. Ogden, R.A. Kiddie, D.P Lunny and D.A. Lane, Assessment of p53 protein in normal, benign and malignant oral mucosa, *J Pathol.* 166:389 (1992).

6. S.W. Lowe and H. Ruley, Stabilization of the p53 tumor suppressor is induced by adenovirus 5 E1A and accompanies apoptosis, *Gene Devel.* 7:535 (1993).

EXPRESSION OF THE E6 AND E7 GENES OF HUMAN PAPILLOMAVIRUSES IN TUMORS OF DIFFERENT DIGNITY

Thomas Iftner,[1] Stephan Böhm,[1] Martin Oft,[1]
Sharon P. Wilczynski,[2] Herbert Pfister[1]

[1] Institut für Klinische und Molekulare Virologie
Friedrich-Alexander-Universität
D-91054 Erlangen
Germany
[2] Department of Pathology
City of Hope
National Medical Center
Duarte
CA 91010
USA

INTRODUCTION

The E6 and E7 genes of genital human papillomaviruses (HPV) immortalize keratinocytes and the E6/7 segment of the viral genome appears to be transcribed in most, if not all, HPV-positive cancers (zur Hausen, 1991). The E6 and E7 proteins are therefore regarded as good candidates for immunotherapy. In situ hybridization studies with HPV16-infected low grade cervical lesions showed only very weak transcription of E6 / E7 in the basal layer, whereas expression strongly increased in the more differentiated layers accompanied by high levels of DNA replication (Dürst et al. 1992; Stoler et al. 1992). In high grade squamous intraepithelial lesions, transcription of the E6 / E7 region appeared derepressed, and in situ hybridization signals were evenly distributed throughout the undifferentiated epithelium. The initial studies did not distinguish between mRNAs specific for E6 and E7. Another potential problem was the use of an anti-sense RNA probe covering the complete ORFs E6 and E7 for the detection of HPV 16 E6 / E7 mRNA. Such probes may hybridize with the 5' ends of E1^4 transcripts, which predominate in HPV 6-induced condylomas (Nasseri et al. 1987), and also seem to exist in low grade HPV 16-infected intraepithelial neoplasias (Higgins et al., 1992). We therefore designed new probes for in situ hybridization which specifically detect transcripts with a coding potential for E6 and E7, respectively, taking into account more recent data on HPV transcription strategies.

High risk genital HPVs like HPV 16 and less oncogenic viruses like HPV 6 or HPV 11 generate the E7-specific mRNA in different ways. E6/E7 colinear transcripts derived from the promoter in front of ORF E6 could encode both E6 and E7, but reinitiation of translation at the E7 AUG is highly unlikely so that these mRNAs are probably E6-specific. Initiation at a separate promoter within ORF E6 of HPV 6 and HPV 11 leads to transcripts with E7 as the first translatable ORF (Smotkin et al., 1989). In HPV 16, expression of E7 is achieved by splicing out introns from the E6/E7 colinear transcripts. Removal of the introns within ORF E6 allows translation of a full length E7 protein and two truncated E6 proteins with no obvious biological activity (Sedman et al., 1991).

DESIGN OF PROBES FOR IN SITU HYBRIDIZATION

To obtain riboprobes specific for individual mRNA species we cloned subgenomic fragments of HPV 6 (Iftner et al., 1992) and HPV 16 into the pBS or pGEM 1 RNA expression vectors, determined their orientation and synthesized in vitro anti-sense RNA. The HPV 6-specific probe 1 detects E6 mRNAs starting at promoter P1, whereas probe 2 recognizes all mRNAs starting at promoter P2 or upstream of it (Fig. 1). The net signal resulting from the E7 mRNA starting at P2 can be obtained by subtracting signals generated by probe 1. The HPV 16-specific probe 3 exclusively covers intron sequences of the spliced E6*-I mRNA (Fig. 1 transcript d) and is therefore specific for unspliced transcripts; probe 4 hybridizes to both unspliced and spliced E6/E7 colinear transcripts and probe 5 allows the identification of mRNAs with 5' ends within ORF E7 (Fig. 1).

EXPRESSION OF VIRAL ONCOGENES IN LOW GRADE GENITAL LESIONS

Serial thin sections of fifteen HPV 6-positive anogenital condylomas were analysed by in situ-hybridisation as described before (Iftner et al., 1992). The E6 probe led to weak signals within the basal layer, whereas the HPV 6 probe 2 gave rise to a more pronounced labelling of all cells within the 2 - 3 lowest epidermal layers (Fig. 2). No E6-specific signal could be disclosed in three cases. In two of these cases labelling with probe 2, which is consequently specific for E7 mRNAs, extended into the stratum granulosum, whereas the third case revealed only focal signals in the upper layers of the epidermis.

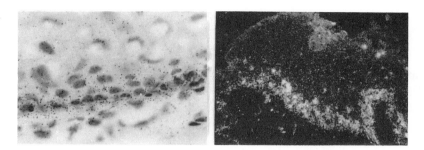

Figure 1. Genetic and transcriptional map of the E6/E7 genomic region of HPV6 (left) and HPV16 (right) and localization of the mRNA-specific probes 1 to 5. The open reading frames (open boxes) and the nucleotide positions of the probe boundaries (at the top) correspond to the published sequence of HPV6b (Schwarz et al., 1983) and HPV16 (Seedorf et al., 1985). Vertical lines within the ORFs represent the first translational start codons. The major transcripts of the early region of HPV6 (a-c) and HPV16 (d-f) are depicted in the lower part (Smotkin et al., 1986; 1989; Doorbar et al, 1990).

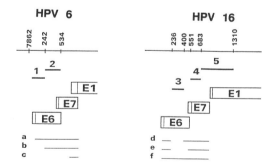

Figure 2. *In situ* hybridisation analysis of a anal condyloma with the HPV6 E6-specific riboprobe 1 (left) showing details of the basal layers in bright-field illumination. The result of hybridization with riboprobe 2 is visualized by dark-field optics (right). The silver grains generated in the film emulsion after exposure to the ^{35}S-labeled probes are seen as dark grains under bright-field and white grains under dark-field illumination.

No viral transcripts could be detected with the HPV 16 probe 3 in two HPV 16-positive low grade vulvar intraepithelial neoplasias. Hybridization with probe 4 led to moderate signals exclusively in the upper third of the epithelium, but much stronger signals were obtained with probe 5 (Fig.3 A-C). These are probably due to a predominant E1^E4 mRNA which could be substantiated by additional in situ hybridizations with subgenomic probes specific for the intron and second exon of this transcript (data not shown). These expression patterns confirm results of previous studies of low grade HPV 16-associated lesions (Dürst et al. 1992, Higgins et al. 1992, Stoler et al. 1992). The comparison of HPV 6 and HPV-16 induced low grade intraepithelial lesions revealed a much more restricted expression of the E6 and E7 genes in the case of HPV 16. This could be explained by a special need to prevent malignant conversion of low grade lesions by avoiding undue expression of the more potent oncoproteins of HPV 16 (Vousden, 1991). According to this hypothesis, a stringent control of oncogene expression is certainly particularly important in proliferation-competent cells of the basal layers.

ONCOGENE EXPRESSION IN GENITAL CANCERS

Seven HPV 16-positive cancers showed no detectable E6-message (unspliced transcripts hybridizing to probe 3) but low to moderate levels of potential E7-mRNAs (identified with probe 4) in the cytoplasm of all tumor cells (Fig. 3 D-F). As the HPV 16-specific probe 3 revealed no signals in any of the investigated cases, we confirmed that this probe works in principle by verifying that clear signals could be obtained with denatured sections of HPV 16 DNA-positive specimens due to hybridization with single stranded DNA (data not shown). As there were no unspliced E6 / E7 transcripts detectable, we consider signals obtained with the anti-sense riboprobe 4 as specific for mRNA encoding the E7 protein.

Like with the intraepithelial neoplasias, signals obtained with probe 5 were consistently stronger than those obtained with probe 4 (Fig. 3 E and F). This points to the existence of transcripts with an exon starting in ORF E7. Five cancers showed comparable labelling with probe 5 and an ORF E4-specific anti-sense riboprobe (data not shown) supporting the presence of an E1^E4 mRNA. In spite of strong probe 5 signals no hybridization was obtained with the E4-specific probe in two cancers, which may be explained by disruption of the early HPV 16 transcription unit due to integration.

The results of this study confirm the general concept that transcription of the E6 / E7 region is derepressed with increasing severity of the tumors (Dürst et al. 1992, Stoler et al. 1992). The differentiation between unspliced and spliced transcripts now demonstrated that the increased levels are mainly due to mRNAs with a coding potential for E7. However, the actual levels of E7-specific RNAs turned out to be considerably lower than anticipated from earlier studies using ORF E6 / E7-specific probes. Our data indicate that the strong signals obtained with such probes are due to hybridization with 5'

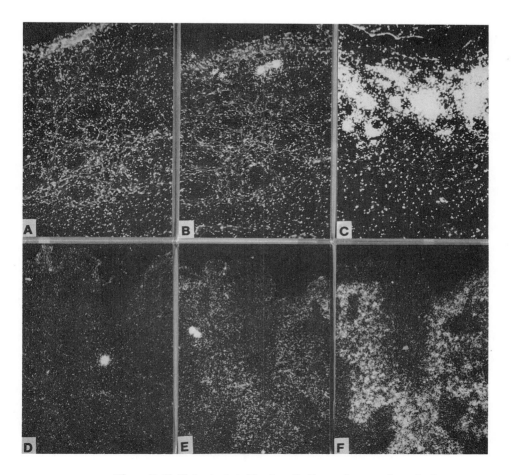

Figure 3. (A-C) *In situ* hybridization of adjacent tissue sections of a low grade vulvar intraepithelial neoplasia with riboprobes 3 (A), 4(B), 5(C). (D-F) *In situ* hybridization of adjacent sections of a vulvar squamous cell carcinoma with riboprobes 3(D), 4(E), 5(F).

sequences of an abundant mRNA class that seems to initiate within ORF E7. We assume that they represent an E1^E4 mRNA (Doorbar et al. 1990, Sherman et al. 1992) which is the major mRNA class of HPV 16 in benign lesions (Higgins et al. 1992) or fusion transcripts of E1 and cellular sequences in the case of integrated HPV 16 DNA. In any case, the major mRNA class of HPV 16 both in benign and malignant tumors would be driven by a promoter within ORF E7.

ACKNOWLEDGEMENTS

We thank Ms. A. Schmitt for excellent technical assistance. This work was supported by grant 89.042.2 from the Wilhelm Sander-Stiftung to T.I. and by Public Health Service grant CA53005 to S.P.W.

REFERENCES

Dürst, M., Glitz, D., Schneider, A. and zur Hausen, H. 1992, Human papillomavirus type 16 (HPV16) gene expression and DNA replication in cervical neoplasia: analysis by *in situ* hybridization. *Virology* 189: 132.

Doorbar, J., Parton, A., Hartley, K., Banks, L., Crook, T., Stanley, M. and Crawford L. 1990, Detection of novel splicing patterns in a HPV16-containing keratinocyte cell line. *Virology* 178: 254.

Higgins, G.D., Uzelin, D.M., Phillips, G.E., McEvoy, P., Marin, R. and Burell, C.J. 1992, Transcription patterns of human papillomavirus type 16 in genital intraepithelial neoplasia: evidence for promoter usage within the E7 open reading frame during epithelial differentiation. *J Gen Virol.* 73:2047.

Iftner, T., Oft, M., Böhm,S., Wilczynski, S.P. and Pfister, H. 1992, Transcription of the E6 and E7 genes of human papillomavirus type 6 in anogenital condylomata is restricted to undifferentiated cell layers of the epithelium. *J Virol.* 66:4639.

Nasseri, M., R. Hirochika, T.R. Broker and T.L. Chow. 1987, A human papillomavirus type 11 transcript encoding an E1/E4 protein. *Virology* 159:433.

Schwarz, E., Dürst, M., Demankowski, C., Lattermann, O., Zech, R., Wolfsperger, E., Suhai, S. and zur Hausen, H. 1983, DNA sequence and genome organization of genital human papillomavirus type 6b. *EMBO J.* 2:223.

Sedman, A.S., Barbosa, M., Vass, W.C., Hubbert, N.L., Haas, J.A., Lowy, D.R. and Schiller, T.J. 1991, The full-length E6 protein of human papillomavirus type 16 has transforming and trans-activating activities and cooperates with E7 to immortalize keratinocytes in culture. *J Virol.* 65:4860.

Seedorf, K., Krammer, G., Dürst, M., Suhai, S. and Röwekamp, W.G. 1985, Human papillomavirus type 16 DNA sequence. *Virology* 145:181.

Sherman, L., N. Alloul, I. Golan and A. Baram. 1992, Expression and splicing patterns of human papillomavirus type 16 mRNAs in precancerous lesions and carcinomas of the cervix, in human keratinozytes immortalized by HPV16, and in cell lines established from cervical cancers. *Int. J. Cancer* 50:356.

Smotkin, D., and Wettstein, F.O. 1986, Transcription of human papillomavirus type 16 early genes in a cervical cancer and a cancer-derived cell line and identification of the E7 protein. *Proc Natl Acad Sci USA* 83:4680.

Smotkin, D., Prokoph, H. and Wettstein, F. O. 1989, Oncogenic and nononcogenic human papillomaviruses generate the E6 and E7 mRNA by different mechanisms. *J Virol.* 63: 1441.

Stoler, M.H., C.R. Rhodes, A. Whitbeck, S.M. Wolinsky, L.T. Chow and T.R. Broker. 1992, Human papillomavirus type 16 and 18 gene expression in cervical neoplasias. *Hum Pathol.* 23:117.

Vousden, K.H. 1991, Human papillomavirus transforming genes. *Seminars in Virol.* 2: 307.

zur Hausen, H. 1991, Human papillomaviruses in the pathogenesis of anogenital cancer. *Virology* 184:9.

DETECTION OF HPV-16 E2 PROTEIN IN CERVICAL KERATINOCYTES

V. Bouvard[1], A. Storey[1], D. Pim[1], E. Baraggino[2], U. Wisenfeld[2] and L. Banks[1]

[1]International Centre for Genetic Engineering and Biotechnology
Padriciano 99
Trieste
Italy
[2]Clinica Obstetrica and Gynaecologica
Ospedale Maggiore
Trieste
Italy

INTRODUCTION

The two major HPV-16 oncogenes, E6 and E7 are transcribed from the viral p97 promoter, the activity of which is modulated by a complex network of transcriptional elements located in the viral Upstream Regulatory Region (URR). Genetic analysis of Bovine Papillomavirus (BPV) has shown that the viral E2 gene product is an important regulator of viral gene expression[1,2] and some studies have shown that the BPV E2 protein will repress transcription from the HPV-16 promoter[3.] A weak transcriptional repressor activity has also been reported for the HPV-18 E2 protein[4]. In many late stage tumours and derived cell lines the HPV DNA Is often integrated into the host genome with concomitant loss of E2 coding sequences[5]. These observations gave rise to a hypothesis which suggested that integration and deletion of E2 regulatory activity was a prerequisite for late stage tumour progression. However, there are now several reports[6,7] of the existence of episomal HPV-16 DNA capable of encoding full length E2 protein in late stage tumours. In addition, a recent HPV-16 isolate defective for keratinocyte immortalisation was shown to contain a mutation in the E2 gene; cotransfecting a wild type E2 restored the immortalising activity of this virus[8].

Here we have attempted to clarify the mechanism of action of the HPV-16 E2 protein. We demonstrate the continued expression of E2 mRNA in immortalised keratinocytes and show expression of the E2 protein in these cells. We also show that the full length E2 protein acts as a potent transcriptional activator in cervical keratinocytes. These studies indicate that disruption of E2 function is not a prerequisite for virus mediated immortalisation of human cells.

RESULTS

Identification of the HPV-16 E2 protein

In order to investigate E2 expression in HPV immortalised keratinocytes northern blot analyses were performed on a number of different HPV-16 immortalised cell lines; W12 cells which contain episomal HPV-16 DNA[9].; T17 and T121[10] which are HPV-16 immortalised oral keratinocytes which contain HPV 16 expressed from the retroviral vector PJ4Ω; AC89/E2 cells8 which were obtained by cotransfecting E2-defective HPV-16 together with wild type E2 in plasmid pJ4Ω.16E2. The results obtained are shown in Figure 1.

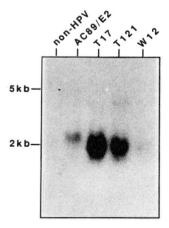

Figure 1. Northern blot analysis of E2 expression in immortalised keratinocytes. Cells used were non HPV containing keratinocytes, AC89/E2, T17, T121 and W12. Molecular weight markers are indicated.

The four HPV-16 containing lines all continue to express E2 mRNA. Considerably higher levels of expression were detected in lines T17 and T121 which contain HPV-16 DNA in plasmid pJ4Ω. The lowest level appeared in the W12 cell line in which the virus is using its own promoter. We were then interested in investigating E2 protein expression. To do this cells were labelled with [^{35}S]-methionine for 1hr and then extracted with RIPA buffer. Proteins were then reacted with an anti E2 polyclonal antibody (kindly provided by Lutz Gissmann) and immune complexes were analysed by SDS PAGE and autoradiography. The results obtained are shown in Figure 2.

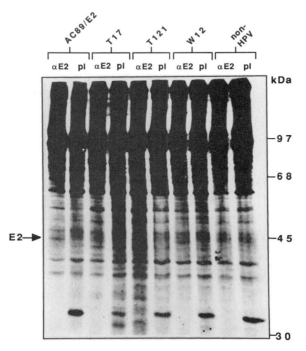

Figure 2. Immunoprecipitation analysis of E2 protein in human keratinocytes. Cells used are indicated above the lanes. Labelled cell extracts were reacted either with a polyclonal anti E2 antibody (αE2) or a rabbit preimmune antibody (pI). Protein corresponding to E2 is arrowed.

A specific polypeptide of 43kd is precipitated from two of the keratinocyte cell lines, W12 and AC89/E2. Interestingly, no E2 protein is detected in the cells where the virus is under the control of an heterologous promoter, even though the Northern analysis would have indicated otherwise. It is apparent from this experiment however that the level of E2 protein expressed in the W12 and AC89/E2 cells is very low.

HPV-16 E2 activates viral transcription in keratinocytes

Having demonstrated the continued expression of the HPV-16 E2 protein in the HPV immortalised keratinocytes, we investigated the transcriptional activity of the protein in these cells. The viral URR was cloned into a CAT reporter plasmid and promoter activity was then measured following cotransfection of normal keratinocytes with pJ4Ω.16E2 and the URR-CAT plasmid. The results obtained are shown in Figure 3. These results show that HPV-16 E2 activates strongly the HPV-16 promoter in normal keratinocytes. The endogenous background level of transcription results in approximately 15% CAT conversion . This contrasts with the 100% conversion upon transfection of 10 µg of the E2

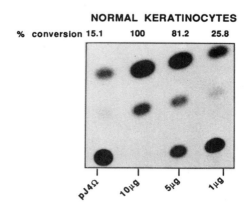

Figure 3. Activation of HPV-16 promoter by full length HPV-16 E2 protein. Cells were co-transfected with URR-CAT plasmid and either pJ4Ω or the indicted amounts of pU4Ω.16E2. Numbers show percentage CAT conversion.

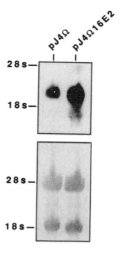

Figure 4. Northern analysis of E7 mRNA in W12 cells following transfection with either pJ4Ω or pJ4Ω.16E2 (upper panel). Bottom panel shows a methylene blue stain of the filter to demonstrate equal loading of RNA. Positions of 28S and 18S RNAs are indicated.

expression plasmid. The specificity of this activity is verified by the titration of the E2 expression plasmid.

Finally we analysed the effect of E2 upon viral transcription in the context of the other viral gene products. To do this W12 cells were transfected with pJ4Ω.16E2 and RNA was isolated after 48hr. Northern blot analysis was then performed for E7 mRNA and the results obtained are shown in Figure 4.

These results demonstrate a significant increase in the level of E7 mRNA expression following transfection of the W12 cells with pJ4Ω.16E2 over that of control transfected cells. This shows that HPV-16 E2 directly increases the level of viral oncogene expression by stimulating viral p97 activity.

DISCUSSION

The results presented here show the continued expression of the HPV-16 E2 protein in two HPV-16 immortalised keratinocyte cell lines, W12 and AC89/E2. Both cell lines are feeder-dependent and continue to express E7 protein (data not shown). The presence of E2 protein in these cells suggests that loss of the E2 gene by viral DNA integration is not a prerequisite for viral mediated immortalisation or for high level E7 expression. It is important to note that E2 protein was only detected in the two lines containing HPV-16 under the control of its homologous promoter and thus presumably responsive to E2 regulation. No E2 Protein was detected in the T17 and T121 lines in which the virus is under the control of the heterologous promoter in pJ4Ω. Further, the increase in E7 mRNA expression detected in the W12 cells following transfection with an exogenous E2 plasmid demonstrates that the HPV-16 promoter in these cells is still responsive to E2. A series of experiments was also done to analyse the transcriptional activity of E2 protein in transient transfections of human keratinocytes. These results show that the HPV-16 E2 protein acts as a potent activator of viral gene expression in normal keratinocytes.

Based on the above observations we conclude that full length E2 upregulates viral gene expression and may function in a positive fashion in the early stages of cell immortalisation by increasing E6 and E7 expression. Recent studies have identified a short spliced form of E2 originating from W12 cells[11] and it will be of interest to analyse the transcriptional activity of this alternatively spliced product. By analogy with BPV[2] it is tempting to speculate that this form of E2 will actually function as a transcriptional repressor. It is possible that the virus is able to express different forms of the E2 protein and can thus modulate the levels of viral gene expression.

In conclusion, HPV-16 E2 protein was detected in HPV immortalised keratinocytes at early passage and was shown to upregulate the level of viral oncogene expression. The cells used in this study are now progressing to feeder independence and it will be of interest to determine the E2 status in these later stages of cell transformation.

REFERENCES

1. B.A. Spalholz, Y.C. Yang and P.M. Howley. Transactivation of a bovine papillomavirus transcriptional regulatory element by the E2 gene product. *Cell* 42: 183 (1985).

2. P.F. Lambert, B.A. Spalholz and P.M. Howley. A transcriptional repressor encoded by BPV-1 shares a carboxy-terminal domain with the E2 transactivator. *Cell* 50: 69 (1987).

3. H. Romanczuk, F. Thierry and P.M. Howley. Mutational analysis of cis elements involved in E2 modulation of human papillomavirus type 16 P97 and type 18 P105 promoters. *J. Virol.* 64: 2849 (1990).

4. B.A. Bernard, C. Bailly, M.C. Lenoir, M. Darmon, et al. The human papillomavirus type 18 E2 gene product is a repressor of the HPV18 regulatory region in human keratinocytes. *J. Virol.* 63: 4317 (1989).

5. E. Schwarz, U.K. Freese, L. Gissmann, W. Mayer et al. Structure and transcription of human papillomavirus sequences in cervical carcinoma cells. *Nature* 314: 111 (1985).

6. M. Rohlfs, S. Winkenbach, S. Meyer, T. Rupp et al. Viral transcription in human keratinocyte cell lines immortalised by human papillomavirus type 16. *Virology* 183: 331 (1991).

7. L. Sherman and N. Alloul. Human papillomavirus type 16 expresses a variety of alternatively spliced mRNAs putatively encoding the E2 protein. *Virology* 191: 953 (1992).

8. A. Storey, I. Greenfield, L. Banks, D. Pim et al. Lack of immortalizing activity of a human papillomavirus type 16 variant DNA with a mutation in the E2 gene isolated from normal human cervical keratinocytes. *Oncogene* 7: 459 (1992).

9. M.A. Stanley, H.M. Brown, M. Appleby and A.C. Minson. Properties of a non-tumorigenic human cervical keratinocyte cell line. *Int. J. Cancer* 43: 672 (1989).

10. C.J. Sexton, C.M. Proby, L.Banks, J.N. Stables et al. Characterization of factors involved in human papillomavirus type 16 mediated immortalization of oral keratinocytes. *J. Gen. Virol.* 74: 755 (1993).

11. J. Doorbar, A. Parton, K. Hartley, L. Banks et al. Detection of novel splicing patterns in a HPV-16 containing keratinocyte cell line. *Virology* 178: 254 (1990).

EVALUATION OF THE HYBRID CAPTURE ASSAY FOR DETERMINATION OF HUMAN PAPILLOMA VIRUS

Klaus F Czerwenka, Yongxian Lu, Friedrich Heuss, Mahmood Manavi,
Josef W Hosmann, Darco Jelencic and Ernst Kubista

Dept of Gynecopathology
University of Vienna
Spitalgasse 23
A-1090 Vienna
Austria

INTRODUCTION

There is growing evidence suggesting that human papillomavirus (HPV) infection is a causal factor, in the development of cervical neoplasias and squamous intraepithelial lesions (SILs) of the anogenital region[1] . This provides an impetus to adapt HPV testing for gynecologic screening.

Since HPV does not replicate in *in vitro* culture systems, the presence of HPV DNA in clinical specimens can only be detected by filter hybridization. All of these available methods are not only cumbersome, but also require radiolabeled probes, although they are considered to have high sensitivity and specificity for HPV types. In order to improve on current methods of HPV DNA detection, we chose to adapt the new chemiluminescent molecular hybridization assay technology i.e. the hybrid capture system, for this purpose.[2] This system is a sandwich capture molecular hybridization assay, that utilizes chemiluminescent detection. It is a new, nonisotopic DNA assay, which makes the sophisticated nucleic acid technology simplified and efficient, without the need for radiolabeled probes. This comprehensive HPV test can identify the presence of the 14 most common anogenital HPV types, and distinguish low risk HPV types (6, 11, 42, 43 and 44), from intermediate and high risk HPV types (16, 18, 31, 33, 35, 45, 51, 52 and 56).

An evaluation of the sensitivity and specificity of this new method for the detection of HPV DNA was necessary, hence a methodologic study has been designed here. In planning this comparison, Dot blot DNA-DNA hybridization is considered to be the current standard assay[3,4,5] because of its well-defined sensitivity, and because of the type specificity provided by combined hybridization. Each of the two methods was performed on the same samples obtained either from native cells by brushing, or cell sediments from paraffin-embedded formalin-fixed tissues from female genital tract and breast tissue.

MATERIAL AND METHODS

One hundred and eleven specimens of different degrees of cervical squamous intraepithelial lesions (SILs) and cervical carcinomas (n=91), endometrial adenocarcinomas (n=9), and Pagets disease of the breast-nipple and the vulva (n=11) have been included in this study. Hybrid capture assay was performed in 91 native cells taken from cervix, and 20 cell sediments in paraffin-embedded, formalin-fixed tissues from endometriums, vulva and breast-nipples, using a Digene Hybrid Capture System Kit (Digene Diagnostics, Inc, Beltsville, MD, USA).

Exfoliated cervical cells were washed into 0,1 PBS buffer, pelleted (at 2500 rpm for 10 min for two times at 15-30^{0}c), and resuspended in 1ml of specimen transport medium. Cell sediments from paraffin blocks were cut in three parallel 5-μm sections and collected in tubes. After DNA was extracted, 100 μl DNA extraction solution from each specimen was added separately, into 1ml specimen transport medium.

Hybrid Capture Assay

The main procedures of hybrid capture assay consist of 5 steps, that is, denature the specimen, hybridize with the probe mix, capture the hybrids, react with the conjugate and detect the hybrid by chemiluminescence. In brief, 500 μl of denaturation reagent was added into each control or specimen tube. After incubation for 45 min in a 65^{0}C water bath, 150ul of denatured control of patient's probe and 50 μl of HPV probe were pipetted into the hybridization tubes, incubated for 60 min in a 65^{0}C water bath, then transferred into capture hybridization tubes, incubated for another 60 min in a 65^{0}C water bath, then shaken on a rotary shaker at 1100 rpm, at 20-25^{0}C for 60 min. After decanting the capture tubes, 250 μl of detection reagent 1 were pipetted into each of these tubes, incubated for 30 min at 20-25^{0}C, followed by five washings with wash buffer. 250 μl of detection reagent 2 were then pipetted into each tube, and immediately measured in a luminometer, after the 30 min incubation. The lower limit of detection in this system is 10pg/ml HPV DNA. The relative light units (RLUS) measured on our luminometer Leader 50 (Gen-Probe, Inc, USA) were equal to or greater than the cut-off value, indicating the presence of HPV DNA sequences in the specimen. To control the quality, three replicates of positive and negative controls were tested for each test run. Only when the coefficient of variation in all control results were <30%, and the PCX (positive control mean)/NCX (negative control mean) ratio <1.5, was the validation of the assay accepted.

Dot Blot Method

The Dot Blot was performed using the Vira Type HPV-DNA typing kit (Digene Diagnostics, Inc, Silver Spring, MD, USA), including ^{32}Plabelled RNA probe sets of HPV-6/11, HPV-16/18, and HPV-31/33/35. Dot Blots were dropped onto three replicate Sure Blot Hybridization membranes, and probed with three distinct ^{32}P labelled RNA probe mixtures for the identification of specific HPV types.

RESULTS

Detection of low risk HPV DNA types

The low risk HPV DNA types 6/11/42/43/44 were detected by hybrid capture assay in 10 specimens, and confirmed with probes against HPV DNA types 6/11 Dot blot in 3 specimens. The results obtained from the two methods were shown in Table 1.

Table 1. Hybrid Capture vs. Dot Blot in low risk HPV DNA.

Hybrid Capture	Dot Blot		Total
	+	-	
+	2	8	10
-	1	100	101
Total	3	108	111

When Dot Blot was taken as the reference method, the relative sensitivity of the Hybrid Capture Assay was 2/3=66.6%, while relative specificity was 100/108=92.6%. So the efficiency of the Hybrid Capture Assay in low risk HPV DNA types was at least 0.92 in our laboratory, taking into consideration that fewer HPV DNA types were measured by Dot Blot.

Detection of high and intermediate risk HPV types

As shown in Table 2, among 104 specimens, Hybrid Capture Assay detected the high and intermediate risk HPV DNA types 16/18/31/33/45/51/52/56 in 44 specimens, and identified with probes specific for HPV types 16/18, 31/33/35 by Dot Blot in 29 specimens.

Table 2. Hybrid Capture vs. Dot Blot in High and intermediate risk HPV DNA.

Hybrid Capture	Dot Blot		Total
	+	-	
+	29	15	44
-	0	60	60
Total	29	75	104

The sensitivity and specificity of our Hybrid Capture Assay for high and intermediate risk HPV DNA were 29/29=100.0%, and 60/75=80.0%, respectively. The efficiency from this data was approximately 0.86.

DISCUSSION

The comparison of the HPV DNA detection systems applied in this methodologic study demonstrated the high sensitivity, specificity and efficiency of the Hybrid Capture Assay. This assay system is a comprehensive HPV test, which identifies the presence of the 14 most common HPV types, with a specific HPV RNA probe cocktail, and can only distinguish low risk HPV types from high and intermediate risk HPV types; the results obtained from the two methods were compared among the two groups, which are divided according to the low and high risk HPV types. Both high and low risk positive cases of our study cohort increased, as shown in Table 1 and 2. This increase in positive rate may not only result from the additional detection of HPV types (other than types 6, 11, 16, 18, 31, 33 and 35 by Dot Blot method), but also from the additional sensitivity of the assay system itself.

Although the lower limit of HPV DNA detection in the Hybrid Capture System is 10pg/ml, higher than 2.5pg/ml by Dot Blot, it requires a specimen less than 1/7 the size of the clinical specimen used by Dot Blot to obtain comparable results. As to specificity, there were a few cases of false-positive cases in both groups of HPV types by Hybrid Capture Assay, compared with Dot Blot. The existence of false-positive results in our study can be ruled out, because three replicates of the negative control in each experiment were always negative for HPV DNA. It must be taken into our consideration that most of the additional positives were HPV types, for which type-specific probes were not available by Dot Blot.

Although our study is just at a preliminary stage, clearly the results obtained from the Hybrid Capture Assay have already showed promise, for HPV DNA detection in gynecologic screening. This new technique has many advantages for routine use. Firstly, one can detect the 14 major HPV types, which account for the most neoplasms in the female genital tract, without the need for radiolabeled probes. Secondly, the Hybrid Capture System makes the HPV DNA detection much easier and significantly faster, resembling an immunoassay procedure. One can get results in less than five hours. Thirdly, this new technique is adaptable to readily available clinical samples, such as swabs, or scrapes taken from the cervix, as well as to paraffin-embedded, formalin-fixed tissues. The Hybrid Capture Assay has, however, its limitations; it will not distinguish among the viral types within the same group. Thus this method is limited in its application as a research method for identifying the association between specific HPV types and different disease severities.

In this preliminary study, we did not analyse the correlation between HPV DNA types, and the histological, and cytological diagnosis. To make a definite evaluation of this new, efficient and nonisotopic HPV DNA type detection method, additional studies will be necessary, with a full series of probes in Dot Blot or Southern Blot. The possible variability must be evaluated in different clinical and histological conditions, and in larger populations.

REFERENCES

1. A.T. Lorincz and R. Reid, Association of human papillomavirus with gynecologic cancer, *Current Opinion in Oncology*, 1:123-132, (1989).

2. M. Garcia et al, Detection of human papillomavirus deoxyribonucleic acid in cervical specimens by a fast, highly sensitive, chemiluminescent assay, 11th International Papillomavirus Workshop, (1992).

3. K.F. Czerwenka, H.J. Schön et al, Reliability of in situ hybridization of smears and biopsies for papilloma virus genotyping of the uterine cervix, *Eur J Clin Chem Clin Biochem.*, 29:139-145, (1991).

4. A.T. Lorincz, W.D. Lancaster and G. Temple, Cloning and characterization of the DNA of a new human papillomavirus from a woman with dysplasia of the uterine cervix, *J Virol.*, 58:225-229, (1986).

5. A.T. Lorincz, A.P. Quinn et al, A new type of papillomavirus associated with cancer of the uterine cervix, *Virology*, 159:187-190, (1987).

UTILIZATION OF A PCR-BASED, MULTIPLE RESTRICTION ENDONUCLEASE DIGEST TECHNIQUE FOR ENHANCED DETECTION AND TYPING OF HPV FROM CLINICAL SAMPLES

Eileen Epsaro[1], Jarrett Burton[2], Sheila Mathieson[1],
Joseph Merola[2], and Jeffrey A. Sands[1]

[1]Department of Molecular Biology
Lehigh University,
[2]St. Luke's Hospital
Bethlehem
PA 18015
USA

INTRODUCTION

The hypothesis that specific types of human papilloma-viruses (HPVs) play a central role in the pathogenesis of invasive cervical cancer and the presumed precursor lesions of invasive cervical cancer (cervical intraepithelial neoplasia CIN 1-3)is well established.[1] Studies have shown that infection with one or more of a large number of HPVs (including HPV 16, 18, 31, 33, 35, 39, 45, 51, 52, 56, 58, 66, 6, 11, 42, 43, and 44) can result in CIN 1, but only a subset of these HPV types (HPV 16, 18, 31, 33, 35, 39, 45, 51, 52, 56, 58, and 66) can be etiologically linked to CIN 2-3 and invasive cancer.[1,2] A recent study by Schiffman et al.[3] further strengthens previous observations about the relationship between HPV and all grades of CIN and supports the hypothesis that CIN 1 and CIN 2-3 are separate entities directly resulting from infection of different epithelia with specific HPV types. Thus, the importance of sensitive methods to detect and type HPV from clinical samples is evident.

In the United States, there is as of 1993 only one FDA approved clinical test, the Virapap test, available for identification and typing of HPV from clinical samples. This is a dot blot nucleic acid hybridization assay to detect the presence of one of seven most prevalent HPV types in clinical samples and identify it as belonging to one of three categories: (1) type 6 or 11, (2) type 16 or 18, and (3) type 31, 33, or 35. The discovery that within this group there exists a wide range of oncogenic potential[4,5,6], in addition to the fact that infection with HPV types other than the seven listed above may be medically significant, led us to initiate a large-scale study comparing the efficiency of the Virapap test and a recently described PCR technique[7] to detect and type HPV from 291 women undergoing a routine gynecological examination. The PCR technique used is based on the highly conserved nature of the L1 open reading frame (ORF) of HPV that allows use of a single primer set of oligonucleotides, 20 base pairs in length, that, when used together, will initiate the PCR amplification of an approximately 450 base-pair HPV product.[8,9] Subsequent digestion of the PCR product with a panel of seven restriction endonucleases and analysis of the HPV type-specific pattern was used to determine the HPV type(s) present in the patient sample.

From January 1992 through March 1993, cervical swabs were obtained from a total of 291 patients who obtained Pap smears as part of a gynecological visit. Patient samples were first screened for the presence of HPV using the Virapap HPV assay kit (Digene Diagnostics Inc., Silver Spring, MD, USA). All samples were further analyzed for the presence of HPV by a PCR-based method and subsequent restriction endonuclease digestion analysis of the PCR product to determine HPV type(s) present. For PCR amplification, two sets of primers were used, one set (MY09/MY11, Perkin-Elmer Corp.) to amplify a 450-base pair region of the HPV L1 gene and a second set (PC04/GH20, Perkin-Elmer) to amplify a 268-base pair region of the cellular β-globin gene, which was used as an internal positive control for the PCR reaction. All amplifications were done for 35 cycles, and negative controls (no DNA added) were routinely included to monitor for contamination. A 10 ul portion of the PCR product was electrophoresed to visualize the 450-base pair L1 and the 268-base pair β-globin bands. The remainder of the PCR product was divided and subjected to restriction endonuclease digestion. Restriction digest patterns from the cellular β-globin fragment were subtracted, leaving the pattern of restriction fragment lengths from the L1 450-base pair PCR product, as shown below for twelve of the major HPV types in Table 1 (generously provided by H. Bauer, Roche Molecular Systems, Alameda CA 94501).

Our analysis of 291 clinical samples has resulted in 53 positive cases (18.2%) as detected by our PCR approach, in contrast to only twenty five (8.6%) detected positive by the Virapap assay system. All samples that tested positive by the Virapap hybridization assay also tested positive in our PCR assay, and in all cases the specific typing identified by restriction digestion of the PCR product fell within the category identified by Vira-type. Thus, this commercial test seemed to have no problem with false positives (none detected), but it missed slightly over half (53%) of the truly positive cases.

Table 1. Specific HPV types and the expected restriction fragment lengths following digestion with each of seven specific enzymes.

HPV Type	BamHI	DdeI	HaeIII	HinfI	PstI	RsaI	Sau3AI
6b	449	382	217	234	449	161	366
		67	124	215		149	63
			108			72	20
						67	
11	366	449	217	234	242	216	366
	83		124	215	207	135	63
			108			72	20
						26	
16	452	452	452	452	216	310	369
					210	72	63
					26	70	20
18	372	432	455	455	242	135	372
	83	23			213	125	63
						85	20
						72	
						38	
31	452	285	328	237	216	380	369
		167	124	215	210	72	63
					26		20
33	449	320	449	234	242	236	267
		77		215	207	102	162
		52				72	20
						39	
35	452	294	269	452	426	177	369
		135	183		26	161	63
		23				72	20
						42	
45	372	324	455	455	242	338	372
	83	131			213	72	63
						45	20
45V	372	324	455	455	242	203	249
	83	131			213	180	123
						72	63
							20
52	449	357	266	449	423	449	366
		92	183		26		63
							20
53	449	206	232	368	449	449	342
		158	217	81			87
		85					20
54	369	452	217	234	452	138	369
	83		127	218		125	63
			108			117	20
						72	

A summary of our results is presented in Table 2 below.

Table 2.   Results of HPV typing.

```
HPV TYPING BY PCR-RESTRICTION DIGESTION (PCR-RD) TECHNIQUE
```

HPV Type:	6b	11	16	18	31	33	35	45	45V	52	53	54	other
Cases* :	5	1	12	1	6	6	1	2	1	1	3	1	5

* In addition, two samples contained mixed HPV types and six samples were too weakly positive to type.

The PCR-RD method offers major advantages over the Virapap hybridization method for the detection of HPV from clinical samples. The increased sensitivity of the PCR-RD assay allows the detection of HPV in specimens determined to be HPV negative by the hybridization assay. Most likely, these hybridization negative but PCR positive cases represent samples with low copy number of viral DNA and/or the presence of HPV types other than the seven types detectable by the hybridization assay. The PCR-RD assay also provides definitive identification of a wide range of HPV types in addition to the seven types detected by the Virapap assay. Finally, the PCR-RD method can be used for the detection of HPV from additional clinical samples (fresh or paraffin-embedded; smears or biopsies; male or female) to provide information on HPV reservoirs and the potential involvement of HPV DNA in human cancers other than cervical.

In summary, we have made use of a PCR/restriction digestion technique that allows very sensitive, accurate, and rapid detection and typing of HPV infection from cervical samples. This technique has allowed us to quantitate the prevalence of the more oncogenic HPV types in our population, to detect infection with less frequent HPV types (such as 45, 52, 53, and 54) and to detect multiple infections and/or cases of infection with untypable or previously unrecognized HPV types.

REFERENCES

1. L.A. Brinton, Epidemiology of cervical cancer - overview in "The Epidemiology of Human Papillomavirus and Cervical Cancer" N. Munoz , F.X. Bosch, K.V. Shah, A. Meheus, eds., IARC Sci Publ No. 119. Lyon. (1992).
2. A.T. Lorincz, R. Reid, A.B. Jenson, M.D. Greenberg, W. Lancaster, and R.J. Kurman, Human papillomavirus infection of the cervix: relative risk associations of 15 common anogenital types, *Obstet Gynecol.* 79:328 (1992).
.3. M.H. Schiffman, Recent progress in defining the epidemiology of human papillomavirus infection and cervical neoplasia, *J Natl Cancer Inst.* 85: 958 (1993).
4. zur Hausen, H., and A. Schneider, *in* N. Salzman and P. Howley, eds., The Papovaviridae, vol. 2, The Papillomaviruses. Plenum Press, New York (1987).

5. A.T. Lorincz, W.D. Lancaster and G.F. Temple, Cloning and characterisation of the DNA of a new human papillomavirus from a woman with dysplasia of the uterine cervix, *J Virol.* 58: 225 (1986).

6. R. Reid, *Am J Obstet Gynecol.* 156:212 (1987).

7. H.M. Bauer, G.E. Greer, J.C. Chambers, C.T. Tashiro, J Chimera, A. Reingold, and M.Manos, Genital human papillomavirus infection in female university students as determined by a PCR method, *Journ Amer Med Assoc.* 265: 472 (1991).

8. Y. Ting and M. Manos, *in* PCR Protocols: A guide to methods and applications, ed. M. Innis, Academic Press, Inc. CA, 356 (1990).

9. M. Schiffman, H.M. Bauer, A.T. Lorincz, M.M. Manos, J.C. Byrne, A.G. Glass, D.M. Cadell, and P.M. Howley, Comparison of Southern blot hybridisation and polymerase chain reaction methods for the detection of human papillomavirus DNA, *J Clin Microbiol.* 29: 573 (1991).

A GENE CASSETTE FOR HIGH LEVEL EXPRESSION OF THE LI CAPSID PROTEIN OF HPV-16 IN HETEROLOGOUS CELLS

Stephen R. Kelsall[1] and Jerzy K. Kulski[2]

Department of Microbiology
[1]University of Western Australia
[2]Royal Perth Hospital
Perth, Western Australia 6000

INTRODUCTION

The L1 major capsid protein of human papillomavirus type 16 (HPV-16) is potentially a useful reagent for studying immune responses to this virus and for the development of a vaccine to control the occurrence of primary infections and HPV-16–associated genital carcinomas[1,2]. However immunological studies utilizing L1 protein have been impeded by the lack of availability of a correctly folded form of the protein. Gene expression technology offers an efficient means for producing large amounts of the protein provided the problems that affect recombinant proteins can be overcome. Since these problems can require the testing of different expression systems, it would be an advantage for the L1 coding sequence to be readily insertable into a variety of expression plasmids and carry sequence characteristics favoring efficient expression in different cellular and genetic environments.

Our aims were: (1) to construct a gene cassette that carries the L1 coding sequence of HPV-16 along with sequence characteristics favouring efficient expression in a variety of cell types, and (2) to test prokaryotic and eukaryotic expression systems for their capacity to produce L1 protein at high levels and in correctly folded form.

CONSTRUCTION AND FEATURES OF THE CASSETTE

The cassette consecutively consists of an 11 nucleotide (nt) 5' noncoding sequence, the L1 coding sequence and stop codon (nts 5637-7154[3]), 72 bp of HPV-16 3' noncoding sequence, the nt sequence GACCTGCAGGCATGC derived from the pUC18/19 multiple cloning site (MCS), and the entire pUC18/19 MCS beginning at the *Hind*III site. Most (~98%) of the L1 DNA was obtained from the cloned HPV16 genomic DNA[4] as two fragments: an *Acc*I-*Bam*HI fragment (nts 5669-6150) comprising only L1 coding sequence, and a *Bam*HI-*Ssp*I fragment (nts 6151-7226) consisting of the 3' L1 coding sequence, the stop codon, and 72 nts of noncoding sequence. The missing 32 nts of 5' coding sequence were supplied by a 43 nt synthetic *Hind*III-*Acc*I gene fragment (Fig. 1A) which also

Immunology of Human Papillomaviruses
Edited by M.A. Stanley, Plenum Press, New York, 1994

contained the 11 nt 5' noncoding sequence. The complete cassette was constructed using a series of standard cloning and fusion steps[5]. The final form of the cassette was as an insert in the plasmid 'pUCL1' (Fig. 1B).

Conservative mutations and mutations to the 5' non-coding sequence were included in the synthetic DNA (Fig. 1A). A *Hin*fI site was conservatively placed within the coding sequence so as to allow insertion of the cassette into vectors carrying an *Nco*I site; other conservative mutations were designed to lower the GC content for efficient translational initiation in prokaryotes. The natural 5' noncoding sequence was mostly replaced: an A was included at position -3 for efficient translational initiation in eukaryotes, and restriction sites for *Hin*dIII and *Xba*I—which are low in Gs and Cs—were included for manipulation of the gene with its methionine codon intact. The three restriction sites present at the 5' terminus can be used alone or in combination with any of several restriction sites present at the 3' terminus to recover the cassette from pUCL1 (Fig. 1B).

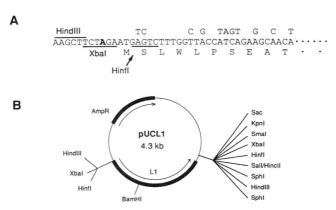

Figure 1. (A) Sequence of modified 5' terminus of cassette showing conservative nucleotide changes (original bases are those above the sequence), restriction enzyme sites, adenine at position -3 (emboldened), and encoded amino acids. (B) Plasmid pUCL1 showing restriction enzyme sites for excision of the cassette.

PRODUCTION AND ANALYSIS OF L1 PROTEINS

Plasmid Constructions and Production of Recombinant Baculovirus

E. coli plasmids were constructed to express the full-length L1 coding sequence either as a fused or unfused protein in *E. coli*, or as an unfused protein in insect cells. Plasmids pGEX2T[6] and pTrc99A[7] were used to construct expression vectors pGEXL1 and pTrcL1 and to produce fused and unfused forms of the L1 protein respectively in *E. coli*. Baculovirus transfer plasmid pVL1392[8] was used to construct the recombinant plasmid pVL16L1 and produce an unfused L1 protein in cultured cells (Sf-21) of the insect *Spodoptera frugiperda* using a baculovirus expression system. Plasmids pGEXL1, pTrcL1 or pVL16L1 were produced by transferring the L1 gene from pUCL1 (Fig. 1) to pGEX2T, pTrc99A or pVL139 respectively, using standard subcloning procedures[5].

Analysis of proteins produced in *E. coli* and insect cells

pGEXL1 or pTrcL1 when expressed in *E. coli* produced a protein of the expected size (83K as a fusion protein or 56K as a nonfusion protein) which reacted with an L1-specific monoclonal antibody (mab), CAMVIR-1[9], and was present in cell lysates at levels of 3-4% of total protein (Fig. 2A, lanes 1 and 2). However, the level of production of the 27.5K protein (Sj26) by pGEX2T at 15% of total cellular protein was markedly greater than that of the 83K fusion protein by pGEXL1 (Fig. 2). The level of production of a truncated form of the L1 fusion protein (65K) by pGEXL1 which lacked ~100 amino acids at the C-terminus also was higher than that of the 83K fusion protein (Fig. 2A, lanes 2 and 3), suggesting a role for the missing amino acids in controlling the level of production of the L1 protein in *E. coli*. In addition, both the fused and unfused proteins produced by pGEXL1 and pTrcL1 respectively, were obtained from cell lysates as inclusion bodies with less than 1% of protein remaining soluble after centrifugation at 10,000 g for 20 minutes (Fig. 2B).

In order to further characterize the 56K protein produced by pTrcL1 in *E. coli* the protein was purified by SDS-PAGE and used as an immunogen to produce mouse mabs (S. Kelsall, M. Cicchini, G. Shellam and J. Kulski, unpublished data). Mabs from 10 different clones reacted with the proteins produced by either pGEXL1 or pTrcL1. The linear epitopes of the L1 protein reacting to these mabs were determined by peptide mapping (J. Zhou, D. Davis and I. Frazer). Five different peptide locations on the L1 protein[2] produced by either pGEXL1 or pTrcL1, were recognized:

KLDDTENASAYAANA (124-138) by antibody MC-12
GTVGENVPDDLYIKG (264-278) by antibodies MC-10 and MC-34
QIFNKPYWLQRAQGH (304-318) by antibody MC-15
FSADLDQFPLGRKFL (454-468) by antibodies MC-14, MC-18, MC-39, MC-40
KAKPKFTLGKRKATP (474-488) by antibodies MC-7, MC-53

The mab CAMVIR-1 which recognises the peptide sequence IQDGDMVHTGFGAMD (194-208) of the L1 protein also reacted with the protein produced by pGEXL1 and pTrcL1.

The recombinant baculovirus, vAc16L1 harbouring the L1 gene cassette, was produced by co-transfecting Sf-21 insect cells with the recombinant baculovirus plasmid, pVL16L1, and the wild type baculovirus (AcNPV) genomic DNA. The presence of the L1 protein produced by vAc16L1 in Sf-21 cells was detected in high yields by indirect immunofluorescence using mab CAMVIR-1 (data not shown). Several proteins, ranging in size between 14K and 56K were identified in extracts of Sf-21 cells infected with vAc16L1 by SDS-PAGE and western immonoblotting with the mab CAMVIR-1 (D. Park, L. Selvey, S. Kelsall and I. Frazer, unpublished data).

CONCLUSIONS

The specificity and utility of the L1 gene cassette was demonstrated by producing high yields of the encoded protein in *E. coli* and in insect cells. The protein produced by the L1 gene cassette was of the expected molecular size and reacted with mabs specific to the L1 protein of HPV-16. These observations confirmed that the 5' terminus of the L1 gene cassette contained signals favouring efficient translational initiation in both prokaryotes and eukaryotes. Further studies of the protein produced by the cassette may help in the development of serological tests and immunogens required for the diagnosis and treatment of HPV-16 infections.

A

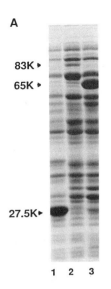

83K ▸

65K ▸

27.5K ▸

1 2 3

B

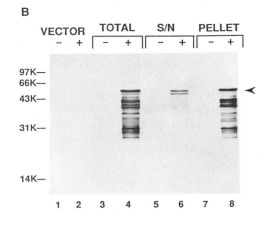

Figure 2. (A) Proteins produced by *E. coli* and pGEX2T (lane 1), pGEXL1 (lane 2), and pGEXL1 carrying the L1 gene with a 3' terminal deletion (lane 3). Proteins detected by SDS-PAGE in a 11% gel stained with Coomassie Blue. Arrowheads indicate positions of fused and unfused proteins. (B) Proteins produced by pTrcL1 in *E. coli* and detected by immunostaining with mab CAMVIR-1 after SDS-PAGE through an 11% gel. Immunoreactive protein produced by pTrcL1 in uninduced (-) and induced cells (+), total protein lysate (lane 3 and 4), 10,000 g supernatants (lane 5 and 6) and pellets (lane 7 and 8). Total protein lysates from uninduced (lane 1) and induced (lane 2) cells harbouring pTrc99A. Arrowhead indicates position of 56K protein. *M*r markers are indicated at left.

REFERENCES

1. D.H. Davies, G.A.J. McIndoe and B.M. Chain, Cancer of the cervix: prospects for immunological control, *Int. J. Exp. Path.* 72:239 (1991).
2. W.F.H. Jarrett, K.T. Smith, B.W. O'Neil, J.M. Gaukroger, L.M. Chandrachud, G.J. Grindlay, G.M. McGarvie and M.S. Campo, Studies on vaccination against papillomavirus: Prophylactic and therapeutic with recombinant structural proteins, *Virology* 184:34 (1991).
3. K. Seedorf, G. Krämmer, M. Dürst, S. Suhai and W.G. Röwekamp, Human papillomavirus type 16 DNA sequence, *Virology* 145:181 (1985).
4. M. Dürst, L. Gissman, H. Ikenberg and H. zur Hausen, A papillomavirus DNA from a cervical carcinoma and its prevalence in cancer biopsy samples from different geographic regions, *Proc. Natl. Acad. Sci. USA* 80:3812 (1983).
5. J. Sambrook, E.F. Fritsch and T. Maniatis. "Molecular Cloning: a Laboratory Manual," Cold Spring Harbor Laboratory, Cold Spring Harbor, New York (1989).
6. D.B. Smith and K.S. Johnson, Single-step purification of polypeptides expressed in *Escherichia coli* as fusions with glutathione *S*-transferase, *Gene* 67:31 (1988).
7. E. Amann, B. Ochs and K.-J. Abel, Tightly regulated *tac* promoter vectors useful for the expression of unfused and fused proteins in *Escherichia coli*, *Gene* 69:301 (1988).
8. V.A. Luckow and M.D. Summers, Signals important for high-level expression of foreign genes in *Autographa californica* nuclear polyhedrosis virus expression vectors, *Virology* 167:56 (1988).
9. C.S. McLean, M.J. Churcher, J. Meinke, G.L. Smith, G. Higgins, M. Stanley and A.C. Minson, Production and characterisation of a monoclonal antibody to human papillomavirus type 16 using recombinant vaccinia virus, *J. Clin. Pathol.* 43:488 (1990).

GENOTYPING OF HUMAN PAPILLOMAVIRUS (HPV) BY SINGLE-STRAND CONFORMATIONAL POLYMORPHISM (SSCP)

Ingeborg Zehbe,[1] Eva Rylander,[2] Jan Sällström,[1] and Erik Wilander[1]

[1]Department of Pathology
[2]Department of Gynaecology and Obstetrics
University Hospital
751 85 Uppsala, Sweden

INTRODUCTION

Nowadays, the polymerase chain reaction (PCR) is the most sensitive and widely used method for the detection of human papillomavirus (HPV) using ethidium bromide gel electrophoresis together with hybridization assays for typing. In this study, we demonstrate single-strand conformational polymorphism (SSCP) as simultaneous detection and typing method for PCR-amplified products. SSCP as first described by Orita et al.[1,2] employs denaturation of double strand DNA into single strand DNA and separation of the products by polyacrylamide gel electrophoresis (PAGE). This method makes possible the detection of HPV-DNA conformational changes resulting in indivual band patterns of the most common HPV-types.

A subset of human papillomaviruses are found in the genital tract. These are further classified into low, medium and high risk types. The most common low risk types 6 and 11 are mainly found in condylomata acuminata and low grade squamous intraepithelia lesions (SILs) whereas the high risk types 16 and 18 are found in a majority of high grade SILs and invasive carcinomas. The medium risk types e. g. 31, 33 and 35 are less frequent in invasive cancers and occur in both high and low grade SILs. Therefore, early recognition of HPV-infections and distinction of HPV-types is of clinical importance.

Immunology of Human Papillomaviruses
Edited by M.A. Stanley, Plenum Press, New York, 1994

MATERIAL AND METHODS

For the analysis of the different HPV type band patterns, we applied PCR-SSCP on HPV-positive paraffin-embedded tissues confirmed by *in situ* hybridization with type-specific genomic nucleic acid probes for HPV-types, 6, 11, 16, 18, 31, 33 and 35 [3,4]. To exclude diverse band patterns within the same HPV genotype, we selected 5 different cases for each HPV-type. Furthermore, all samples were run 10 times under the same conditions and resulted always in the same band patterns. All cases were double-checked by ethidium bromide gel electrophoresis and the correlation of the tested cases was 100%.

DNA-extraction was performed according to Lungo et al.[5] and DNA-amplification was done according to Walboomers et al.[6] using the consensus primers GP5 and GP6 from the L1 region resulting in a 150 bp PCR-product. 50 µl amplification mixture consisted of 50 mM KCl, 10 mM Tris-HCL, 3.5 mM MgCl$_2$, 200 µM of each dNTP, 25 pmol of each primer, 1 unit *Taq* polymerase (Perkin Elmer Cetus) and 10-20 µl DNA overlaid with 50 µl light mineral oil (Sigma). Forty amplification cycles were performed on a PHC-3 thermal cycler (Techne): 1 min denaturation at 94 °C, annealing 1 min 30 sec at 40 °C and extension 2 min at 72 °C.

The analysis of the PCR-products was run on PhastSystem (Pharmacia Biotechnology LKB) which offers a semi-automated electrophoresis on pre-made 12.5% homogenous acrylamid gels and buffer strips combined with silver-staining. One µl of the PCR-product and 1 µl of the denaturation mixture (99% formamide, 0.05% bromophenol blue and 0.05% xylene cyanol) were denatured and subsequently pipetted onto a sample-comb which was fitted on holders of the PhastSystem instrument above the gel. Initially, the gel was pre-run at 400 V 10.0 mA 4.0W 10°C 100 AVh and sample loading was programmed at 102 AVh. Another 150 AVh were run under the same conditions. 16 specimens including Ø-X 174 DNA marker may be run at the same time.

Gels were stained in the development chamber of the PhastSystem as follows: 20% trichloroacetic acid (TCA) 5 min at 20 °C, 8.3% glutaraldehyde in dH$_2$O 5 min at 20 °C, Milli-Q-water 2x2 min at 50 °C, 0.5% silver nitrate 8 min at 40 °C, Milli-Q-water 2x30 sec at 30 °C, developer (sodium carbonate and formaldehyde), 1x30 sec and 1x4 min at 30 °C, 5% acetic acid 2 min at 50 °C and 5% acetic acid/5% glycerol 3 min at 50 °C.

RESULTS

SSCP allows the distinction of the conformational change pattern from the denatured PCR-products of HPV-types 6, 11, 16, 18, 31, 33 and 35 corresponding to the amplification products of the GP5 and GP6 consensus primers (figure 1). Low risk types can be clearly distinguised from medium and high risk types demonstrating diverse band patterns. This application of a non radioisotopic HPV-detection and typing method of PCR-amplified products provides a fast alternative to the standard and work-intensive ethidium bromideØØ gel electrophoresis with differential hybridization assays. The time for the SSCP-anlaysis is approximately 2 hours and should make it possible to screen large quantities of samples.

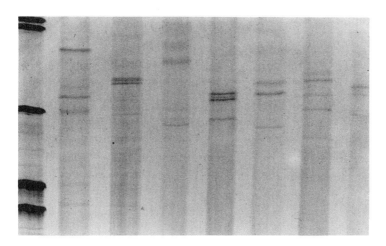

Figure 1. DNA marker Ø-X 174 and the individual band patterns of the most common HPV types: 6, 11, 16, 18, 31, 33 and 35

DISCUSSION

The proposed assay for the simultaneous detection and typing of HPV has shown that it is possible to distinguish the most common HPV-types. SSCP is a reliable and reproducable method and applicable for both prospective and retrospective studies. The type of specimen could be cervical lavages, Papanicolaou smears, frozen or formalin-fixed biopsies. The advantage to use previously diagnosed smears or biopsies for the detection of HPV is the possibility to compare the cyto- or histopathological diagnosis with the molecular biological finding.

There is still a range of less frequent or even novel HPV-types to be tested. Another consideration would be how multiple HPV-infections manifest themselves on the acrylamide gels. In our hands, the sensitivity of SSCP is comparable to the detection with ethidium bromide gel electrophoresis. However, this applies only to known HPV-positive cases analyzed by *in situ* hybridization and has to be tested further, preferably on previously negative biopsies morphologically showing HPV-suspicious lesions.

ACKNOWLEDGEMENTS

This study was sponsored by the Swedish Cancer Foundation and Lion's Cancer Foundation.

REFERENCES

1. M. Orita, H. Iwahana, H. Kanazawa, K. Hayashi and T. Sekiya, Detection of polymorphisms of human DNA by gel electrophoresis as single-strand conformational polymorphism, *Proc Natl Acad Sci USA.* 86:2755 (1989).

2. M. Orita, Y. Suzuki, T. Sekiya and K. Hayashi, Rapid and sensitive detection of point mutations and DNA polymorphisms using the polymerase chain reaction, *Genomics* 5:874 (1989).

3. I. Zehbe, E. Rylander, A. Strand and E. Wilander, Biotinylated cDNA probes for the detection of human papillomavirus (HPV) in gynaecological biopsies, *Anticancer Research* 12:1383 (1992).

4. I. Zehbe, E. Rylander, A. Strand and E. Wilander, Use of Probemix and Omniprobe biotinylated cDNA probes for detecting HPV infection in biopsy specimens from the genital tract, *J Clin Pathol.* 46:437 (1993).

5. O. Lungo, Jr. T. C. Wright, amd S. Silverstein, Typing of human papillomavirus by polymerase chain reaction amplification with L1 consensus primers and RFLP analysis, *Mol Cell Probes* 6:145. (1992).

6. J. M. M. Walboomers, P. W. J. Melkert, A. J. C. van den Brule, P. Snijders and C. J. L. M. Meijer, The polymerase chain reaction for human papillomavirus screening in diagnostic cytopathology of the cervix, *in*: "Diagnostic molecular pathology. A practical approach," vol. 2, ed. C. S. Herrington and J. O'D Mc Gee, Oxford University Press, Oxford, New York, Tokyo (1992).

HUMAN PAPILLOMAVIRUS INFECTION IN WOMEN WITH CERVICAL CANCER BUT WITHOUT CYTOLOGICAL ABNORMALITIES IN THE PRECEDING YEARS

Martine Chabaud,[1] Nubia Munoz,[2] Marie Claude Cottu,[1] Pierre Coursaget,[1] Philippe Anthonioz,[1] Nicolas Day[3],Elizabeth MacGregor[4]

[1]Institut De Virologie et Laboratoire de Pathologie cellulaire
2 bis Bd Tonnelle
37042 Tours cedex
France
[2]Unit of Field and Intervention Studies
International Agency for Research on Cancer
69372 Lyon cedex 08
[3]MCR Biostatistics Unit
Institute of Public Health
Cambridge
UK
[4]Department of Pathology
Aberdeen
UK

INTRODUCTION

Human papillomavirus (HPV) have been recognized as the aetiological agent of squamous carcinoma of the cervix (Munoz et al., 1992). Existing data suggest that HPV type affects the malignant potentiel of HPV associated lesions, low risk being associated with types 6 and 11 and high risk with types 16 and 18 (Lorincz et al, 1992). During a retrospective study to determine the prevalence of cytological abnormalities before cancer, Pap smears were collected from women with cervical cancer from the area of Aberdeen in the period 1974-1985. Some carcinoma of the cervix were observed in women who were diagnosed cytologically negative over the period of 1-10 years before cancer diagnosis. The absence of cytological abnormalities could indicate the absence of HPV infection. Thus, we have investigated the role of HPV in such carcinomas. The polymerase chain reaction was used to search for the presence of HPV 6, 11, 16, 18, 31 and 33 in cervical tissue from these carcinomas and *in situ* PCR was utilised to localise viral DNA in the cervical tissues.

MATERIALS AND METHODS

Patients

Tissue sections from formalin fixed and paraffin embedded surgical tumor specimens were obtained from 25 women aged 28 to 70 years with normal cytological smears in the years preceding the diagnosis of the cancers. Squamous intraepithelial lesions were not observed one year or more before carcinoma detection in 20 women; however Pap smears taken less than one year before the cancer diagnosis were cytologically positive. The five remaining women were always diagnosed cytologically negative before cancer diagnosis.

PCR Amplification

Eight 5μm sections were cut from paraffin blocks and were lysed. Total cellular DNA was prepared by proteinase K digestion, phenol-chloroform extraction, and ethanol precipitation. DNA extracted from tissue section was subjected to PCR amplification with sets of primers corresponding to sequences in the L1 region of the HPV 6, 11, 16, 18, 31 and 33 genomes and consensus primers. The samples were subjected to 30 cycles of amplification using a DNA Thermal Cycler (Perkin-Elmer-Cetus, Norwalk, USA). For each cycle, denaturation was at 94^{0}C for 30 secs, annealing of primers at Tm-5^{0}C for 30 secs, and elongation at 75^{0}C for 1 min. After amplification, the DNA was visualized by ethidium bromide staining. Subsequently amplified DNA were transferred onto a nylon membrane and hybridized with a digoxigenin labelled probe obtained by random primer incorporation of digoxigenin-dUTP. The hybrids were detected by enzyme-linked immunoassay using an antidigoxigenin alkaline phosphatase conjugated and subsequent enzyme catalysed colour reaction (DNA labelling and detection kit, Boehringer Mannheim, F.G.R.).

In situ PCR

Oligonucleotide primed *in situ* amplification of HPV DNA was done simultaneously with the labelling of the newly synthesised DNA by incorporation of digoxigenin-dUTP, followed by *in situ* hybridization and detection of specific DNA complex with labelled antidigoxigenin antibodies according to the method described by Mayelo et al. 1993.

RESULTS

At least one HPV was detected in 92% of the tumor sections from women cytologically negative before the cancer diagnosis (Table 1). HPV 16 and HPV 18 were detected in 65 % and 30 % respectively of patients with a positive Pap smear during the last year preceding the diagnosis of carcinoma. Cytologically negative women during all the period were HPV-DNA positive. It must be noted that 8 out of 23 HPV-DNA positive samples were positive for both HPV 16 and HPV 18. HPV 6, 11, 31 and 33 were not found in such women. HPV DNA was detected only with consensus primers in four cases. Two patients (8%) were found to be HPV DNA negative.The detection of the virus by *in situ* PCR in 8 of these cases shows that in the great majority of them, only few cells contained HPV-DNA, in both the epithelium and the lamina propria in one case.

DISCUSSION

HPV 16 and HPV 18 were detected in 68% and 40% respectively of the cervical cancer from patients diagnosed cytologically negative over the period of 1-10 years before cancer diagnosis. Milan et al (1986) found HPV 16 and HPV 18 in respectively 36% and 10,5% of cervical cancer from the west of Scotland as determined by southern blot technique using radioactively labelled probe. HPV 16 is the predominant HPV genotype detected in cervix cancer around the world. However, we found a high frequency of HPV 18 among the cytologically negative women.The results show that in 92% of patients without abnormalities in archival Pap smears cancer is associated with HPV infection, as generally observed in patients who developed carcinomas after diagnosis of cervical intraepithelial lesions in Pap smear. In a 5 year follow up study, De Villiers et al. (1992) found that 19 of 2928 patients (0.65%) with normal cytology at the first visit developed lesions of carcinoma *in situ* or invasive carcinoma. HPV was evident in 12 of them (63%). In our study, the patients with normal Pap smears developed carcinoma one year after the last cytologically negative smear and five had no positive Pap smears. This suggests a very fast evolution of the HPV infection. The absence of HPV in two cases of cervical cancers indicates that such tumours may also arise without HPV infection or that HPV is not detected. In support of the first possibility there is the report of Yee et al.(1985) showing that two cell lines derived from cervical carcinoma were negative for HPVs.

Table 1. Detection of HPV-DNA in scottish women with cervical cancer but without cytological abnormalities in the preceding years.

Patients cytologically negative	types of papillomavirus				HPV positive
	16	18	16 and 18	X	
one year or more before carcinoma (20)	8(40%)	1(5%)	5(25%)	4(20%)	18(90%)
during the years before carcinoma (5)	1(20%)	1(20%)	3(60%)	0(0%)	5(100%)
Total (25)	9(36%)	2(8%)	8(32%)	4(16%)	23(92%)

It must be noted that few cells contained HPV DNA as detected by *in situ* PCR and as it is clear that cytological evaluation on the basis of Pap smear cannot guarantee that genital mucosa does not harbour an HPV infection, this could explain the cytologically negative diagnosis of these patients.

REFERENCES

DeVilliers, E.M., Wagner, D., Schneider, A., Wesch, H., Munz, F., Miklaw, H., Zur Hausen, H., 1992, Human papillomavirus DNA in women without and with cytological abnormalities: results of a 5-year follow up study, *Gynecol Oncol.* 44:33.

Lorincz, A., Reid, R., Bennet Jenson, A., Greenberg, MD., Lancaster, W., Kurman, R.J., 1992, Human papillomavirus infection of the cervix: relative risk associations of 15 anogenital types, *Obstet Gynecol.* 79:1.

Mayelo, V, Coursaget, P., Jallais, L., Lhuintre, Y., Anthonioz, P., 1993, Detection of papillomavirus type 16 and type 18 in formalin-fixed tissues by mean of *in situ* gene amplification associated to direct labelled, submitted to publication.

Milan, D.W.M., Davis, J.A., Torbert ,T.E., Campo, M.S., 1986, DNA sequences of human papillomavirus types 11, 16, and 18 in lesions of the uterine cervix in the West of Scotland, *Brit Med J.* 293:93.

Munoz, N., Bosch, RX., de Sanjose, S., Tafur, L., Gili, M., Viladiu,P., Navarro, C., Ascunce, N., Gonzalez, L.C., Kador, J.M., Guerrero, E., Lorincz, A., Santamaria, M., Alonzo de Ruiz, P., Aristizabal, N., Shah, K., 1992, The causal link between human papillomavirus and invasive cervical cancer: a population-based case-control study in Colombia and Spain, *Int J Cancer* 52:743.

Yee, C., Krishnan-Hewlett, Z., Baker, C.C., Schlegel, R., Howley, P.M., 1985, Presence and expression of human papillomavirus sequences in human cervical carcinoma cell lines, *Am J Pathol.* 119:361.

HPV INFECTION AND CARCINOMAS OF THE LARYNX

Olaf Arndt[1], Josef Brock[2], Ingrid Bauer[2], and Günter Kundt[3]

[1]HNO Abteilung des Marienkrankenhauses Hamburg
Alfredstrasse 9
22087 Hamburg
Germany
[2]Institut für Biochemie der Medizinischen Fakultät der Universität Rostock
Schillingallee 70
18057 Rostock
Germany
[3]Institut für Medizinische Statistik der Medizinischen Fakultät der Universität
Rostock
Heydemannstr 9
18057 Rostock
Germany

INTRODUCTION

The laryngeal carcinomas are the most important tumors of ENT. Particularly, men are most frequently affected by precancerous lesions and carcinomas of the larynx. The worldwide ratio of women to men is 1 to 10. In the last years a backward trend in this predominance was seen. This may be a reflection of increased cigarette smoking in women.[1] On the basis of diminishing the sex ratio difference in the development of laryngeal cancer, direct hormonal influences were discussed. As in most neoplasms, an ancestral or genetic pre-condition can be observed for laryngeal cancers too.

There is agreement amongst most authors with regard to the important role played by tobacco abuse in the development of precancerous lesions and also cancers of the

Immunology of Human Papillomaviruses
Edited by M.A. Stanley, Plenum Press, New York, 1994

larynx. About 95% of the patients are smokers of varying quantity. The risk of a heavy smoker is 30 times than that of a non-smoker. Benzpyrene and benzanthracene are carcinogenic parts of cigarette smoke which have an interaction with the DNA of epithelial cells. Different studies on patients with laryngeal cancers showed a significantly higher risk by additional exposure to alcohol. Alcohol is only a co-carcinogen, but regular consumption might lead to a secondary deficiency in various important nutrients. In addition, it exerts an influence on detoxifying enzymatic systems. Statistically, there is a moderate synergy between alcohol and tobacco in increasing the risk by about 50% more than predicted if these effects were simply additive.

The role of viral infections in the genesis of laryngeal carcinomas is not clearly defined. A high detection rate of herpes simplex virus is not able to explain the carcinogenesis. The papillomavirus etiology of recurrent respiratory papillomatosis has recently been firmly established. A high rate of detection of HPV6/11 has been found using sensitive detection techniques such as Southern blotting and the polymerase chain reaction. Malignant conversion of those papillomas was not seen without the additional influence of nicotine and/or x-rays. There was no detection of HPV 16/18 in these lesions.[2] On the other hand, in squamous cell carcinomas of the larynx the oncogenic HPV types 16/18 have been most frequently detected. [3,4,5,7-13,16-18]

The reaction of the mucosa is relatively uniform. In the multistep process of the development of laryngeal cancer, primarily we see mild or moderate grades of epithelial dysplasia. The rate of malignancy in this group is about 2 to 5%. In contrast there is a HPV 16/18 detection rate of between 15 and 20%. Middle grades of dysplasia have a HPV 16/18 detection rate of about 35%. Biopsies from patients with severe dysplasia have a HPV detection rate of about 80%. The rate of malignancy is 20% or more. About 90% of all malignant tumours of the larynx are squamous cell cancers. It is possible that in these cases HPV viral DNA is integrated in the host cell genome and the transforming proteins E6 and E7 could interact with host genes. Influencing differentiation could bring about a blockade of known tumor suppressor genes p53 and/or p105 RB and it is possible that progression to laryngeal cancer could occur as a result. There is an important similarity when compared to the development of cervical cancer.

The history of HPV detection with different methods is shown in Table 1. In 1982 Syrjänen was the first who analyzed a series from laryngeal carcinomas for HPV capsid antigen: in 36% of the cases there was a positive result.[3] Abrahamson[4] could detect HPV 16 related sequences in laryngeal cancers by southern blotting. One year later laryngeal carcinomas were examined by Kahn also using Southern blotting and proved positive for HPV[5] and Kashima could in 70% of the examined cases detect the capsid antigen.[8] Furthermore Brandsma could detect HPV 16 related sequences in verrucous carcinomas of the larynx;[9] subsequently Scheurelen, Syrjänen and Löning detected HPV [7,10,11] using a range of techniques. However De Villiers and Ishibashi were not able to detect HPV sequences with these types of carcinomas.[6,14]

Table 1 History of HPV Detection in laryngeal carcinomas.

AUTHOR	YEAR	TYPE	TECHNIQUE
SYRJÄNEN[3]	1982	not defined	capsid antigen
ABRAHAMSON[4]	1985	HPV 16 related	Southern blot
KAHN[5]	1986	HPV 30	Southern blot
DE VILLIERS[6]	1986	not detected	Southern blot
SCHEURELEN[7]	1986	HPV 16	Southern blot
KASHIMA[8]	1986	not defined	capsid antigen
BRANDSMA[9]	1986	HPV 16 related	Southern Blot
LÖNING[10]	1987	HPV 16/18	Dot blot
SYRJÄNEN[11]	1987	HPV 6/11/16	ISH
BRANDSMA[12]	1989	HPV 11, 16 related	Southern blot
KIYABU[13]	1989	HPV 16	E6 - PCR
ISHIBASHI[14]	1990	not detected	Southern blot
ARNDT[15]	1991	HPV 16/18	Dot blot
MORGAN[16]	1991	HPV6/11, 16, 33	E7 - PCR
WATTS[17]	1991	HPV 11, 16, 18	E6 - PCR
WATTS[17]	1991	HPV 11, 16/18	Southern blot
ARNDT[18]	1992	HPV 16, 18	E6 - PCR

In the recent past there have been many studies using the polymerase chain reaction (PCR). Kiyabu[13] had a detection rate of 40% using primers specific for HPV 16 E6 and using E7 specific primers 50% of cases were positive in the study by Morgan[16] for at least one type of HPV 6/11, 16 or 33. In 75% of all cases Watts[17] could locate E6 specifically by PCR.

RESULTS

Our own studies showed the following results. We examined biopsies of laryngeal cancer from 150 patients, 15 women and 135 men. The age was on average 59 years. The most patients were in the fifth decade of life. In all cases the histological finding were the same: SQUAMOUS CELL CANCER with different keratinization and differentiation.
The vocal cords were found to have 67 (44.7%) of all carcinomas examined: the most common location in our study was in the supraglottic region - 83 cases 3.3%). Only in 20 tumors was there no keratinization. There were no significant differences in the laryngeal locations.

Primary the external influences were tobacco use and alcohol. Only eleven patients (7.3%) were non-smokers, and 44 (29.3%) did not regularly consume alcohol. Overall in only ten patients (6.7%) could no external factor be identified. A single external factor could to be found in 37 patients; the remaining patients were exposed to two external agents. When the nicotine and alcohol levels were graded as shown in table 2 and 3 we were able to derive an equation level or risk factor (rf).

Table 2. Grading of the smoking levels of the patients.

Level of nicotine consumption	Quantity of cigarettes/day
1	non-smoker
2	<20
3	circa 20
4	>20

Table 3 Grading of alcohol consumption.

level of alcohol consumption	quantity of alcohol/day
1	no regular alcohol consumption
2	w - < 60g, m - <75g
3	w - ca 60g, m - ca 75g
4	w - > 60g, m - >75g

w = women   m = men

From the data in Tables 2 and 3 the risk factor - **rf** = level of alcohol consumption x level of nicotine consumption - could be calculated for each case

In table 4 are shown the different rates of HPV detection by PCR using E6 specific primers. The amplification products were proved by hybridization with a commercial oligonucleotide.

In the glottic carcinomas that we found we had a HPV detection rate of 65%. On the other hand only 14.5% of the cancers with a supraglottic location were proved positive for the types looked for under the same conditions. This is a significant difference. For HPV 6/11 alone, two were glottic; three others were supraglottic cancers. This is a detection rate of about 3% in both locations of the larynx. Only one biopsy was positive for an oncogenic HPV type and this was HPV 18. Twenty four (35.8%) of all glottic

Table 4. Results of the E6 specific PCR.

PCR	normal epithelium	glottic location		supraglottic location	
			* #		* #
TOGETHER	15	W	8 / 57	W	7 / 61
		M	59 / 58	M	76 / 58
POSITIVE	1	W	6 / 55	W	0
		M	35 / 59	M	12 / 58
NEGATIVE	14	W	2 / 60	W	7 / 61
		M	24 / 57	M	64 / 58
6/11	1	W	2 / 53	W	0
		M	0	M	3 / 54
16	0	W	3 / 57	W	0
		M	21 / 59	M	4 / 60
18	0	W	0	W	0
		M	0	M	1 / 52
16+18	0	W	0	W	0
		M	10 / 58	M	2 / 54
6/11+16	0	W	1 / 54	W	0
		M	3 / 58	M	1 / 63
6/11+18	0	W	0	W	0
		M	0	M	1 / 66
6/11+16+18	0	W	0	W	0
		M	1 / 63	M	0

W - women. M - men, *quantity.   #age

carcinomas were positive for HPV 16 only but only 4 biopsies of supraglottic cancers showed the same result - a ratio of 7:1.

In the glottic group 10 cases (15%) had a double infection i. e. HPV 16 and 18. On the other hand 2.4% of the supraglottic cancers were HPV 16 and 18 positive. Benign and oncogene virus types were detect together in 5 glottic (7.5%) and in 2.4% of the supraglottic cancers. It would appear that detection of HPV in cancers of the glottic area was four times higher than that of the supraglottic one.

The connection between the age, the risk factor and the HPV 16/18 detection rate in the different locations of the carcinomas as follows. The HPV negative patients were about 56 years old. They have had a risk factor of 5.32. The HPV 16/18 positive group had a risk factor of 7.31 whilst the patients were about 2 years older. When compared to the supraglottic cases there were some similarities. The HPV 16/18 positive group had a significantly higher risk factor - rf 10.7 - and the patients were also about 2 years older (mean age 60.7 years). The HPV negative patients were about 58 years old and they had a rf of 6.6. Furthermore the HPV 16/18 positive group had a significantly higher rf. One could speculate that mucosal changes due to the influence of environmental promoters and/or carcinogens are a precondition for infection with HPV.

The results demonstrate the importance of HPV 16 in the development of glottic carcinomas; 58% of the carcinomas from this laryngeal area showed a positive result to the detection of this HPV type.

The risk factor comparison between the patients of both groups showed a significantly higher rate in the supraglottic group. It is possible that external factors like nicotine and alcohol are initiating factors in the development of supraglottic carcinomas. The rf showed similarities to patients with carcinomas of hypopharynx, tonsils and tongue but, the detection rate of HPV 16/18 is higher one in these cancers and indeed is similar to the rate in the glottic region.[15] The question remains however why is there a significantly lower detection rate of HPV in carcinomas of the supraglottic region? This issue must be addressed with further work.

REFERENCES

1. E. Meyer-Breiting, A. Burkhardt, *Tumours of the larynx* Springer, Berlin-Heidelberg-New York (1988)
2. J. E. Levi, R. Delcelo, V. N. Alberti, H. Torloni, L. L. Villa, Human papillomavirus DNA in respiratory papillomatosis detected by in situ hybridization and polymerase chain reaction, *Am J Pathol.* 135:1179 (1989)
3. K. J. Syrjänen, S. M. Syrjänen, S. Pyrhonen, Human papillomavirus antigens in lesions of laryngeal sqamous cell carcinomas, *ORL* 44:323 (1982)
4. A. Abrahamson, J. Steinberg, B. Steinberg, B. Winkler, Verrucous carcinoma of the larynx: Possible human papillomavirus etiology, *Arch Otolaryngol.* 111:709 (1985)
5. T. Kahn, E. Schwarz, H. zur Hausen, Molecular cloning and charactrization of the DNA of new human papillomavirus (HPV 30) from a laryngeal carcinoma, *Int J Cancer* 37:61 (1986)
6. L.-E. de Villiers, H. Weidauer, H. Otto, H. zur Hausen, Papillomviren in benignen und malignen Tumoren des Mundes und des oberen Respirationstraktes, *Laryngol Rhinol Otol.* 65:177 (1986)
7. W. Scheurelen, A. Stremlau, L. Gissmann, D. Hahn, H. P. Zenner, H. zur Hausen, Rearrenged HPV 16 molecules in anal and laryngeal carcinoma, *Int J Cancer* 38:671 (1986)
8. H. Kashima, P. Mounts, F. Kuhajda, M. Goodstein, F. Lowry, Demonstration of HPV capsid antigen in carcinoma in situ, *Laryngoscope* 97:347 (1987)
9. J. L. Brandsma, B. M. Steinberg, A. L. Abrahamson, Presence of human papillomavirus type 16 related sequences in verrucous carcinoma of the larynx, *Cancer Res.* 46:2185 (1986)
10. T. Löning, M. Meichsner, K. Milde-Langosch, H. Heinze, I. Orlt, K. Hörmann, K.Sesterhenn, J. Becker, P. Reichert, HPV DNA detection in tumours of thehead and neck: A comparative light microscopy and DNA hybridization study, *Otol Rhinol Laryngol.* 49:259 (1987)
11. S. M. Syrjänen, K. J. Syrjänen, R. Mäntyjärvi, Y. Collan, J. Karja, Human papillomavirus in squamous cell carcinomas of the larynx demonstrated by in situ DNA hybridization, *ORL* 49:175 (1987)
12. J. L. Brandsma, A. L. Abramson, Association of papilloma virus with cancer of head and neck, *Arch Otolaryngol Head Neck Surg.* 63:1708 (1989)

13. M. T. Kiyabu., D. Shibata, N. Arnheim, W. J. Martin, P. L. Fitzgibbons, Detection of human papillomavirus in formalin-fixed, invasive squamous carcinomas using the polymerase chain reaction, *Am J Surg Pathol.* 13:221 (1989)

14. T. Ishibashi, S. Matsushima, Y. Tsunkawa, M. Asai, Y. Nomura, T. Sugimura, M.Terada, Human papillomavirus DNA in squamous cell carcinoma of the upperaerodigestive tract, *Arch Otolaryngol Head Neck Surg.* 116:294 (1990)

15. O. Arndt, I. Bauer, J. Brock, Nachweis humaner Papillomvirus (HPV) DNA inmalignen Tumoren des Oropharynx mittels Dot Blot Technik, *Laryngol Rhinol Otol.* 70:142 (1991)

16. D. W. Morgan, V. Abdullah, R. Quincy, Human papillomavirus and carcinoma of the laryngopharynx, *J Laryngol Otol.* 105:288 (1991)

17. S. L. Watts, E. E. Brewer, T. L. Fry, Human papillomavirus DNA types in squamous cell carcinomas of the head and neck, *Oral Surg Oral Med Oral Pathol.* 71:701 (1991)

18. O. Arndt, I. Bauer. K. Zeise, J. Brock, Der Nachweis humaner Papillomvirus DNA in formalinfixierten invasiven Plattenepithelkarzinomen des Larynx mit der Polymerase Chain Reaktion, *Otol Rhinol Laryngol.* in press (1993)

PERINATAL TRANSMISSION AND PERSISTENCE OF THE CANCER ASSOCIATED HUMAN PAPILLOMAVIRUSES

Farzin Pakarian,[1] Jeremy Kaye,[2] John Cason,[2] Barbara Kell,[2]
Richard Jewers,[2] Kankipati S. Raju,[1] Jennifer M. Best,[2]

Department of Obstetrics and Gynaecology
and Richard Dimbleby Laboratory of Cancer Virology
UMDS
St Thomas' Campus,
London SE1 7EH
U.K.

INTRODUCTION

There is currently an increasing interest in developing prophylactic and therapeutic vaccines against the human papillomavirus types (HPV 16, 18, 31, 33) associated with cervical cancer.[1] Although techniques are available to produce such HPV-16 vaccines, knowledge of the natural history of these infections is required before rational vaccination programmes can be designed. Perinatal transmission of HPV types 6 and 11 has been demonstrated.[2] This may occasionally lead to the development of the juvenile respiratory papillomatosis. However, the perinatal acquisition and possible persistence of the cancer associated HPV types have been largely ignored.

METHODS

Eighteen pregnant women, attending antenatal clinics at St Thomas' Hospital were recruited. Ten of these women had a previous history of abnormal smears and/or genital warts

Immunology of Human Papillomaviruses
Edited by M.A. Stanley, Plenum Press, New York, 1994

and were selected in order to obtain a high prevalence of HPV infection in our study population. Seventeen women had single births and one had twins. Cell scrapes from the cervix and posterior vaginal vault were collected from these women between 28 and 38 weeks gestation. Swabs were taken from the mouth and external genitalia of the 19 neonates at 24 hours and from 18 at six weeks post delivery. These samples were put in 5 mls of distilled water and stored at -20 C until processed for HPV-DNA.

All samples were initially tested for HPV-DNA by the polymerase chain reaction (PCR) using consensus primers[3] which amplify a conserved region within the L1 opening reading frame of many types of HPV. 450 base pair amplicons were visualized after electrophoresis on a 2% agarose gel by ethidium bromide staining (Figure 1). Samples that were HPV positive were then typed by PCR using HPV type specific primers.[4] That samples contained sufficient DNA for PCR was confirmed using a beta globin PCR.

RESULTS

Six of the eighteen (33%) women were positive for HPV-DNA prior to delivery. At 24 hours, 9 of the 19 infants (47%) had HPV-DNA in either buccal or genital samples. Seven (one set of twins) of the 9 HPV-DNA positive infants were delivered to 6 mothers who were HPV-DNA positive. At six weeks, six of the 18 (33%) infants tested were HPV-DNA positive; 4 of these infants were born to HPV-DNA positive mothers and were positive at 24 hours and two infants had HPV-DNA negative mothers and were HPV-DNA negative at birth.

Table 1. Distribution of HPV types detected in maternal cervical cells and infant buccal or genital swabs at birth and six weeks.

Hpv type	Number positive		
	Maternal	At birth	At six weeks
6/11	0	1	0
16	3	4	4
16/18	2	3	0
18	1	1	2

When the type of HPV was investigated, 4 of the 9 infants who were HPV-DNA positive at 24 hours were HPV-16 positive, 3 had HPV-16/18 dual infections, one had HPV-18, and one HPV-11 (Table 1). At 24 hours, identical HPV types were detected in samples from 7 mothers and their infants, including dual infections in 2 mother-infant pairs (one set of twins). At six weeks, 4 infants were HPV-16 positive and 2 were HPV-18 positive.

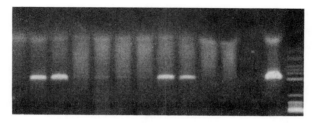

Figure 1. Showing 450 base pair amplicons after electrophororesis on a 2% agarose gel by ethidium bromide staining

DISCUSSION

We have demonstrated that HPV types 16 and 18 may be transmitted from mother to infant. Although it is probable that HPV infection was acquired during passage through an infected birth canal, we cannot exclude transmission *in utero* or postnatally. The fact that 4 HPV positive children (at both birth and at six weeks) had HPV negative mothers may be due to postnatal acquisition of HPV or alternatively be explained by the well recognised fact that single point measurements may underestimate a woman's HPV status. [5] It seems unlikely that these results represent false positives since all standard precautions were taken to prevent contamination of PCR reactions. [6]

We have also demonstrated the persistence of HPV-16 and 18 to six weeks post delivery in 4 of the 9 (44%) infants who were positive at 24 hours. Whilst at 24 hours HPV infections in the infants were equally distributed between buccal and genital sites, at six weeks HPV infections were nearly all restricted to the buccal mucosa. It should be noted that it was not possible for us to sample the internal genital mucosa, although this may have also been infected.

Immunological tolerance may result from infection with other viruses during the prenatal and neonatal period. Whether perinatal acquisition of HPV or resulting immunological tolerance to HPV predisposes to an increased risk of cervical intraepithelial neoplasia in later life remains to be established.

REFERENCES

1. J. Cason, S. Khan, J.M.Best, Towards vaccines against human papillomavirus type-16 genital infection, Vaccine 11: 603 (1993).
2. L. Gissmann, L. Wolnick, H. Ikenberg, Human Papillomavirus types 6 and 11 DNA sequences in genital and laryngeal papillomas and in some cervical cancers, Proceeding of the National Academy of Sciences USA, 80: 560 (1983).

3. M. Manos, Y. Ting, D. Wright, A. Lewis, T. Broker, S.Wolinsky, Use of polymerase chain reaction amplification for the detection of genital Human Papillomaviruses, Cancer cells, 7: 209 (1989).

4. A. van den Brule, C.Meijer, V.Bakels, P. Kenemans, J.Walboomers, Rapid detection of Human Papillomavirus in cervical scrapes by combined general primer mediated and type specific polymerase c hain reaction, J Clin Micro. 28: 2739 (1990).

5. A. Schneider, T. Kirchhoff, G.Meinhardt, L. Gissmann, Repeated evaluation of human papillomavirus type 16 status in cervical swabs of young women with a history of normal Papanicolaou smears, Obstet Gynecol. 79: 683 (1992).

6. P.Muir, F.Nicholson, M. Jhetam, S. Neogi, J.E. Banatvala, Rapid diagnosis of enterovirus infections by magnetic bead extraction and polymerase chain reaction detection of enterovirus RNA in clinical specimens, J Clin Micro. 31: 31(1993).

HPV-DNA ON COLPOCYTOLOGICAL SMEARS FROM HIV POSITIVE FEMALES

Roberto Zarcone

Univeristy of Naples
Federico II
Faculty of Medicine and Surgery
Departement of Gynaecology and Obstetrics

INTRODUCTION

Latest statistics about AIDS cases in Italy show a progressive increase of heterosexuals (Table 1 and 2). 20% of AIDS cases among females and 4% among males

Table 1   AIDS : Cases in Italy

31/03/89		30/09/92
16,6%	homosexual	15%
68,8%	drug addict	66,8%
3,0%	homosex. and drug add.	2,5%
1,8%	hemophilia	1,1%
1,5%	transfusion	1,4%
5,9%	heterosexual intercourses	7,1%
3,0%	uncertain factors	6,1%

transmitted by heterosexual intercourse. In Europe, heterosexual transmission represents 12% of the total figure, and 33% among AIDS affected females. A slight decrease of AIDS

Immunology of Human Papillomaviruses
Edited by M.A. Stanley, Plenum Press, New York, 1994

Table 2 Distribution of aids cases among
heterosexuals on 30/09/92

drug addict partners	58,4%
partners coming from zones at risk	15,5%
uncertain partners	21,4%
others	4,0%
prostitution	0,7%
TOTAL	100%
	1029

cases as a consequence of hemophilia, transfusions and drug addiction has been recorded.
In 34% of AIDS pediatric cases, the mother has contracted infection through sexual
transmission.

By defining "AIDS" in the context of other pathologies, such as cervical cancer, a
higher number of females will be affected by the disease. Considering that the transmission
mechanism male to female is more efficient than female to male, in future, it could well be
that there will be a higher proportion of female cases which can be attributed to
heterosexual transmission among AIDS patients and the ratio male : female among HIV
carriers will tend to parity.

MATERIAL AND METHODS

Analysis of HPV-DNA on cervico vaginal tissue samples has been carried out on 18
HIV positive females from 1 to 8 years and aged between 18 and 37. Assay and typing was
carried out by *in situ* hybridization using the Enzo PathoGene DNA Probe Assay. This
technique uses three probes: 6-11 (A); 16-18 (B); 31-33-51 (C) bound covalently to biotin.

Table 3 Initial prognostic and diagnostic aspects

	AGE	DIAGNOSIS	CD4	CD4/CD8	β2MICROGLOBULIN
1)	20	HPV vulvar	440	0,61	3,48
2)	24	HPV vulvar	480	0,58	3,27
3)	29	HPV vulvar + VIN1	500	0,63	3,50
4)	27	CIN1 - HPV	407	0,58	3,60
5)	25	CIN2 - HPV (6-11)	443	0,58	3,60

Patients presenting with viral pathology and/or neoplastic pathology of the inferior genital tract were examined, in accordance with standards of other research centers. At first presentation patients exhibited the following profile:-

CDA > 400 cells/mm^3 (n.v. 800/1200mm) ;

WBC > 6000 cells/mm^3;

HB > 13 gr%;

Bet.2 Microglobulin < 4 µg%;

Hepatic functionality indices were within normal limits (Table 3).

Three patients had been treated with Zidovudine (AZT) at a dosage of 500 mg/die two times a day.

Therapy with natural Alfa Interferon (Alfa Wassermann) from normal human leukocytes was carried out on 5 patients, with a regime of 1 Million Units (M.U.) three times a week for three months in patients presenting vulvar HPV and/or VIN. Patients presenting with CIN and/or HPV were treated with a two phase therapy as follows:-:

induction therapy: 1 M.U.three times a week for 3 cycles

maintenance therapy: 1 M.U three times a week for 3 months.

RESULTS

5 patients had suffered from hepatitis B, 7 patients were drug addicts of duration 1 to 14 years, 3 patients suffered from vulvocondylomas and one of them suffered from vulvocondylomas associated to VIN II (Bowen disease), one suffered from CIN II, four patients were pregnant and one patient was voluntarily aborted, while three patients delivered through partus caesareus. Parity was 0 to 5 : the number of spontaneous abortions was 0 to 3. (Table 4). 11 patients out of 18, (i.e. 61%) have tested positive at all three probes. One pregnant patient, in her first trimester, has not tested positive with probe C .

Table 4 Anamnesis and number of examined patients

HIV postive females	18
range	18-37
vulvoconylomas	3
CIN 1-2	1
V.C.E.	2
pregnants	4

One patient, initially has tested negative and successively has tested positive at probe A + B. The successive check-ups have been confirmed (Table 5 and 6).

Table 5 Results at DNA probe

1 patients has tested positive at "A" probe

6 patients have tested positive at "C" probe

2 patients have tested positive at "A" + "B" probes

2 patients have tested positive at "A" + "C" probes

1 pregnant patient has tested negative at probe C

1 patient has tested negative and subsequently
   positive at probes A + B

Table 6 Distributions of HIV positive females

HIV positive females	pregnants	menopause patients
A = 27,27%	A = 54,54%	A = 39,28%
B = 18,18%	B = 30,30%	B = 28,57%
C = 72,72%	C = 54,54%	C = 64,28%

A vulvar biopsy has been also carried out on 3 patients suffering from vulvocondylomas; two of them have tested negative and one has tested positive with probe A. In all three patients presenting with vulvar lesions, a complete regression has been recorded after 3 months of treatment (as showed in Tables 7 and 8). In one patient presenting with florid condylomas, physical therapy was also performed. Patients presenting with cervical lesions have given a complete response after 3 months and the successive check-ups have confirmed this response (average follow-up 50 weeks). Slight

Table 7 Therapeutic prospects

VULVOCONDYLOMAS:	1.000.000 I.U. three times a week for three months
CERVICOCONDYLOMAS:	two-phase therapy
a)	induction therapy: 1.000.000 I.U. three times a week for three cycles
b)	maintenance therapy: 1.000.000 I.U. three times a week for three months

Table 8 Immunologic aspects during the follow-up of the patients treated with α ifn

	beginning	3 month	6 month
CD4	454	491	521
CD4/CD8	0,60	0,64	0,64
β2M	3,37	3,34	2,81

collateral effects such as fever and debility have been recorded; however, they have spontaneously disappeared.

DISCUSSION

HIV could act as a cofactor in increasing HPV manifestation since HIV positive females show a higher HPV and/or CIN and/or VIN incidence due to a presumptive immunodeficit. Indeed there is evidence that there is an increase of Langerhans cells and helper T Lymphocytes in treated tissues after IFN therapy. AZT is the most effective antiviral drug in inhibiting viral growth and prolonging survival.

L'IFNα (Alfa Wassermann) has been used, in our study in the treatment of HPV viral lesions. Antiviral, antiproliferous and immunomodulating actions have been attributed to natural alpha Interferon. and all these properties can be used to reduce the replication of HIV, increase the number of Helper T Lymphocoytes and possibly delay the onset of AIDS.

On the other hand, AZT therapy cannot be used on patients presenting with collateral effects such as leucopenia, anemia, thrombocytopenia (which depend upon the duration of therapy) or because there are some contra-indication such as anemia, thrombocytopenia, high level of transaminase, use of methadone, poor general health or because they have refused therapy: Nonetheless it is necessary to use alternative drugs which have a bio-inhibiting effect, until an alternative immunotherapy, such as a vaccine, is available. Studies carried out among patients that have been treated with AZT in addition to αIFN, are very reassuring because they show significant improvements especially if the two therapies are associated. It would be useful to examine the role of the decline of immunocompetence in the pathogenesis of CIN among HIV positive females.

REFERENCES

1. B. Spurret, D.S. Iones, G. Stewart. Cervical dysplasia and HIV infection. *Lancet*1:237-8 (1988).

2. S. Brown, E.K. Snekjian, A.G. Montag. Cytomegalovirus infection of the uterine cervix in a patient with acquired immunodeficiency syndrome. *Obstet Gynaecol.* 71:489-91 (1988).

3. I. De Vincenzi, R. Ancelle-Park, J.B. Brunet et al. Transmission heterosexulle du HIV: une etude multicentrique europeenne. *Bullettin Epidemiologique Hebdomedaire* 33:130-1 (1988).

4. Gruppo di studio europeo: Risk factors for male to female transmission of HIV. *B M S.* 298:401 (1989).

5. R.J.S. Hawthorn, A.B. MacLean. Langerhans cell density in the normal exocervical epitherlium and in thecervical intrepithelial neoplasia. *Br J Obstet Gynaecol.* 94: 815-6 (1987).

6. O.J. Iversen, S. Engen. *Epidemiology Community Health.* 41:55-8 (1986).

7. A.H. Johnson, H. Lage. Heterosexual transmission of human immunodeficiency virus. *AIDS* 2s:49-56 (1988).

8. T.C. Quinn, D. Glasser, R.O. Cannon et al. Human immunodeficiency virus infection among patients attending clinics for sexually transmitted disease. *N Engl J Med.* 318:197-203 (1988).

9. B. Spurret, D.S. Iosen, G. Stewart. Cervical dysplasia and HIV infection. *Lancet* 1:237-8 (1988).

10. R. Zarcone, G. Cardone, T. Mancino, R.I. Voto, et al. Quadri citologicic cervicali nelle pazienti sieropostive per HIV: primi dati. *In Atti III Convegno Nazionale Aids e sindromi correlate.* Napoli 841 (1989).

11. R. Zarcone, G. Cardone, V. Grande, R.I. Voto, et al. Trasmissione eterosessuale dell' HIV: *progetto di studio Co Fe Se.* 17 (1990).

12. A. Cardone, D. Addonizio, A. Zarcone. Applicazione di un nuovo metado di ibridazione in situ su strisci colpocitologici. *In Atti 5¤ Congr Naz Sc Gin Ost.* Isola d'Elba ETS ed. Pisa 1991, pag.102.

13. R. Zarcone. Diagnostica virale in Ginecologia ed Ostetricia mediante tecnica di ibridizzazione in situ su materiale citologico. *VI Conv Nazio della Soc Ital di Colp e Patol Cerv Vag.* Taormina 10-11-12 ottobre 1991.

HUMORAL IMMUNE RESPONSE TO GENITAL HUMAN PAPILLOMAVIRUS INFECTIONS

Lutz Gissmann

Department of Obstetrics and Gynecology
Loyola University Medical Center
Maywood IL 60153
USA

It is generally accepted that infection with particular types of human papillomaviruses such as HPV 16 or HPV 18 is the most important event in the development of cervical cancer and hence diagnosis of and interference with HPV infection is expected to be of relevance for cancer detection and control. Because of the high prevalence of asymptomatic genital HPV infection, the daignostic value of HPV DNA detection in clinical materials has still to be evaluated. Serology of HPV infections, on the other hand is so far only poorly developed becuase of the lack of suitable experimental systems for virus replication and production of viral proteins that can be used as antigens in serological assays. This restriction is particularly important in case of the mucosotropic HPV types since also in clinical lesions their replication is very low thus prepartion of viral proteins in sufficient quantities has been impossible. With the advances of recombinant DNA technology the genomic clones of all different HPV types became available and expression of individual genes can be achived in a variety of prokaryotic and eukaryotic systems such as E.coli, yeast, Baculovirus and Vaccinia. A description of the vectors used and a critical evaluation of the assays currently employed for the detection of HPV-specific antibodies are given elsewhere [1]. The initial information about the humoral immune response against genital papillomavrisues were obtained when fusion proteins expressed in E.coli were used in Western blot assays [2,3]. Subsequently, in the majority of studies the ELISA technique was employed taking advantage either of synthetic peptide or, more recently of complete viral proteins. Another approach to measure HPV-specific antibodies directed against conformational epitopes was introduced by Müller et al[4] who used viral proteins which were produced by an in vitro transcription/translation system for radio-immunoprecipitation (RIPA). A careful comparison of the different assays in terms of sensitivity and specificity still has to be done. Specificity of the antigen-antibody reactions is a major concern in view of the fact that different papillomarviruses do show a considerable amount of amino acid sequence homology. Cross-reaction of the antigens with antibodies which arose as response to a different HPV type may be difficult to exclude in all instances. In fact, the results which were obtained by different investigators are in part still controversial which may be explained by the variety of reagents and methods used by the individual laboratories thus the introduction of standardized procedures is urgently needed. For example, because of the high degree of sequence homology in the structural proteins between different human papillomaviruses it is unclear to what extent antibodies to the late viral proteins are measured in a type-specific manner and whether such antibodies indicate a current or past virus-producing lesion in this particular patient. There is, however, an agreement between different laboratories that antibodies directed to the E6, E7 (and possibly also the E2 and E4) proteins of HPV16 are more frequently found in sera from cervical cancer patients than in healthy women. Depending on the test employed these antibodies occur in 10-43% (anti-E4), 16-47% (anti-E6) and 20-79% (anti-E7), respectively, of the patients sera, whereas only 0-13%, 2 - 4% and 0 - 15% of sera obtained from age-matched controls were positive [2, 4, 5, 6, 7, 8]. Similar observations have been made in case of HPV 18 E6- or E7-specific antibodies but the number of sera from HPV 18 positive cervical cancer patients which were tested so far is much smaller. Although the antibodies to the early HPV proteins mentioned before can be considered as a marker of cervical cancer, the biological processes leading to these immune responses are far from being understood. Antibodies to the E4 protein, for instance, are not expected to be prevalent in cancer patients since this protein seems to be involved in virus particle production [9] which is not existing in the tumor cells. It remains to be elucidated whether in those patients the E4-specific antibodies simply indicate a past papillomavrius infection or whether the E4 protein may sometimes be expressed in cervical cancer biopsies even in the absence of virus replication. The E6 and E7 proteins, on the other hand are constantly epxressed in cervical cancer cells and the enhanced E6- and E7-specific antibody response in such patients can easily be explained by the long exposure of the immune system to these proteins especially since the antibody titers were shown to rise with tumor stage and seem to drop after treatment of the disease [10]. Therefore, the available data clearly demonstrate that HPV-positive cervical cancer is immunogenic and thus may represent a target for immune surveillance mechanisms. It remains to be seen, however, whether the antibodies to early viral proteins are only a marker for tumor growth or whether they by themselves influence the outcome of the disease. In fact, only a proportion of patients develop measurable antibodies even if an HPV 16 or HPV 18 infection was proven by the presence of the viral DNA within their tumor biopsies. Amongst other possible reasons for this phenomenon which were discussed elsewhere [11,12], it is worth considering that antibody development may be dependent on the HLA type of the patient. This option is of particular interest in view of the fact that a recent study demonstrated an increased risk to develop cervical cancer in women of the HLA DQw3 haplotype[13]. Alternatively, some patients may have become tolerant to the HPV proteins E6 and E7 due to exposure to the virus early in life. In fact, recent data suggest that infections by HPV16 in young children may be more common than generally assumed[2,10,14] but it may be very difficult to establish a correlation between early infection and a negative immun response later in life. In contrast to the strong association of HPV-specific antibodies with cervical cancer, the development of the humoral immune response during natural infections is completely unknown and hence the significance of antibodies directed to the HPV proteins as found in a small number of healthy individuals (see above) is also a matter of future research. It is generally accepted, however, that papillomavirus infections are surveilled by the immune system but humoral antibodies are probably less relevant than the T-cell mediated responses as was concluded both from observations in humans and from experimental animal systems (for review see [15]). Thus, Bonnez and colleagues [16] demonstrated that antibodies directed against complete particles of the human papillomavirus type 11 were present in patients suffering from recurrent respiratory papillomatosis which is known to be induced by this type of virus. Therefore, HPV 11 virus-specific antibodies do not seem to prevent the recurrence of this disease at least not at titers which were measured in this study. It would be interesting to analyze the cellular immune responses within such patients in comparison to healthy individuals as well as to patients with regressing papillomas.

REFERENCES

1. L. Gissman, M. Müller. Serological immune response to HPV. In: P. Stern and M. Stanley (eds), Human Papillomaviruses and Cervical Cancer. Oxford University Press, in press.

2. I. Jochmus-Kudielka, A. Schneider, R. Braun, R. Kimming, et al. Antibodies against the human papillomavirus type 16 early proteins in human sera: Correlation of anti-E7 reactivity and cervical cancer. *J. Natl. Cancer Inst.* 81:1698-1704 (1989).

3. H.G. Köchel, M. Monazahian, K. Sievert, M. Hoehne, et al. Occurrence of antibodies to L1, L2, E4 and E7 gene products of human papillomavirus types 6b, 16 and 18 among cervical cancer patients and controls. *Int. J. Cancer* 48: 682-688 (1991).

4. M. Müller, R.P. Viscidi, Y. Sun, E. Gurerrero, et al. Antibodies to HPV 16 E6 and E7 proteins as markers for HPV 16-associated invasive cervical cancer. *Virology* 187: 508-514 (1992).

5. V.M. Mann, S. Loo de Lao, M. Brenes, L.A. Brinton, et al. Occurrence of IgA and IgG antibodies to select peptides representing human papillomavirus type 16 among cervical cancer cases and controls. *Cancer Res.* 50: 7815-7819 (1990).

6. T. Kanda, T. Onda, S. Zanma, T. Yasugi, et al. Independent association of antibodies against human papillomavirus type 16 E1/E4 and E7 proteins with cervical cancer. *Virology* 190: 724-732 (1992).

7. Nindl Ingo and L.G., unpublised data.

8. J. Dillner, L. Dillner, J. Robb, J. Willems, et al. A synthetic peptide defines a serologic IgA response to a hyman papillomarvirus-encoded nuclear antigen expressed in virus-carrying neoplasia. (1989).

9. J. Doorbar, S. Ely, J. Sterling, C. McClean, et al. Specific interaction between HPV 16 E1-E4 and cytokeratin results in collapse of the epithelial intermediate filament network. *Nature* 352: 824-827 (1991).

10. L.G. et al, unpublished data.

11. L. Gissmann, C. Bleul, I. Jochmus, M. Müller. Detection of anttibodies to human papillomarvirus 16 and 18 proteins in human sera. *Cervix* 10: 115-117 (1992).

12. L. Gissmann. The current role of HPV serology. In: G. Gross and G. von Krogh (eds), Human papillomavirus infections in dermatovenereology. CRC Press, Boca Raton, in press.

13. R. Wank and C. Thomssen. High risk of squamous cell carcinoma of the cervix for women with HLA-DQw3. *Nature* 352: 723-725 (1991).

14. S.A. Jenson, X-P. Yu, J.M. Valentine, L.A. Koutsky, et al. Characterization of human antibody-reactive epitopes encoded by human papillomavirus types 16 and 18. *J. Virol.* 65: 1208-1218 (1992).

15. C. Benton, H. Shahidullah, J.A.A. Hunter. Human papillomavirus in the immunosuppressed. *Papillomavirus Report* 3: 23-26 (1992).

16. W. Bonnez, H.K. Kashima, B. Leventhal, P. Mounts, et al. Antibody response to human papillomavirus (HPV) type 11 in children with juvenil-onset recurrent respiratory papillomatosis (RRP). *Virology* 188: 384-387 (1992).

HPV16 ANTIBODIES IN CERVICAL CANCER PATIENTS AND HEALTHY CONTROL WOMEN

V. Vonka[1], E. Hamsiková[1], J. Novák[1], V. Hofmannová[1], N. Munoz[2], S. de Sanjosé[2], K. Shah[3] and Z. Roth[4]

[1]Institute of Hematology and Blood Transfusion
Prague
Czech Republic
[2]I.A.R.C.
Lyon
France
[3]Johns Hopkins University
Baltimore
Md
USA
[4]National Institute of Health
Prague
Czech Republic

INTRODUCTION

Because papillomaviruses (PV) cannot be grown in tissue culture systems and virus-induced lesions are a very limited source of viral antigens, in most serological studies on human PV (HPV) either synthetic peptides or bacterially produced fusion proteins have been used. Most of the attention has been paid to HPV16 which is most frequently implicated in the pathogenesis of cervical cancer (CC). This communication reports data recently obtained in our laboratory when testing sera obtained from CC patients and healthy individuals for antibodies against seven HPV16 derived peptides.

Immunology of Human Papillomaviruses
Edited by M.A. Stanley, Plenum Press, New York, 1994

MATERIALS AND METHODS

Sera originated from a collection created in the course of the I.A.R.C. study on CC carried out in Spain and Colombia[1,2]. Healthy control subjects were matched with the patients by age and area of living.

2. ELISA

The peptides used are shown in Table 1. They were synthetized as described[3]. IgG-specific ELISA was performed in principle as in the previous studies[4]. The cut-off value between positivity and negativity was the mean absorbance value (A) plus 3 SDs as determined in children's sera; the outliers had been eliminated before the calculations were made. The positive results were clasified on a scale of + to +++, i.e. weakly, intermediately and strongly positive.

Table 1. List of HPV16-derived peptides used

Peptide	Sequence	Reference
E2-245	HKSAIVTLTYDSEWQRDQ-C	5
E4/6	QSQTPETPATPLSCCTETQW	6
E7/1	MHGDTPTLHEYMLDLQPETT	3
E7/2	YMLDLQPETTDLYCYEQLND	-"-
E7/3	DLYCYEQLNDSSEEEDEIDG	-"-
L1	TSQAIACQKHTPPAPKEDPLK	7
L2	PMDTFIVSTNPNTVTSSTPI	-"-

3. Polymerase chain reaction (PCR)

PCR was performed as described[1].

RESULTS AND DISCUSSION

The serological results obtained with the seven HPV16 derived antigens are summarized in Figure 1. More patients than controls displayed reactivity with all HPV16 antigens. The most marked were the differences in the prevalence of antibodies against the three E7 peptides used ($p<0.001$). Also the difference in the prevalence of E2 was highly significant ($p=0.005$). The differences in the prevalence of L1, L2 and E4 antibodies did not attain statistical significance.

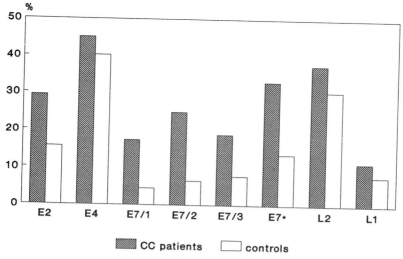

Fig.1. Antibody presence to HPV16-derived peptides in cervical
cancer patients and healthy control subjects

As indicated in Table 2 the difference in the prevalence of E7 and E2 antibodies were not age-dependent. As concerns the L2 antibody, its age distribution indicates that the overall higher prevalence of this antibody in patients than in controls (see Fig.1) was mainly due to the different L2 antibody status of the youngest age-group (20-40 yrs). In this group the prevalence of L2 antibody in patients was significantly higher than in controls. This finding may imply that women with an early HPV infection are at an increased risk for developing CC and, if so, that in young women monitoring the presence of antibody to the epitope(s) in the peptide used may be of some diagnostic and prognostic value.

Table 2.   Age distribution of antibodies to HPV16 peptides in cervical cancer patients and healthy control subjects

Age (yrs)	Group	No	Antibody presence to indicated peptide			
			E2	E7/1,2,3	E4	L2
21-40	Patients	33	18.2	33.3	33.3	51.5+
	Controls	35	8.6	20.0	37.1	25.7
41-60	Patients	63	34.9+	34.99++	46.0	38.1
	Controls	58	17.4	11.6	38.4	32.2
≥61	Patients	37	29.7	32.4+	54.1	24.3
	Controls	33	18.2	12.1	48.5	30.3

+ $p < 0.05$ ++ $p < 0.01$

As indicated in Fig.2, in addition to being more frequent (Fig.1), the reactivity of the patients sera with E7 protein tended to be broader than the reactivity of control sera. Twice as many E7 antibody positive CC sera than control sera were reactive with more than one E7 peptide and three times as many CC than control sera were reactive with all three E7 peptides. These results corroborate our previous observation in Czech patients[8]. There was also a difference between patients and controls in the occurrence of antibodies to various E7 peptides. It may also be of interest that the presence of E7/3 antibody alone was much more frequent in the control sera than in the patients sera. This finding may imply that the solitary presence of E7/3 antibody is a marker of non-malignant HPV16 infection. However, it may also indicate that E7/3 antibody frequently develops earlier after infection than antibodies to other E7 epitopes.

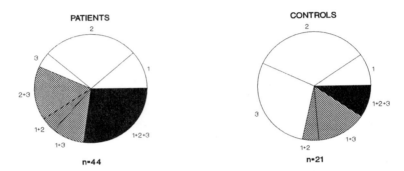

Fig.2. Antibody presence to various HPV16 E7-derived peptides in E7-antibody positive sera from cervical cancer patients and control subjects (1=E7/1, 2=E7/2, 3=E7/3)

In 133 patients and 154 control subjects who were tested serologically, exfoliated cells were tested for the presence of HPV-DNA by PCR. These results are summarized in Table 3. Although HPV16 E7 antibodies were detected more frequently in HPV16 DNA-positive patients than in patients who were PCR-negative or in whom other HPV DNAs were present, the prevalences of HPV16 E7 antibodies in the latter groups of patients were higher than in control subjects (not shown). In addition, the reactivity of E7-antibody in

Table 3.   HPV DNA presence in exfoliated cells as determined by PCR

Group	No tested	Neg	HPV16	HPV18	HPV31	HPV33	HPV35	HPVn.i [1]
Patients	133	29.3	44.4	6.8	4.5	5.3	0.8	9.0
Controls	154	91.6	5.2	0.6	0.6	0.6	0.6	0.6

[1] n.i. - not identified

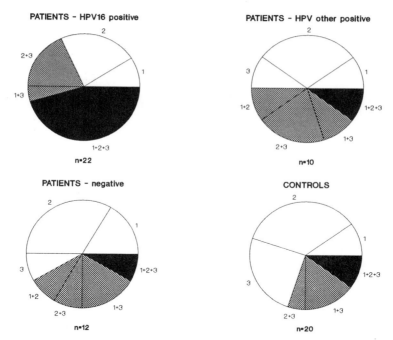

Fig.3. Relationship between antibody presence to various E7–derived peptides and results of PCR

HPV16-positive sera of these patients tended to be broader than in the other patients. This is shown in Fig. 3. Most remarkably, nearly half of the E7-antibody positive sera from HPV16-positive patients were reactive with all three peptides, while such a reactivity was only exceptionally observed in other groups of patients or controls. This observation seems to indicate that the simultaneous presence of antibodies to all three E7 peptides is a marker of HPV16-associated CC.

Table 4. Correlation between presence of antibodies toHPV16-derived peptides and presence of HPV DNA as determined in exfoliated cells [v1)]

HPV type	No	Antibody presence						
		E2	E4	E7/1	E7/2	E7/3	L1	L2
16	67	0.11[+]	0.09	0.16[++]	0.21[+++]	0.18[+++]	0.02	-0.05
18	10	0.15[++]	-0.03	0.01	0.09	-0.07	0.01	-0.00
31	7	0.03	0.05	0.02	-0.01	0.01	-0.05	0.03
33	8	0.01	-0.06	-0.06	0.05	0.00	-0.05	0.01
35	2	0.06	0.01	-0.03	-0.04	0.09	-0.03	0.03

[+] $p < 0.05$ [++] $p < 0.01$ [+++] $p \leq 0.0001$
1) expressed as correlation co-efficients

Finally, the correlation between the results of PCR and the presence of antibodies to all seven HPV16-derived antigens was analysed, as shown in Table 4. HPV16 DNA+ status strongly correlated with the presence of antibodies reactive with all three E7 peptides and weakly with E2 antibody but not with the presence of the other antibodies. The presence of HPV 18, 31, 33 or 35 DNA did not correlate with the presence of HPV16 E7 antibodies. This seems to indicate the type specificity of the E7 antibodies relative to at least these HPV types.

REFERENCES

1. N. Munoz, F.X. Bosch, S. de Sanjosé, L. Tafur, I. Izarzugaza, M. Gili, P. Viladiu, C. Navarro, C. Martos, N. Ascunce, L.C. Gonzales, J.M. Kaldor, E. Guerrero, A. Lörincz, M. Santamaria, P. Alonso de Ruiz, N. Aristizabel and K. Shah, The causal link between human papillomavirus and invasive cervical cancer: a population-based case-control study in Colombia and Spain, *Int J Cancer*, 52:743-749 (1992).
2. F.X. Bosch, N. Munoz, S. de Sanjosé, I. Izarzugaza, M. Gili, P. Viladu, M.J. Tormo, P. Moreo, N. Ascunce, L.C. Gonzalez, L. Tafur, J.M. Kaldor, E. Guerrero, N. Aristizabal, M. Santemaria, P. Alonzo de Ruiz and K. Shah, Risk factors for cervical cancer in Columbia and Spain, *Int J Cancer*, 52:750-758 (1992).
3. V. Krchnák, J. Vágner, A. Suchánková, M. Krcmár, L. Ritterová and V. Vonka, Synthetic peptides derived from E7 region of human papillomavirus type 16 used as antigens in ELISA, *J Gen Virol.*, 71:2719-2724 (1990).
4. E. Hamsíková, H. Závadová, L. Kutinová, V. Ludvíková, V. Krchnák, S. Nemecková and V. Vonka, Priming effect of recombinant vaccinia virus coding for the middle hepatitis B sruface antigen, *Arch. Virol.*, 113:283-289 (1990).
5. J. Dillner, L. Dillner, J. Robb, J. Willnes, I. Jones, W. Lancaster, R. Smith and R. Lerner, A synthetic peptide defines a serological IgA response to human papillomavirus-encoded nuclear antigen expressed in virus-carrying cervical neoplasia, *Proc Natl Acad Sci USA*, 86:3834-3841 (1989).
6. A. Suchánková, V. Krchnák, J. Vágner, E. Hamsíková, M. Krcmár, L. Ritterová and V. Vonka, Epitope mapping of the human papillomavirus type 16 E4 protein by means of synthetic peptides, *J Gen Virol.*, 73:429-432 (1992).
7. A. Wikström, C. Eklund, G. von Krogh, P. Lidbrink and J. Dillner, Levels of immunoglobulin G antibodies against defined epitopes of the L1 and L2 capsid proteins of human papillomavirus type 6 are elevated in men with history of condylomata acuminata, *J Clin Microbiol.*, 30:1795-1800.
8. A. Suchánková, M. Krcmár, V. Krchnák, E. Hamsíková, J. Kanka, J. Vágner and V. Vonka, Range of HPV16 E7 antibodies in cervical cancer patients and healthy subjects, *Int J Cancer*, 51:837-838 (1992).

PREVALENCE OF ANTIBODIES AGAINST DEFINED HPV EPITOPES AMONG INCIDENT CASES OF CERVICAL NEOPLASIA: CURRENT STATUS AND CONCEPTS

Lena Dillner and Joakim Dillner

Department of Virology
Karolinska Institute
Stockholm
Sweden

CONFORMATIONAL EPITOPES: AN ADVANTAGE?

Much of the recent discussion on HPV serology has focussed on the distinction between linear and conformational epitopes, with the difference being that the conformational epitopes are sensitive to conformational changes, whereas the linear ones are not. In practice, this has amounted to that assays using immunoblotting or synthetic peptides are generally classified as linear epitope assays, whereas various other assays including immunofluorescence, immunoprecipitation and ELISAs using whole proteins are claimed to be conformational epitope assays. In many respects, this distinction between linear and conformational epitopes is misleading, since it erroneously implies that epitopes displayed in immunoblotting or in synthetic peptides are devoid of conformation and since it does not point out that assays using e.g. whole proteins will display both linear and conformational epitopes. Furthermore, there exist no theoretical grounds to assume that conformational epitopes would be more specific than linear epitopes. On the contrary, conformational epitopes are, by definition, more sensitive to conformational change and assays based on such epitopes are therefore likely to have greater assay variability problems. Although there is convincing evidence demonstrating that intact HPV particles contain immunodominant and type-specific epitopes that are sensitive to conformational change[1,2], there are no grounds for extrapolation of these findings into believing that conformational epitopes would be more immunodominant or type-specific also in other proteins.

A further disadvantage of the linear/conformational epitope nomenclature is that it lumps together synthetic peptide-based assays, where serological results have been very promising, with fusion protein immunoblotting assays, where the results have mostly been confusing[3,4]. Compared to synthetic peptide-based assays, fusion protein immunoblotting has a lower sensitivity. The non-HPV-part of the fusion protein may also cause masking of epitopes, either by steric hindrance or by adversely affecting the conformation of the HPV part of the protein. Certain serological studies using fusion protein immunoblotting[3,4] have reported that antibodies that are type-specific for HPV 6/11, 16 and 18 have no association with the diseases caused by these viruses. At first glance, these conclusions seem to defy the principle that if A=B and B=C, then A=C. There could thus be 3 different explanations for these findings: 1) Condylomas and cervical neoplasias are not caused by HPV. Although it is not quite clear, this explanation appears to be the one favoured by these authors[4]. In this scenario, genital-type HPV is not sexually transmitted and the HPV-associated diseases must then be due to some sexually transmitted cofactor. Since there is such an enormous amount of data to indicate the contrary[5,6], we will not discuss this possibility further. 2) The studied HPV antibodies do associate with HPV-associated disease, but these authors failed to detect the association. Such a failure could e.g. be due to incorrect epidemiological matching of cases and controls, to interassay variation problems or to the use of an assay that is only semiquantitative and may not detect differences in antibody titers. 3) The antibodies measured are not HPV type-specific, as claimed. This explanation is probably the most likely. There are more than 70 HPV types, most of which are not sexually transmitted and not malignancy-associated. Failure to detect crossreactivity among 4 tested types does not imply that there are no crossreactivities with the remaining 66 types. The semiquantitative nature of the assay may have resulted in failure to detect crossreactives that are of only slightly lower affinity. Also, the non-HPV part of the fusion protein may have caused epitope masking for some HPV types, but not for others. We also have experimental evidence to indicate that some of these epitopes are indeed broadly cross-reactive[7]. We found that hyperimmunization of guinea pigs with purified papillomavirus particles from both cows, dogs and chaffinches regularly induced antibodies reactive with an L1 peptide[7] that had previously been reported by Jenison et al[4] to be HPV 6/11 type-specific. We also have preliminary evidence to suggest that the HPV 16 "type-specific" L2 epitope reported by Jenison et al[8] is closely related to the group-specific antigen which is exposed on disrupted BPV[unpublished observation].

PAPILLOMAVIRUS GROUP-SPECIFIC RESPONSES IN HUMAN SERA

It has long been known that broadly cross-reactive epitopes exist on papillomavirus virions and are exposed after disruption of intact particles[9,2]. Most of these epitopes are positioned in the L1 protein and several of them have been mapped[10,7]. There is also an abundant antibody response to such cross-reactive epitopes in human sera. With optimally disrupted virions, 85-90% of human sera will react with disrupted BPV particles, at a mean ELISA titer of 1:300[11,12]. In our first papers using this antigen, we employed disruption of virus by repeated freeze-thawing[13,14], which is not optimally effective. We have compared the disruption methods in use[7] and have found that disruption using high pH carbonate buffer (as presently used by us) gives about equal results as the method of Baird[15] of treating virions with SDS and beta-mercaptoethanol at room temperature. Also boiling the sample will, however, reduce antigenicity, resulting in that human group-specific antibodies are harder to detect by immunoblotting[3,16]. The laboratories of Christensen and A.B. Jenson utilize high pH carbonate buffer treatment in conjunction with reduction, which also seems very effective[16]. Since the human group-specific antibodies are broadly cross-reactive among HPV types, they are not likely to be extremely disease-specific. We have, however, found significantly elevated anti-BPV antibodies among patients with HPV-associated diseases[13,14] and the laboratories of Christensen and Baird have reported very strong disease-specificity of these antibodies[15,16]. None of these studies used an epidemiologically controlled selection of cases and controls, however, and in recent well-controlled studies we found only a weak association of these antibodies with cervical cancer (Relative risk=1.6)[11]. It should be kept in mind, however, that the human group-specific antibodies are very abundant and that these epitopes of the virions may be exposed after mere freeze-thawing or changes in pH. This is a serious caveat for so-called "type-specific" assays based on whole virions or virus-like particles.

DEFINED EPITOPES AND COMPOSITE ANTIGENS

Considering the large number of HPV types that exist, that different epitopes may have different patterns of cross-reactivity between HPV types, that the induction of antibodies during the course of HPV-induced disease may be different for different epitopes and that the immunological memory for different epitopes may be different, it seems evident that serological results will be different, both with regard to type-specificity and disease-association, depending on the epitope(s) that are studied. Rather than making a distinction between linear and conformational epitopes, it would seem more appropriate to classify serological assays according to whether or not they are based on defined epitopes or on composite antigens containing multiple epitopes. In assays based on defined epitopes, it is possible to separate epitopes to which there is an HPV-type-specific response and/or HPV-associated disease-specific response from those epitopes that have limited or no type-specificity or disease-specificity.

The use of composite antigens containing a multitude of epitopes, such as whole proteins, wart extracts, virus-like particles etc, is not likely to provide informative results, unless the composite antigens contain a few dominant epitopes that are all type-specific/disease-specific. Indeed, in the case where composite antigen serological assays have provided the most well characterized and clear-cut disease-specificity, namely assays based on whole E7 protein[17, 18, 19, 20], the E7 response has been shown to be highly related to the response to a defined epitope (peptide E701) in the E7 aminoterminus[18, 20].

THE MAJOR DEFINED EPITOPES IN HPV

There are a large amount of studies that have defined individual HPV epitopes reactive with antibodies in human sera. The genomic positions of some of the major, characterized defined epitopes is summarized in Figure 1. Both E6 and E7 contain several different epitopes for which a cervical cancer-association of their antibody responses has been reported. The most extensively studied peptide is situated close to the aminoterminus of E7 and is here termed E701(Mueller)[18]. The antigenic reactivity of this peptide is virtually the same as for peptides E7/2(Vonka)[20] and E7:2(Dillner)[21] that map to the same region of E7. Antibodies against several E7 epitopes regularly decline following treatment for cervical cancer[22,unpublished observation]. A few epitopes have been found in E1[21], but have as yet not been further characterized. E2 contains several epitopes, two of which have been extensively characterized (peptides 245 and E2:9). The antibody response against peptide 245 from HPV 16 (245:16) is elevated among patients with CIN[23,24,25,26] and cervical cancer[11,12,19,25,27]. Titers decline after treatment for CIN[24,28] and, for IgA, also after cervical cancer treatment[27]. The antibodies against the homologous peptide from HPV 18 (245:18) also have an association with cervical cancer[11,12,29], which appears to be particularly high among patients with cervical adenocarcinoma[11,29]. The response to E2:9 is also elevated in cervical cancer[12] and E2:9 is the only epitope to which the antibody response has been found to be elevated also in anal cancer[30]

In E4, there are 3 major defined epitopes reported by 3 groups. The E4:4(Dillner)[21] epitope overlaps the E4/6(Vonka)[31] epitope by 16 residues, but the 2 epitopes are only moderately crossreactive. Only moderate disease-association has been reported for the E4 epitopes[17,21,31].

In L2, peptide L2:49[32,33] is positioned close to the L2(Galloway)[8] epitope, but they do not crossreact. The L2(Galloway) epitope has no disease-association[3,8]. The L2:49 response is also not associated with cervical cancer, but rather with benign condylomas[32]. In a poorly conserved region in the L2 carboxyterminus, Lehtinen et al described a type-specific epitope to which an IgA response is preferentially found among patients with HPV 16-carrying CIN[34]. These antibodies disappear concomitantly with spontaneous regression of the cervical lesion[34].

In the L1 region there are two major epitopes in the middle region (L1:13 and L1:16) to which an antibody response is preferentially seen in cervical cancer[11,33]. In contrast, a highly reactive epitope in the carboxyterminal part of L1 (L1:31) has no disease-association[11,32,33].

APPLICABLE SPECIFICITY CRITERIA FOR HPV-SEROLOGICAL ASSAYS

Since it is not possible to define a population of individuals that have never been exposed to HPV and should be seronegative, HPV-serological assays have to be evaluated for specificity using alternative criteria. The major ones that have been applied are:

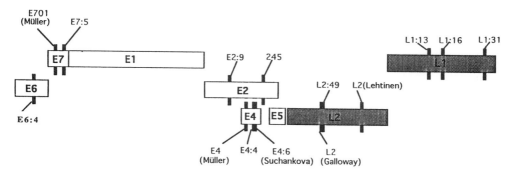

Figure 1. The genomic positions of the major defined HPV 16-derived epitopes characterized to date.

1) Seropositivity against several different HPV-derived antigens is strongly correlated, implying that these antibodies were induced by the same virus. E.g., the antibody responses against the L1:13, L1:31 and L2:49 epitopes are strongly related to each other[11,12]. Also among the epitopes from the early region is there a strong interrelatedness of certain epitopes, most notably between the E701, 245:16 and E2:9 epitopes[11,12] (Figure 2).

2) Seroconversions against several different HPV epitopes occur at the same time. New HPV infections are frequently detectable concomitantly with seroconversion.

When a cohort of 65 men and 111 women with >5 sexual partners per year were followed up with serum sampling and swabs for PCR taken from multiple locations at regular intervals for a follow-up of up to 20 months, 16 seroconversions were detected. The seroconversions against multiple epitopes had occured at the same time and in 5/16 cases a new HPV infection was detectable concomitantly with seroconversion[35].

3) Affinity purified human antipeptide antibodies react with the homologous HPV-encoded protein[23].

4) Several antibody responses against HPV-derived peptides decline following treatment for CIN or cervical cancer, or following spontaneous regression.

This has been found both for peptide 245[24,27,28], for several E7-derived peptides[22,unpublished observations] as well as for IgA to the L2(Lehtinen) peptide[34].

5) Several antibodies against HPV-derived peptides are strongly related to HPV-associated diseases.

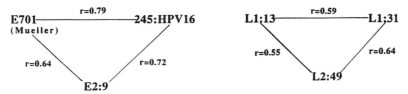

Figure 2. Interrelatedness of the antibody response against defined HPV 16-derived epitopes. The correlation coefficients (r-values) between the antibody responses against the different epitopes are shown. Data based on analysis of more than 1000 sera (mostly the studies by J. Dillner et al[11] and by L. Dillner et al[12]). As can be seen, the antibody responses to the 3 early region epitopes to the left are interrelated, as are the antibody responses against the 3 late region epitopes to the right.

Table 1 summarizes the results of some of the major studies that have demonstrated promising disease-related responses in peptide-based serological assays.

Although there are many epitopes for which most of the specificity criteria apply (or even all of these criteria as in the case of epitope 245:16), it should also be noted that there are several epitopes for which none of these specificity criteria apply[3,4,8]. Far-reaching conclusions about near-ubiquitous and non-sexual transmission of oncogenic genital HPVs is not warranted from any of the serological data obtained to date.

A population-based seroepidemiological study of cervical cancer[11]

We analyzed sera from 94 incident, pretreatment cases of cervical cancer from Northern Sweden that were matched for sex, age and area of residence against 188 controls derived from the Västerbotten Project, a population-based blood bank containing samples from more than 30000 residents (about 80% attendance rate) in Västerbotten county in Northern Sweden. The sera were analyzed for IgG and IgA against 12 synthetic peptide antigens derived from HPV types 6, 11, 16 or 18 as well as against herpes simplex virus 1 and 2, C. trachomatis, cytomegalovirus, Epstein-Barr virus and disrupted bovine papillomavirus. Significantly increased relative risks (RRs) were found for IgG to several HPV 16 or HPV 18-derived antigens, namely L1:13 (RR=3.1), 245:16 (RR=2.8), 245:18 (RR=9.1), E701(Mueller) (RR=3.8) and E7:5 (RR=2.7). For IgA, an increased prevalence was also found for several HPV 16 or 18-derived antigens, namely L1:13 (RR=2.0), 245:16 (RR=3.2), 245:18 (RR=2.3) and E6:4 (RR=2.7). An increased risk was also found for IgG to C. trachomatis (RR=1.7, Confidence intervals(CI)=2.8-1.1). Antibodies to herpes simplex 2 were not significantly associated with cervical cancer (RR=1.4), neither were the broadly crossreactive PV antibodies against disrupted BPV virions (RR=1.6).

Analysis of interactions showed that several responses were related. For example, the response against 245:16 was related to the response against 245:6 (derived from the homologous region of HPV 6), presumably due to crossreactivity. Compensating 245:16 IgA for the interaction term with 245:6 IgA resulted in a relative risk of 16.4 (CI=4.7-56.8). Similarly, compensating the L1:13 IgG response for the interaction term with the L1:31 response yielded a relative risk of 7.1 (CI=3.2-15.7).

ANALYSIS OF THE PRESENCE OF ANTIBODIES AGAINST DEFINED HPV-EPITOPES AND HPV DNA STATUS AMONG INCIDENT CASES OF CERVICAL CANCER[12]

Sera from 233 incident, pretreatment cases of invasive cervical cancer that occured in the Stockholm area during 1989-1992 and from 157 healthy age and sex-matched blood donors attending the same hospital were analyzed for the presence of IgG and IgA antibodies against a panel of previously described HPV-derived peptide antigens and against carbonate-disrupted bovine papillomavirus particles. 10 different serological variables were found to be significantly associated with cervical cancer. The most interesting were IgG to E2:9 (51% pos. cases, 25% pos. controls), IgG to L1:13 (55% pos. cases, 18% pos. controls) and IgA to 245:18 (45% pos. cases, 20% pos. controls). Comparison with the population-based study from Northern Sweden that was analyzed in parallel showed mostly similar results, but discrepancies were noted. In particular, IgG to the E7 peptide E701 had no association with cancer in this study, and IgG to 245:18 was associated with cervical cancer also in this study (p<0.001), but at a much lower level than in the population-based study. The differences between the 2 studies were mostly due to a lower antibody prevalence among controls in the population-based study, suggesting that the difference was attributable to the more stringent epidemiologic design in that study. For the cancers that occured during 1989, we also collected fresh biopsies from the tumors which were then analyzed by Southern blotting and PCR. The tumors from 31/46 patients were HPV-positive in Southern blotting and 41/44 tumors were HPV-positive by PCR. The most common type was HPV 16, found in about 70% of cases. The mean age of HPV-negative and HPV-positive women (as defined by Southern blotting) was identical (54 years). Interestingly, the 3 women that had HPV 33-carrying cancers had a mean age of 72 years. HPV carrier status, as determined by Southern blotting, had no significant effect on prognosis after a 3-year follow-up. 3/44 tumors were also HSV-2 positive by PCR.

Table 1. Summary of major reports in the literature that have found serum antibodies against HPV-derived peptides to be associated with incident cases of cervical cancer (CxCa), cervical intraepithelial neoplasia (CIN) or anal cancer (AnalCa). "HPV16CxCa" indicates that only HPV 16-carrying cervical cancers were studied. The studies marked with an asterisk have used an epidemiologically valid selection of cases and controls (cohort study or population-based controls), the other studies have mostly used some type of hospital patients or blood donors as controls (age and sex-matching was performed in almost all studies). The study marked "*?" used both population-based controls and hospital patient controls.

Epitope and Antibody Class	Disease Studied	Relative Risk	Study Size(n)	p-value	Reference Number
E701, IgG	HPV16CxCa	4.1	277	<0.00001	(18)*
E701, IgG	CxCa	6.2	140	<0.02	(20)
E701, IgG	CxCa	3.8	282	0.000	(11)*
E701, IgG	CxCa	1.0	390	NS	(12)
E701:HPV18, IgG	CxCa	Infinite	232	<0.001	(35)
E7:1, IgG	HPV16CxCa	2.5	90	<0.03	(21)
E7:5, IgG	CxCa	2.7	282	0.016	(11)*
E7:5, IgG	CxCa	2.9	390	<0.001	(12)
245:HPV16, IgA	CIN	3.4	61	<0.002	(23)
245:16, IgG	CIN	2.1	61	<0.005	(23)
245:16, IgA/IgG	CIN	6.0	77	0.007	(26)*
245:16, IgA	CxCa	9.5	122	<0.03	(27)
245:16, IgA	CxCa	5.0	88	<0.005	(29)
245:16, IgA	CxCa	3.2	282	0.000	(11)*
245:16, IgG	CxCa	1.9	358	<0.03	(19)*?
245:16, IgG	CxCa	2.8	282	0.000	(12)*
245:HPV18, IgG	CxCa	4.3	88	<0.0005	(29)
245:18, IgG	CxCa	9.1	282	0.000	(11)*
245:18, IgG	CxCa	1.8	192	<0.001	(12)
245:18, IgA	CxCa	2.8	88	<0.0005	(29)
245:18, IgA	CxCa	2.3	282	0.001	(11)*
245:18, IgA	CxCa	2.2	390	<0.001	(12)
E2:9, IgG	CxCa	2.0	390	<0.001	(12)
E2:9, IgA	CxCa	1.9	390	<0.001	(12)
E2:9, IgA	AnalCa	3.7	143	<0.0001	(30)
E6:4, IgA	CxCa	2.7	282	0.008	(11)*
Any E6, IgG	HPV16CxCa	4.0	277	<0.0001	(18)*
L1:13, IgG	HPV16CxCa	3.4	90	<0.0001	(33)
L1:13, IgG	CxCa	3.1	282	0.000	(11)*
L1:13, IgG	CxCa	3.1	228	<0.001	(12)
L1:16, IgA	HPV16CxCa	6.6	90	<0.0001	(33)
L2/Lehtinen, IgA	CIN	4.0	58	<0.05	(34)
E4/6, IgG	CxCa	3.2	60	<0.01	(31)
E4/6, IgG	CxCa	0.9	228	NS	(11)*
E4:4, IgA	HPV16CxCa	2.2	90	<0.0001	(21)
Combinations:					
Four E6/E7 peptides, pos. for >2	HPV16CxCa	11.0	277	<0.0001	(18)*
245:HPV16, IgA minus 245:HPV6, IgA	CxCa	16.4	282	0.000	(11)*
L1:13, IgG minus L1:31, IgG	CxCa	7.1	282	0.000	(11)*

VARIABILITY BETWEEN STUDIES

As can be seen from the Table 1, although a large number of studies have demonstrated significant associations of HPV serology with cervical neoplasia, the relative risk estimates vary. The two major causes of differences in Relative Risk estimates between studies are assay variations (methodological errors) and different methods for selection of cases and controls (epidemiological errors). Both these sources of error are important. E.g., whereas the Lehtinen laboratory has found similar or higher relative risks for 245:16 IgA than found by our laboratory[11,12,23,24,26,27,29], Lehtinen et al consistently report a comparatively lower relative risk for 245:16 IgG[11,12,23,24,26,27,29]. We performed a parallel analysis of the same study[11,27] and found reasonable agreement for 245:16 IgA (kappa koefficient of 0.6 for cases, 0.4 for controls; both laboatories found high disease-specificity), but poor correlation for 245:16 IgG (disease-specificity only found by our laboratory).

We also have evidence to show that the epidemiological source of error is at least as important as the methodological one. Thus, in our large (n=282) population-based study[11], we found relative risks for E701 IgG at 3.8 (CI=2.01-7.23; p=0.000) and for 245:HPV18 IgG of 9.1 (CI: 4.3-19.2; p=0.000). In our parallel study of 233 cases of incident cervical cancer from Stockholm and 157 healthy blood donors from the same hospital[12], we found a relative risk for E701 IgG of 1.0 (no difference) and for 245:18 IgG of 1.8 (p<0.001), even though the assays for the 2 studies were performed using identical methods (coefficient of variation <10%), including the use of the same positive and negative reference sera on all plates. Most of the antigens that were tested in both studies yielded rather similar results, however (confer Table 1). As summarized in Table 1, most studies have not used epidemiologically valid formats, such as population-based controls or cohort studies, but have mostly used some sort of hospital outpatients as controls.

CONCLUSION

There are by now a large number of studies of HPV serology that have demonstrated that the antibody responses against several different defined HPV-derived epitopes are associated with cervical neoplasia. Since peptide-based tests are very inexpensive, simple and reliable, it should now be possible to combine the most disease-specific epitopes into a useful HPV-serological test with a high predictive value for HPV-associated disease.

REFERENCES

1. N.D. Christensen and J.W. Kreider, Antibody-mediated neutralization in vivo of infectious papillomavi–ruses, *J Virol.* 64:3151 (1990).

2. J. Dillner. Immunobiology of papillomavirus. Prospects for vaccination, *Cancer J.* 5:181 (1992).

3. D.A. Galloway and S.A. Jenison, Characterization of the humoral immune response to genital papillomaviruses, *Mol Biol Med.* 7:59 (1990).

4. S.A. Jenison, X.P. Yu, J.M. Valentine, A. Koutsky, A.E. Christiansen, A.M. Beckmann, and D.A. Galloway, Evidence of prevalent genital-type human papillomavirus infections in adults and children, *J Infect Dis.* 162:60 (1990).

5. H. zur Hausen, Viruses in human cancers, *Science* 254:1167 (1991).

6. M.H. Schiffman, Recent progress in defining the epidemiology of human papillomavirus infection and cervical neoplasia, *J Natl Cancer Inst.* 84:394 (1992).

7. L. Dillner, P. Heino, J. Moreno-Lopez, and J. Dillner, Antigenic and immunogenic epitopes shared by human papillomavirus type 16 and bovine, canine, and avian papillomaviruses, *J Virol.* 65:6862 (1991).

8. S.A. Jenison, X.P. Yu, J.M. Valentine, and D.A. Galloway, Characterization of human antibody-reactive epitopes encoded by human papillomavirus types 16 and 18, *J Virol.* 65:1208 (1991).

9. G. Orth, F. Breitburd, and M. Favre, Evidence for antigenic determinants shared by the structural polypeptides of (Shope) rabbit papillomavirus and human papillomavirus type 1. *Virology* 91:243 (1978).

10. S.A. Jenison, X.P. Yu, J.A. Valentine, and D.A. Galloway, Human antibodies react with an epitope of the human papillomavirus type 6b L1 open reading frame which is distinct from the type-common epitope, *J Virol.* 63:809 (1989).

11. J. Dillner, P. Lenner, M. Lehtinen, C. Eklund, P. Heino, F. Wiklund, G. Hallmans and U. Stendahl, A population-based seropeidemiological study of cervical cancer, *Cancer Res.* In press 1994.

12. L. Dillner, P. Heino, E. Åvall, A. Zellbi, C. Pettersson, O. Forslund, B.G. Hansson, M. Grandien, P. Bistoletti and J. Dillner, Analysis of the presence of antibodies against defined HPV epitopes and HPV DNA status among incident cases of cervical cancer, In preparation.

13. L. Dillner, Z. Bekassy, N. Jonsson, J. Moreno-Lopez, and J. Blomberg, Detection of IgA antibodies against human papillomavirus in cervical secretions from patients with cervical intraepithelial neoplasia, *Int J Cancer* 43:36 (1989).

14. L. Dillner, J. Moreno-Lopez, and J. Dillner, Serological responses to papillomavirus group-specific antigens in women with neoplasia of the cervix uteri, *J Clin Microbiol.* 28:624 (1990).

15. P.J. Baird, Serological evidence for the association of papillomavirus and cervical neoplasia, *Lancet* ii:17 (1983).

16. N.D. Christensen, J.W. Kreider, K.V. Shah, and R.F. Rando, Detection of human serum antibodies that neutralize infectious human papillomavirus type 11 virions, *J Gen Virol.* 73:1261 (1992).

17. I. Jochmus-Kudielka, A. Schneider, R. Braun, R. Kimmig, U. Koldovsky, K. E. Schneweis, K. Seedorf, and L. Gissman, Antibodies against the human papillomavirus type 16 early proteins in human sera: Correlation of anti-E7 reactivity with cervical cancer, *J Nat Cancer Inst.* 81:1698 (1989).

18. Muller, M., R. P. Viscidi, Y. Sun, E. Guerrero, P. M. Hill, F. Shah, F. X. Bosch, N. Munoz, L. Gissmann, and K. V. Shah. 1992. Antibodies to HPV-16 E6 and E7 proteins as markers for HPV-16 associated invasive cervical carcinoma. *Virology* 187:508-514.

19. V.M. Mann, S. Loo de Lao, M. Brenes, L.A. Brinton, J.A. Rawls, M. Green, W.C. Reeves, and W.E. Rawls, Occurrence of IgA and IgG antibodies to select peptides representing human papillomavirus type 16 among cervical cancer cases and controls, *Cancer Res.* 50:7815 (1990).

20. A. Suchankova, L. Ritterova, M. Krcmar, V. Krchnak, J. Vagner, I. Jochmus, L. Gissman, J. Kanka, and V. Vonka, Comparison of ELISA and Western blotting for human papillomavirus type 16 E7 antibody determination, *J Gen Virol.* 72:2577 (1991).

21. J. Dillner, Mapping of linear epitopes of human papillomavirus type 16: The E1, E2, E4, E5, E6 and E7 open reading frames. Int J Cancer 46:703 (1990).

22. J. Dillner, Disappearance of antibodies against HPV 16 E7 following treatment for cervical cancer, *Lancet* 341:1594 (1993).

23. J. Dillner, L. Dillner, J. Robb, J. Willems, I. Jones, W. Lancaster, R. Smith, and R. Lerner, A synthetic peptide defines a serologic IgA response to a human papillomavirus-encoded nuclear antigen expressed in virus-carrying cervical neoplasia, *Proc Natl Acad Sci. USA* 86:3838 (1989).

24. M. Lehtinen, P. Parkkonen, H. Luoto, A. Ylä-Outinen, U. Romppanen, I. Rantala, and J. Paavonen, Antipeptide IgA antibodies to a human papillomavirus type 16 E2 derived synthetic peptide predict the natural history of cervical HPV infection, *Serono Symposia Publications* 78:509 (1990).

25. W.C. Reeves, J.A. Rawls, M. Green, and W.E. Rawls, Antibodies to human papillomavirus type 16 in patients with cervical neoplasia, *Lancet* i:551 (1990).

26. H. Strickler, M.H. Schiffman, and J. Dillner, Unpublished observation.

27. M. Lehtinen, A. Leminen, T. Kuoppala, M. Tiikkainen, T. Lehtinen, P. Lehtovirta, R. Punnonen, E. Vesterinen, and J. Paavonen, Pre- and posttreatment serum antibody responses to HPV 16 E2 and HSV 2 ICP8 proteins in women with cervical carcinoma, *J Med Virol.* 37:180 (1992).

28. K. Elfgren, P. Bistoletti, L. Dillner, and J. Dillner, Unpublished observation.

29. M. Lehtinen, A. Leminen, J. Paavonen, P. Lehtovirta, H. Hyöty, E. Vesterinen, and J. Dillner, Predominance of serum antibodies to synthetic peptide stemming from HPV 18 open reading frame E2 in cervical adenocarcinoma, *J Clin Pathol.* 45:494 (1992).

30. P. Heino, S. Goldman, U. Lagerstedt, and J. Dillner, Molecular and serological studies of human papillomavirus among patients with anal epidermoid carcinoma, *Int J Cancer* 53:377 (1993).

31. A. Suchankova, V. Krchnak, J. Vagner, E. Hamsikova, M. Krcmar, L. Ritterova, and V. Vonka, Epitope mapping of the human papillomavirus type 16 E4 protein by means of synthetic peptides, *J Gen Virol.* 73:429 (1992).

32. A. Wikström, C. Eklund, G. von Krogh, P. Lidbrink, and J. Dillner, Levels of immunoglobulin G antibodies against defined epitopes of the L1 and L2 capsid proteins of human papillomavirus type 6 are elevated in men with a history of condylomata acuminata, *J Clin Microbiol.* 30:1795 (1992).

33. J. Dillner, L. Dillner, G. Utter, C. Eklund, A. Rotola, S. Costa, and D. DiLuca. 1990. Mapping of linear epitopes of human papillomavirus type 16: The L1 and L2 open reading frames. *Int J Cancer.* 45:529 (1990).

34. M. Lehtinen, J. Niemelä, J. Dillner, P. Parkkonen, T. Nummi, E. Liski, P. Nieminen, T. Reunala, and J. Paavonen, Evaluation of serum antibody responses to a newly identified B-cell epitope in the minor nucleocapsid protein L2 of human papillomavirus type 16, *Clin Diagn Virol.* 1:153 (1993).

35. A. Wikström. G. van Doornum, L. Pronk, and J. Dillner, Unpublished observation.

36. C. Bleul, M. Muller, R. Frank, H. Gausepohl, U. Koldovsky, H.N. Mgaya, J. Luande, M. Pawlita, J. ter Meulen, R. Viscidi, and L. Gissmann, Human papillomavirus type 18 E6 and E7 antibodies in human sera:Increased anti-E7 prevalence in cervical cancer patients, *J Clin Microbiol.* 29:1579 (1991).

SEROLOGICAL RESPONSE TO HPV16 INFECTION

Anna Di Lonardo[1], M. Saveria Campo,[2] and M. Luisa Marcante[1]

[1] Lab. of Virology - C.R.S. - Regina Elena Institute for Cancer Research
00158 Rome
Italy
[2] The Beatson Institute for Cancer Research - CRC Beatson Laboratories
Glasgow G61 1BD
UK

INTRODUCTION

HPV infection of squamous epithelium of female genital tract results in a variety of clinical diseases. HPV types 6 and 11, are generally associated with benign proliferative lesions such as condylomata acuminata, while numerous "high risk" HPV types are involved in the development of cervical dysplasia that can progress to malignancy. In particular HPV type 16 is one of the most important etiological agent in cervical squamous carcinoma. Several studies have demonstrated that HPV16 infection can elicit a humoral immune response. Serological assays using different sources of HPV16 antigens, such as synthetic peptides, or protein expressed in prokaryotic or eukaryotic systems, have shown a significant correlation between the presence of antibodies to some HPV16 proteins and cervical cancer. Antibodies against the transforming protein E6 and E7 have been detected frequently and with high seroprevalence in cervical cancer cases[1,2,3]. In contrast little is known about the serological response to the virus throughout the different stages of the infection to the development of the tumour.

To investigate this aspect, we have collected cervical biopsies and corresponding sera from patients with cervical carcinoma, various stages of Cervical Intraepithelial Neoplasia

(CIN), genital condylomas, latent HPV infections and unaffected people. Cervical biopsy specimens have been analysed for the presence of HPV16 /18 DNA by Southern Blot. Sera have been tested for antibodies against HPV16 E6, E7 and L1 proteins by Western Blot to E. coli derived β-galactosidase fusion proteins. Preliminary data indicated a seroreactivity to the E6 and E7 transforming proteins in cervical cancer. In contrast antibodies to the late L1 protein have been detected very frequently in early genital lesions. Further analyses are in progress to confirm these results and to build a complete serological picture of HPV16 infection.

MATERIALS AND METHODS

Samples

Sera and biopsies were collected from women attending the Gynaecological Clinic or the Blood Transfusion Centre of Regina Elena Cancer Institute - Rome.

Antigen Preparation

Recombinant plasmids containing the HPV16 ORFs E6 (nt 112-551), E7 (nt 562-875) and the 3' end of L1 (nt 6150-6818) were used for the expression of β-gal fusion proteins. 100 μg of purified β-gal fusion proteins E6, E7,and L1, were run on 7,5% polyacrylamide gels, transferred to nitrocellulose membranes and used in Western Blot analyses.

Western Blot

The nitrocellulose strips were blocked (50mM Tris HCl pH7.2, 1M NaCl, 0.1% Tween) and then incubated with sera (pre-absorbed with E. coli bacterial lysate containing the β-gal protein) at a 1:250 dilution. After washing, rabbit anti-human IgG (1:1500) was added to the strips followed by biotinylated F (ab')$_2$ fragment of swine anti-rabbit (1:1000). The strips were incubated with streptavidin biotinylated peroxidase and the complexes were visualised by adding DAB substrate. As a control for the specificity of each reaction, a strip with β-gal protein was always included.

Southern Blot

Biopsies were analysed for the presence of HPV-16/18 DNA by Southern blot hybridisation.

RESULTS AND DISCUSSION

A total of 36 serum samples from healthy women or women with different grades of cervical lesions have been tested for the presence of IgG antibodies against HPV16 E6, E7 and L1 proteins using Western Blot analysis. All the women with the exception of the control group 2 were referred for clinical, colposcopical and cyto-hystological evaluation of the cervix. Most of them had a history of seropositivity to herpes simplex virus type 2 (HSV2). From cyto-hystological diagnoses, cervical biopsies were

Table 1. Distribution of antibodies to HPV 16 proteins in patients with genital lesions

			Antibodies		
Diagnosis	Patient numbers	HPV DNA positive	E6	E7	L1
Cervical carcinoma	10	2#	3	2	2
CINII/HPV	3	1	0	0	1
Cervical condyloma	4	2	1	0	1
Vulval/vaginal condyloma	3	1	3	1	3
Control group n1*	8	2	2	0	6
Control group n2^	8	na	2	1	1

Only two biopsies tested
*   Patients from the Gynaecological Clinic of
     Regina Elena Cancer Institute, normal by
     clinical/cytological examination
^   Individuals from the Blood Transfusion Center of
     Regina Elena Cancer Institutena
na   not applicable

classified as 10 cases of cervical carcinoma, 3 of CINII, 4 of cervical condyloma, and 3 of vulval-vaginal condyloma (Table 1). The biopsies were examined for the presence of HPV16/18 DNA by Southern Blot hybridisation. Two different sources of control individuals were used: the first group comprised 8 women attending the Gynaecological Clinic and reported normal by clinical-cytological examination, the second group comprised 8 female blood donors with unknown history of HPV infection or cervical diseases.

Antibodies against HPV16 E7 protein were more frequent in cervical cancer patients and had a higher titre in the most advanced cases (Table 1 and Figure 1). On the contrary, E7 could not be detected in sera from patients with benign or moderate dysplastic lesions, as well as in the control groups. The serological response to HPV16 E6 protein appeared to be quite different. Antibodies to E6 were detected in almost all disease grades and in both control groups, and frequently simultaneously with L1 antibodies; however E6 antibodies were absent in dysplastic lesions (Table 1). The differences in seroreactivity to E6 and E7 may be due to the presence of the two proteins at different stages of infection or to a different degree of immunogenicity. We have also observed a significant seroprevalence to L1 protein in people affected by vulval-vaginal condylomas and in control group 1 (Table 1).

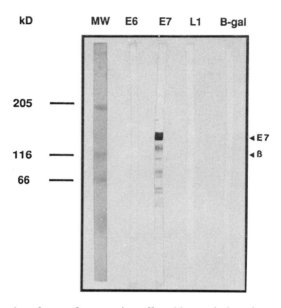

Figure 1. Immunoreaction of serum from a patient affected by cervical carcinoma stage IV against the HPV 16 β-gal fusion protein E6, E7, L1 and β-gal alone. Positive reaction to E7 protein.

Mapping of linear epitopes in the HPV16 L1 protein has lead to the identification of a major immunogenic region (aa 167-271) with a very high homology between different types of Human Papillomavirus and two minor regions which react preferentially with sera from patients with HPV16-associated neoplasia[4]. In addition, rabbit polysera to a HPV16 bacterial fusion L1 have been shown to react against HPV11 disrupted virions in Western Blot assays, as well as in paraffin sections of condylomas[5]. The C-terminus of L1 in our fusion protein contains part of the conserved region; for this reason, given the strong association of HPV6 and 11 infection with genital condylomas, we cannot exclude a cross reaction between antibodies against HPV6/11 L1 in the sera of patients with genital condylomas and HPV16 L1. The increased occurence of L1 antibodies in women attending the Gynaecological Clinic in comparison with the other control group is probably attributable to differences in the populations analysed. Although women in control group 1 were normal by clinical and cytological examination, all of them had a previous history of sexual transmitted disease (such as HSV2), and HPV16/18 DNA was detected in two cervical biopsy samples.

Immune responses against the HPV16 proteins have been observed in both patients and controls also when no HPV DNA was detected in cervical biopsies. This may be due to levels of viral DNA too low to be detected by Southern Blot hybridization.

Despite the limited number of serum samples tested our results are in agreement with those of other groups[1,2], namely that antibodies to L1 and E6 are more frequent during early infection, while antibodies to E7 appear later when the cancer is well established.

ACKNOWLEDGEMENTS

This work was supported by a grant from the Associazione Italiana Ricerca sul Cancro (AIRC) 1992/93 , the CNR ACRO 1992/93 and the CRC. We are also grateful to Dr Gary Sibbet for generous help in preparing this manuscript.

REFERENCES

1. M. Muller, R.P. Viscidi, Y. Sun, E. Guerrero, P.M. Hill, F. Shah, F.X. Bosch, N. Munoz, L. Gissmann and K.V. Shah, Antibodies to HPV-16 E6 and E7 proteins as markers for HPV-16 associated invasive cervical cancer, *Virol.* 187:508-514 (1992).
2. A.K. Ghosh, N.K. Smith, S.N. Stacey, S.S.Glew, M.E. Connor, J.R. Arrand and P.L. Stern, Serological responses to HPV 16 in cervical dysplasia and neoplasia: correlation of antibodies to E6 with cervical cancer, *Int J Cancer* 53:591-596 (1993).
3. S.N. Stacey, J.S. Bartholomew, A. Ghosh, P.L. Stern, M. Mackett and J.R. Arrand, Expression of human papillomavirus type 16 E6 protein by recombinant baculovirus and use for detection of anti-E6 antibodies in human sera, *J Gen Virol.* 73:2337-2345 (1992).
4. J. Dillner, L. Dillner, G. Utter, C. Eklund, A. Rotola, S. Costa and D. Di Luca, Mapping of linear epitopes of human papillomavirus type 16: the L1 and L2 open reading frames, *Int J Cancer* 45:529-535 (1990).
5. N. D. Christensen, J.W. Kreider, N.M. Cladel and D.A. Galloway, Immunological cross-reactivity to laboratory produced HPV-11 virions of polysera raised against bacterially derived fusion proteins and synthetic peptides of HPV-6b and HPV-16 capsid proteins, *Virol.* 75:1-9 (1990).

DETECTION OF ANTIBODIES TO LI, L2, AND E4 GENE PRODUCTS OF HUMAN PAPILLOMAVIRUS TYPES 6, 11, AND 16 AMONG HPV INFECTED PATIENTS AND CONTROLS

Pierre Le Cann,[1] Didier Leboulleux,[2] Catherine Bernard,[3] Cecile Calvet,[4] Marie Christine Legrand,[5] Gerard Lesage,[1] Edith Postec,[5] Christine Mougin,[3] Jose Afoutou,[2] and Pierre Coursaget[1]

[1]Institut de Virologie
Tours
France
[2]Faculte de Medecine
Dakar
Senegal
[3]Laboratoire de Virologie
Centre Hospitalier Regional
Besancon
[4]Institut Regional pour la Sante
Tours
[5]Laboratoire de Virologie
Centre Hospitalier Regional
Brest

INTRODUCTION

Today little is known about the immune response to HPV infections, and no simple and inexpensive method for HPV detection and typing is yet available for mass screening programmes. An alternative to the molecular techniques currently used would be the immunoassays capable of detecting type specific anti-HPV antibodies in sera from patients and healthy subjects.

For this purpose, we tested sera from different population groups from Senegal and France. Antibodies against the L1, L2 and E4 proteins of HPV 16, L1 protein of HPV 6b, and E4 protein of HPV 11 were investigated by ELISA using synthetic peptides.

MATERIAL AND METHODS

Antibodies against epitopes of HPV were searched for by means of ELISA using synthetic peptides designed from those described in the literature (Cason et al., 1989; 1992; Beiss et al., 1991; Dillner et al., 1990; Muller et al., 1990; Jenison et al., 1989; Brown et al., 1991). Sera were tested at 1/10 dilution and antibodies were detected with horse-radish peroxidase labelled monoclonal anti-human IgG.

Anti-HPV were searched for in sera from 96 women with cytological evidence of HPV infection and from 97 women with no cytological evidence of HPV infection (controls). HPV diagnosis was made by polymerase chain reaction using Pap smears.

RESULTS

Three peptides tested: HPV 16 L2 (Dillner et al.1990), HPV 6 L1 (Cason et al.,1992) and HPV 11 E4 (Brown et al., 1991) did not evidence any reactivity, and two peptides: HPV 16 L1 (Cason et al., 1989; 1992) gave a weak reactivity. One of the peptides corresponding to epitopes located within the L1 protein of HPV 6b was very reactive (Jenison et al., 1989). However no significant difference was observed between HPV infected patients (88%) and controls (77%). The other results are shown on table 1. Anti-HPV 16 L2 were observed in 27% of HPV 16 infected women compared to only 7% of other HPV infected women and in 10% of controls. Anti-HPV 16 E4 were detected in 17% of HPV 16 infected women, in 5% of other HPV infected women and in 5% of controls.

DISCUSSION

One peptide located on HPV 6b L1 protein was found to be highly reactive but could not be used for diagnostic purpose since it was shown not to be type specific and because of the high prevalence of anti-HPV 6b antibodies in the general population . Two peptides located on HPV 16 L2 and E4 proteins were found to be type specific but the inability to detect antibodies against these peptides in 3/4 of HPV 16 infected patients limit the application of this methodology to the monitoring of HPV infection.

Table 1. Prevalence of HPV antibodies in different population groups

	HPV 16 peptides			
	L2 (Beiss et al. 1991)		E4 (Müller et al., 1990)	
	N	%	N	%
HPV 16 infected women (40)	11	27%	7	17%
Other HPV infected women (56)	4	7%	3	5%
Controls (97)	10	10%	5	5%

REFERENCES

Beiss, B. K., Heimer, E., Felix, A., Burk, R.D., Ritter, D.B., Mallon, R.G., and Kadish, A.S., 1991, Type specific and cross reactive epitopes in human papillomavirus type 16 capsid proteins, *Virology*, 184: 460.

Brown, D.R., Bryan, J., Rodriguez, M., Rose, R.C., and Strike, D.O., 1991, Detection of human papillomavirus types 6 and 11 E4 gene products in condylomata acuminatum, *J Med Virol.*, 34: 20.

Cason, J., Patel, D., Naylor, J., Lunney, D., Shepherd, P.S., Best, J.M., and McCance, D.J., 1989, Identification of immunogenic regions of the major coat protein of human papillomavirus type 16 that contain type restricted epitopes, *J Gen Virol.*, 70:2973.

Cason, J., Kambo, P.K, Best, J.M., and McCance, D.J., 1992, Detection of antibodies to a linear epitope on the major coat protein (L1) of human papillomavirus type 16 in sera from patients with cervical intraepithelial neoplasia and children, *Int J Cancer*, 50: 349.

Dillner, J., Dillner, L., Eklund, C., Rotola, A., Costa, S., and Diluca, D., 1990, Mapping of linear epitopes of human papillomavirus type 16: the L1 and L2 open reading frames, *Int. J. Cancer*, 45: 529.

Jenison, S.A., Yu, X.P., Valentine, J.M., and Galloway, D.A., 1989, Human antibodies react with an epitope of the human papillomavirus type 6b L1 open reading frame which is distinct from the type-common epitope, *J Virol.*, 63: 809.

Muller, M., Gausepohl, H., De Martynoff, G., Frank, R., Brasseur, R., and Gissman, L., 1990, Identification of seroreactive regions of the human papillomavirus type 16 proteins E4, E6, E7 and L1, *J Gen Virol*, 71: 2709.

IgG ANTIBODIES TO HUMAN PAPILLOMAVIRUS TYPE 16 AND SERUM RETINOL MAY JOINTLY PROTECT AGAINST CERVICAL NEOPLASIA

M. Lehtinen,[1,5] J. Dillner,[2] A. Aromaa,[3] R-K. Aaran,[1] T. Hakulinen,[4] P. Knekt,[3] P. Leinikki,[5] T. Luostarinen,[6] J. Maatela,[3] J. Paavonen,[7] and Hakama [8]

Depts. of [1]Biomedical Sciences and [8]Public Health
University of Tampere
Finland
Depts. of [4]Cancer Epidemiology and [2]Virology
Karolinska Institute
Stockholm
Sweden
[3]Social Insurance Institution, Helsinki and Turku
[5]National Public Health Institute, Finland
[6]Finnish Cancer Registry
[7]Dept. of Obstetrics and Gynecology
University Central Hospital
Helsinki
Finland

INTRODUCTION

Inadequate supply of dietary vitamin A is a risk factor of cervical neoplasia (LaVecchia et al. 1984), and retinoic acid or beta-carotene administration might protect against the effects of such risk factors of cervical neoplasia as human papillomavirus (HPV), and smoking (Winkelstein 1991). Since HPV infections are common and vitamin A intake is vital, it is necessary to try to define their possible interactions. At least three subsidiary interactions exist: 1. Lack of dietary vitamin A increases susceptibility to

Immunology of Human Papillomaviruses
Edited by M.A. Stanley, Plenum Press, New York, 1994

infections (Sommer 1993) and impairs the subsequent immune response (Ross 1992). 2. HPV replication takes place in intermediate and superficial keratinocytes (Howley 1990), the differentiation of which is largely determined by retinoic acid (Gorodeski et al. 1990). 3. Retinoic acid receptors downregulate expression of early HPV genes including the viral oncogenes E6 and E7 (Khan et al. 1993), while in the papillomavirus transformed cells and cervical neoplasia expression of cellular retinol and retinoic acid binding proteins is upregulated (Hillemanns et al. 1992).

We have studied levels of serum retinol in women who during a follow-up of 12 years developed cervical cancer (Knekt et al. 1990). We now report on the combined analysis of serum retinol and IgG antibodies to HPV in the same study population.

MATERIAL AND METHODS

Identification of cases and controls is described in detail elsewhere (Hakama et al. 1993). Briefly, the Finnish Social Insurance Institution carried out a multiphasic screening examination during 1966-1972. Thirty different population groups from various parts of Finland (big cities excluded) were screened. More than 30.000 women (aged 15 years or more) were invited and 85 per cent of them took part in a general health examination, including a questionnaire on medical history and smoking habits, and blood sample (stored at -20°C). The population-based Finnish Cancer Registry receives reports of cancer cases from hospitals, pathology laboratories, and medical practitioners in Finland. Less than 200 cases each of carcinoma in situ (CIS) and invasive cervical carcinoma (ICC) have been reported per year. All persons who had donated blood to the serum bank and were free of cancer at the baseline, and all those who had CIS or ICC diagnosed after the blood sample was drawn (by the year 1981) were identified by linkage of the data files of the serum bank and the cancer registry. Altogether 32 cases with cervical neoplasia and 61 controls (matched individually for sex, age and municipality) were identified, and available for the study.

Serum analyses

Retinol levels were determined by high-pressure liquid chromatography with UV absorption detectors (Knekt et al. 1990). All the IgG antibody analyses were performed by previously described ELISA methods (Dillner et al. 1989, 1990, 1991, Lehtinen et al. 1993). Ultracentrifugation purified, disrupted bovine papillomavirus (BPV) virions were used. Synthetic peptides representing the HPV 16 E2 (HKSAITVTLTYDSEWQEDQ-C), L1 (LCLIGCKPPIGEHWGKGSP-C) and L2 (SGYIPANTTIPF-GGC) proteins were made by t-boc chemistry. As cut-off levels averages of case and control means were used.

Statistics

Risk of or protection against (odds ratios, OR with 95 % confidence interval, CI) cervical neoplasia was estimated by conditional logistic regression, and by the exact methods for contingency tables (Mehta et al. 1985). Joint effects were estimated from the conditional logistic regression model with interaction term included.

RESULTS AND DISCUSSION

In the whole material above mean (high) levels of serum retinol suggested a decreased risk of cervical neoplasia (Table 1). Also high levels of antipeptide IgG antibodies to a structural L2 protein of HPV16 and antivirion (BPV) antibodies suggested a protection comparable to that seen with serum retinol. This was especially true for patients with CIS among whom the odds ratio related to the three factors ranged between 0.27 and 0.22.

Table 1. Odds ratios (OR) related to different types of cervical neoplasia, for high serum retinol and high levels of IgG antibodies to HPV with 95 % confidence intervals (95 % CI), and number of cases (ca) and controls (co) with high level of the variable.

Variable	CIS & ICC			CIS			ICC		
	ca/co	OR	(95% CI)	ca/co	OR	(95% CI)	ca/co	OR	(95%,CI)
Retinol	9/27	0.39	(0 14, 1.14)	4/14	0.27	(0.06, 1.36)	5/13	0.55	(0.13, 2.3)
BPV	10/30	0.53	(0.22, 1.27)	3/16	0.26	(0.07, 1.02)	7/14	1.00[1]	(0.25, 4.1)
HPV16 L1	8/17	0.81	(0.30, 2.2)	3/9	0.47	(0.09, 2.3)	5/8	1.27	(0.33, 4.9)
HPV16 L2	9/25	0.62	(0.26, 1.48)	2/13	0.22	(0.05, 1.07)	7/12	1.26	(0.40, 4.0)
HPV16 E2	8/19	0.69	(0.26, 1.9)	2/5	0.64	(0.12, 3.4)	6/14	0.71	(0.21, 2.5)

[1]Calculated using exact inference methods for contingency tables

The HPV16 L1 peptide has previously been shown to be type-common in nature (Dillner et al. 1990, 1991), whereas the HPV16 L2 peptide is at least partially type-specific (Heino et al. in preparation, Lehtinen et al. 1993). Next we wanted to evaluate the joint effects of the different modes of HPV IgG antibody responses and retinol supply (Table 2).

Table 2. Odds ratios (OR with 95% confidence intervals, 95% CI) related to cervical neoplasia for high levels of HPV antibodies or non-smoking in individuals with high or low serum retinol.

Variable	High serum retinol		Low serum retinol	
	OR	(95 % CI)	OR	(95 % CI)
BPV	1.2	(0.20, 6.6)	0.44	(0.15, 1.3)
HPV16 L1	2.9	(0.52, 16)	0.29	(0.06, 1.55)
HPV16 L2	0.34	(0.06, 1.8)	0.94	(0.30, 2.9)
HPV16 E2	0.41	(0.07, 2,4)	1.0	(0.27, 3.8)
Non-smoking	0.74	(0.11, 4.8)	0.72	(0.20, 2,6)

The concomitant presence of high levels of serum retinol and IgG antibodies to the HPV16 E2 and L2 peptides indicated 59% and 66% protection compared to a situation where low levels of antibodies were detectable (Table 2). High levels of IgG antibodies to the HPV16 E2 and L2 did not indicate similar protection among individuals with low serum retinol. Among individuals with low levels of serum retinol IgG antibodies to the type-common HPV16 L1 peptide or antivirion antibodies were related to 71% and 56% protection against cervical neoplasia. The corresponding analyses with smoking habits and serum retinol levels showed no differences of the kind.

In the interaction analysis (Table 3) we noted a synergistic protective effect of high serum retinol and high levels of IgG antibodies to HPV16 peptides L2 and E2. The opposite was true for the type-common antibodies, since concomitant presence of high levels of serum retinol and type-common antibodies indicated a reduction in the protective effect.

High levels of IgG antibodies to HPV16 peptides L2 and E2 together with serum retinol seems to protect against cervical neoplasia. Since papillomavirus replication takes place in differentiating epithelium, proteins necessary for the replication (E1 and E2) and structural components of the virion (L1 and L2 proteins) are made only in the upper layers of the epithelium (Li et al. 1988, Dillner et al. 1989, 1991, Kadish et al. 1992). Besides that retinoic acid action is a prerequisite for the described expression of HPV antigens, adequate vitamin A supply is necessary also for the subsequent immune response (Ross 1992). The protective joint effect of high levels of serum retinol and IgG antibody response to the more or less type-specific L2 and E2 peptides could reflect successful immune response against replicating HPV16 in women with adequate retinol supply.

High levels of type-common IgG antibodies may protect against cervical neoplasia, but only among individuals with low levels of serum retinol. The antivirion antibodies are directed against conformational (neutralizing) epitopes, a good number of which are present in different papillomaviruses (including the genital HPV types). Besides that most people have antibodies to HPV1 (Pfister and zur Hausen 1978) majority of women acquire

Table 3. Odds ratios (OR) of cervical neoplasia for simultaneous exposure to high levels of HPV antibodies and retinol and to non-smoking and high level of retinol: the observed ratios (obs.) for those with both factors present and expected ratios (exp.) assuming a multiplicative joint effect of the factors.

Variable		CIS & ICC		CIS		ICC	
		OR[1]	(95% CI)	OR[1]	(95% CI)	OR[1]	(95% CI)
BPV	obs.	0.28	(0.06, 1.25)	0.09	(0.01, 1.19)	0.82	(0.11, 5.9)
	exp.	0.11		0.06		0.22	
HPV16 L1	obs.	0.45	(0.09, 2.3)	0.46[2]	(0.01, 5.9)	0.76	(0.07, 8.5)
	exp.	0.05		-		0.29	
HPV16 L2	obs.	0.22	(0.04, 1.20)	-	$(-, 1.7^2)$	0.75	(0.09, 5.9)
	exp.	0.61		0.31		1.24	
HPV16 E2	obs.	0.17	(0.03, 1.01)	-	$(-, 3.0^2)$	0.32	0.03, 3.0)
	exp.	0.42		Ñ		0.33	
Non–smoking	obs	0.30	(0.08, 1.21)	0.25	(0.04, 1.7)	–	$(-,3,7^2)$
	exp.	0.30		0.11		Ñ	

[1]Unit risk was defined for those smoking or with low level of antibodies, and with low level of retinol

[2]Calculated using exact inference methods for contingency tables

genital HPV infection during their sexually active life (Schiffmann et al. 1992). The fact that concomitant infections with multiple HPV types appear to be rare (Koutsky 1991) suggests that there is a booster effect in these women. Thus, high levels of type-common antibodies to HPV could reflect resistance against HPV16 infection and would also explain how individuals without adequate retinol supply became protected.

Retinol or retinoic acid do not have antioxidative properties, which is the characteristic anticarcinogenic feature of their dietary precursor beta-carotene (Tsuchiya et al. 1992). Since serum retinol levels give practically no evidence of the individual beta-carotene intake, it is not surprising that interactions with smoking were not revealed. Unlike retinol retinoic acid is not stored (Blomhoff et al. 1990) and serum retinol levels might have a direct effect on its relative abundance within the infected cell.

In conclusion, the mechanisms of possible interplay between retinol supply, retinoic acid metabolism, HPV gene expression in the differentiating epithelium and immune response remained open, and larger prospective studies are needed to address the multiple interactions of protective factors and causes of cervical neoplasia.

REFERENCES

Blomhoff, R., Green, M., Berg, T., and Norum, K., 1990, Transport and storage of vitamin A, *Science* 250:399.

Dillner, J., Dillner, L., Robb, J., et al., 1989, A synthetic peptide defines a serologic IgA response to a human papillomavirus-encoded nuclear antigen expressed in virus-carrying cervical neoplasia, *Proc Natl Acad Sci USA*. 86:3838.

Dillner, J., Dillner, L., Utter, G., Eklund, C., Rotola, A., Costa, S., and DiLuca, D., 1990, Mapping of linear epitopes of human papillomavirus type 16: The L1 and L2 open reading frames, *Int J Cancer* 45:529.

Dillner, L., Heino, P., Moreno-Lopez, J., and Dillner J., 1991, Antigenic and immunogenic epitopes shared by human papillomavirus type 16 and bovine, canine, and avian papillomaviruses. *J Virol*. 65:6862.

Gorodeski, G.I., Eckert, R.L., Utian, W.H., Shean, L.A., and Rorke, E.A., 1990, Cultured human ecto-cervical epithelial cell differentiation is regulated by the combined direct actions of sex steroids, gluco-corticoids and retinoids, *J Clin Endocrinol Metabol*. 70:1624 (1990).

Hakama, M., Lehtinen, M., Aromaa, A., et al., 1993, Serum antibodies and subsequent cervical neoplasms. A prospective study with 12-years of follow-up, *Am J Epidemiol*.137:273 (1993).

Hillemanns, P., Tannous-Khuri, L., Koulos, J.P., Talmage, D., Wright, T.C.Jr., (1992) Localization of cellular retinoid-binding proteins in human cervical intraepithelial neoplasia and invasive carcinoma, *Am J Pathol*. 141:973.

Howley, P.M., 1990, Papillomaviridae and their replication, *in* "Virology 2nd Edition" B.N. Fields, and D.M. Knipe, eds., Raven Press Ltd. New York.

Kadish, A.S., Hagan, R.J., Ritter, D.B., et al., 1992, Biologic characteristics of specific human papillomavirus types predicted from morphology of cervical lesions, *Hum Pathol*. 23:1262.

Khan, M.A., Jenkins, R., Tolleson, W.H., Creek, K.E., and Pirisi, L., 1993, Retinoic acid inhibition of human papillomavirus type 16-mediated transformation of human keratinocytes, *Cancer Res*. 53:905 (1993).

Knekt, P., Aromaa, A., Maatela, J., et al., 1990, Serum vitamin A and subsequent risk of cancer: cancer incidence follow-up of the Finnish Mobile Clinic Health Survey, *Am J Epidemiol*. 132:857.

Koutsky, L.A., 1991, Role of epidemiology in defining events that influence transmission and natural-history of anogenital papillomavirus infections, *J Natl Cancer Inst*. 83:978.

La Vecchia, C., Franceschi, S., Decarli, A., et al., 1984, Dietary vitamin A and the risk of invasive cervical cancer, *Int J Cancer* 34:319.

Lehtinen, M., Niemelä, J., Dillner, J., et al., 1993, Evaluation of serum antibody response to a newly identified B-cell epitope in the minor nucleocapsid protein L2 of human papillomavirus type 16, *Clin Diagn Virol*.

Li, C-Ch., Gilden, R.W., Showalter, S.D., and Shah, K.V., 1988, Identification of the human papillomavirus E2 protein in genital tract tissues, *J Virol*. 2:606.

Mehta, C.P., Patel, N.R., and Gray, R., 1985, Computing exact confidence intervals for the common odds ratio in several 2x2 contingency tables, *J Am Stat Assoc*. 80:969.

Pfister, H., and zur Hausen, H., 1978, Seroepidemiological studies on human papillomavirus (HPV-1) infections, *Int J Cancer* 21:161.

Ross, C.A., 1992, Vitamin A status: Relationship to immunity and the antibody response, *Proc Soc Exp Biol ed*.200:303.

Schiffman, M.H., 1992, Recent progress in defining the epidemiology of human papillomavirus infection and cervical neoplasia, *J Natl Cancer Inst*.84:394.

Sommer, A., 1993, Vitamin A, Infectious disease and childhood mortality: A 2 Solution, *J Infect Dis*.167:1003.

Tsuchiya, M., Scita, G., Freisleben, H-J., Kagan, V.E., and Packer, L., 1992, Antioxidant radical-scavenging activity of carotenoids and retinoids compared to α-tocopherol, *Meth Enzymol*.213:460.

Winkelstein, W., 1991, Smoking and cervical cancer - current status: a review, *Am J Epidemiol*.131:945.

PROGNOSTIC SIGNIFICANCE OF ANTIBODIES TO HPV-16 E7 / E4 PROTEINS AND FRAGMENTS OF CYTOKERATIN 19 IN INVASIVE CERVICAL CARCINOMA

K.N. Gaarenstroom,[1] J.M.G. Bonfrer,[2] G.G. Kenter,[1] C.M. Korse,[2] Th.J.M. Helmerhorst,[3] and J.B. Trimbos[1]

[1]Department of Gynecology of Leiden University Medical Center
Leiden
The Netherlands
[3]Depts of Gynecology and [2]Clinical Chemistry of the Netherlands Cancer
Institute Amsterdam
The Netherlands

INTRODUCTION

The objective of this study was to search for new markers with prognostic potential in invasive carcinoma of the uterine cervix. Sera of 78 patients with cervical cancer were tested for the presence of Ig-G antibodies to human papillomavirus (HPV) type 16 E7/1 and E4/1 proteins and for the presence of fragments of cytokeratin 19 (CK 19) in serum to determine the relationship between these parameters, tumor stage and prognosis.

It is noteworthy that this study is one of the first, which has focused on the relationship between the presence of antibodies to HPV peptides at particular stages of disease and the effect on the prognosis. The presence of fragments of CK 19 in patients with invasive cervical carcinoma was not investigated at all thus far.

PATIENTS AND METHODS

The study group comprised 78 patients with squamous cell cervical cancer who

Immunology of Human Papillomaviruses
Edited by M.A. Stanley, Plenum Press, New York, 1994

was 82 %, 74 % and 62 %. Variables tested for with stepwise Cox analysis were age, FIGO stage, presence of antibodies to respectively, HPV-16 E7, E4, E7 and/or E4 peptides. In the univariate analysis a significant relation was found between survival and FIGO stage (p < 0.001) as well as the Cyfra 21-1 value (p < 0.001). There was some indication for such a relation with respect to age (non-linear, p = 0.035). Controlling for Cyfra 21-1, the p-value for FIGO stage deteriorated markedly, losing its statistical significance (p = 0.18). Age, viewed non-linearly, still seemed to have an independent relation with survival (p = 0.013). Controlling for age as well, Cyfra 21-1 still remained strongly significant (p <

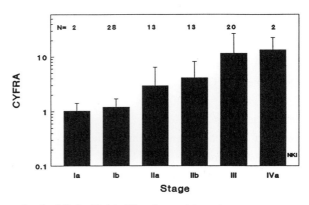

Figure 1. Mean serum level of Cyfra 21-1 in 78 patients with cervical carcinoma related to FIGO stage.

0.001), while the p-value for FIGO stage increased still further (p =0.33). No other variable, reached the 0.05 limit.

Figure 2 shows the survival curves for the patient group with antibodies to HPV 16 E7/1 and/or E4/1 proteins compared to the antibody-negative group. No significant difference was found between these two groups with respect to survival. Figure 3 shows the survival curves for 3 groups according to Cyfra 21-1 level. As shown, patients with increased Cyfra 21-1 level had a significantly worse 5-year survival.

were treated at the Netherlands Cancer Institute, Amsterdam, between 1984 and 1988. Two patients with Figo stage Ia had been treated by cone biopsy of the uterine cervix, the other 76 patients had been treated by either radical hysterectomy and pelvic lymphadenectomy or radiation therapy (40 - 45 Gy in 4 to 5 weeks). Clinical data were obtained from the medical files. Pretreatment sera of the carcinoma cases and 198 age- and sex-matched controls (healthy blooddonors of the bloodbank of Leiden) were tested in enzyme immunoassays (ELISA) for reactivity with HPV-16 E7/1 (peptide PTLHEYMLDLQPETTDLYCYEQLNDSSEEE) and E4/1 (peptide KPSPWAPKKHRRLS) synthetic peptides as described by Müller[1,2]. All sera were tested in duplicate and for each serum an absorbance value was calculated. The mean absorbance value of the controls + three standard deviations was taken as cut-off value[1]. Individual sera of patients with invasive carcinoma were scored as antibody-positive or -negative for each peptide, using a cut-off absorbance value of 0.18 for anti-E7/1 and 0.08 for anti-E4/1.

To measure quantitatively CK 19 fragments in serum of patients with cervical carcinoma, a double determinant enzyme-immunoassay, referred to as Cyfra 21-1, was used. In this test two monoclonal antibodies (MoAb) were used in an assay based on the simultaneous sandwich principle. Polystyrene beads were coated with KS 19.1, while the tracer was a ^{125}I labeled BM 29.21 mouse MoAb.

For statistical analysis the χ^2 test and one way analysis of variance was used to compare the presence of antibodies to HPV peptides or fragments of CK 19 with tumor stage. A stepwise procedure using Proportional Hazard regression analysis was used to identify prognostic factors with respect to survival (all causes of death). Three categories for Cyfra 21-1 level were defined with limits chosen so that approximately equally sized groups were created. A p-value < 0.05 was regarded as indicating a significant difference. Life-table calculations were performed using the product-limit method of Kaplan and Meier.

RESULTS

The mean age of the patient group was 52 years (range 22-83) and the mean follow-up period was 56 months (range 6-97). Forthy-three patients were diagnosed with low stage disease (FIGO Ia, Ib, IIa) and 35 patients with advanced stage carcinoma (FIGO IIb, III, IV).

Antibodies to HPV-16 E7/1 and/or E4/1 peptides were found in, respectively, 29 of the 198 (15%) controls, 15 of the 43 (35%) patients with low stage disease and in 16 of the 35 (46%) patients with advanced stages. Significantly more antibodies were found among patients with cervical cancer compared to the control group (p < 0.001). However, no significant difference was found between low and advanced tumor stage. In contrast, a high serum Cyfra 21-1 level was associated with advanced tumor stage (p < 0.05) (Figure 1).

Twenty-seven of the 78 patients died during follow-up. Survival at 1, 2 and 5 years

CONCLUSIONS

Antibodies to HPV 16 E7/1 and/or E4/1 peptides were more frequently found in patients with cervical carcinoma compared to controls (p < 0.05). However, the presence of these antibodies was not related to tumor stage or survival. In contrast, a high serum Cyfra 21-1 level was associated with advanced tumor stage and a worse prognosis. In conclusion, Cyfra 21-1 seems to be a better marker for cervical cancer compared to antibodies to HPV-16 E7 or E4 peptides.

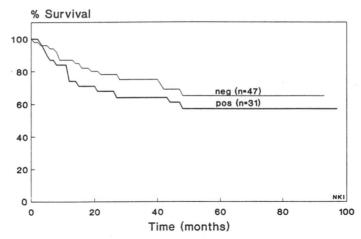

Figure 2. Five-year survival of 78 patients with cervical carcinoma. The patient group with antibodies to HPV-16 E7 and/or E4 peptides was compared to the antibody-negative group.

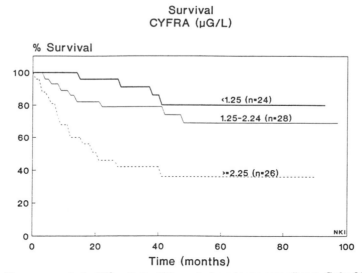

Figure 3. Five-year survival of 78 patients with cervical carcinoma according to Cyfra 21-1 level.

ACKNOWLEDGEMENTS

The authors are grateful to Dr. L. Gissmann and Dr. M. Müller for the analysis of HPV antibodies.

REFERENCES

1. M. Müller, R.P. Viscidi, Y. Sun, E. Guerrero, P.M. Hill, F. Shah, F.X. Bosch, N. Muñoz, L. Gissmann, and K.V. Shah, Antibodies to HPV-16 E7 proteins as markers for HPV-16 associated invasive cervical cancer, *Virology* 187: 508 (1992)
2. M. Müller, H. Gausepohl, G. de Martynoff, R. Frank, R. Brasseur, and L. Gissmann, Identification of seroreactive regions of the human papillomavirus type 16 proteins E4, E6, E7 and L1, *J Gen Virol.* 71: 2709 (1990)

DEVELOPMENT OF SEROLOGICAL ASSAYS FOR DETECTION OF ANTI-HPV-16 E6 AND E7 ANTIBODIES

Anna K. Ghosh, Simon N. Stacey, Leticia Rocha Zavaleta, Nigel K. Smith, John R. Arrand, and Peter L. Stern

CRC Departments of Immunology and Molecular Biology
Paterson Institute for Cancer Research
Christie Hospital NHS Trust
Manchester M20 9BX
UK

INTRODUCTION

The majority of squamous cell carcinomas of the cervix (60 to 80%) contain human papillomavirus (HPV) 16 or 18 DNA, and infection with these viruses is believed to be a major factor in the pathogenesis of the disease. These tumours tend to retain and actively transcribe HPV early region open reading frames (ORFs). The E6 and E7 proteins have been implicated in tumorigenesis owing to their prevalence in cervical tumours and cell lines derived from them (Smotkin and Wettstein, 1986; Seedorf et al., 1987), transforming activity *in vitro* (DiMaio, 1991), and their ability to bind to the product of the tumour suppressor genes p53 and Rb, respectively (Dyson et al., 1989; Werness et al., 1990).

Although the molecular properties of HPV-encoded proteins have been extensively studied, an aspect of the biology of HPV which is still poorly understood is the immune response to the virus. Analysis of serological responses to HPV proteins may help to elucidate the relationship between infection and disease, and have diagnostic potential. Evaluation of antibody responses in patients exposed to high risk HPV type infection has been hampered by lack of appropriate target antigens for use in serological assays. HPVs have not yet been successfully propagated by *in vitro* cell-culture techniques and therefore, no reliable source of authentic viral proteins are readily available. To circumvent this difficulty many investigations have used prokaryotic gene expression systems or synthetic peptides as target antigens in Western blot and ELISA assays. In general, investigations of HPV antibody status using these reagents have given inconsistent results. An exception is the finding that antibodies to HPV-16 E7 are associated with invasive cervical cancer (Jochmus-Kudielka et al., 1989; Kochel et al., 1991; Mann et al., 1990). The frequency of seropositivity rarely exceeds 40% of carcinoma patients, however, which is far less than would be expected based on the expected frequency of HPV-16 DNA. A limitation of the above techniques to detect antibody responses may be the nature of the reagents used as antigens. Synthetic peptides represent short regions of the protein and display linear epitopes, whilst recombinant proteins are often denatured during their purification or use in Western blot assays. Antibodies targeted to non-linear epitopes would not be measured, thus restricting assay sensitivity, and specificity might be reduced by exposure of potentially cross-reactive epitopes which are normally hidden in the native protein. The true serological picture might better be revealed using assays which allow the detection of conformation dependent antibody specificities.

This paper summarises our experience of detecting antibody responses in patients with pre-neoplastic and neoplastic cervical lesions and control populations, to HPV-16 proteins. An initial study investigated antibodies to HPV early proteins E4, E6 and E7 and the major capsid protein L1 by Western blot analysis of recombinant HPV proteins. The assay allowed the detection of anti-E6 antibodies , which were found to associate significantly with cervical cancer. In order to generate improved serological target antigens that allow detection of conformational epitopes, recombinant baculovirus vectors expressing the HPV-16 E6 and E7 ORFs were constructed. These constructs were used in radioimmunoprecipitation assays (RIPA) for detection of antibodies in sera from cervical carcinoma patients and controls. Further assays are being developed for large scale serological screening.

SEROLOGICAL RESPONSES TO HPV-16 PROTEINS

Western blot assays

The aim of this study was to examine antibody responses in patients with cervical cancer, cervical intraepithelial neoplasia (CIN), non-genital cancers and healthy individuals, directed against HPV-16 L1, E4, E6 and E7 gene products expressed in *E. coli* as MS-2 replicase fusion proteins.

Serum samples were collected from: a) 92 patients with histologically diagnosed cervical carcinoma prior to treatment of their disease by radiotherapy; of these patients , 67 were typed for HPV-16 DNA, as described by Connor and Stern (1990); b) 90 patients attending a colposcopy clinic (28 patients with CIN I and/or condylomatous changes and 62 patients with CIN II and/or CIN III ; c) 41 patients with non-genital cancer and d) 123 healthy individuals.

The pEx-MS-2 replicase expression vectors containing HPV-16 ORFs, L1, E4, E6 and E7 were constructed by Seedorf et al., (1987). The preparation of fusion proteins from bacterial extracts and Western blot analysis were as described in Ghosh et al., (1993).

Table 1 summarises the prevalence of antibodies to HPV-16 proteins among the study groups. A more detailed description is found in Ghosh et al., (1993) and only the responses to E6 and E7 will be discussed here. The principal findings were: (i) anti-E6 antibodies were significantly associated with cervical cancer; (ii) the incidence of anti-E7 antibodies is significantly higher in cervical-cancer patients than in cervical dysplasia patients and healthy individuals, but similar to the prevalence in patients with non-genital cancers; (iii) antibodies to L1 are associated with the early phase of cervical dysplasia; and (iv) the prevalence of anti-E4 antibodies is similar in cases of cervical dysplasia, cervical cancer and in non-genital cancer types. There was no correlation between seropositivity and presence of HPV-16 DNA.

The high prevalence of anti-E6 antibodies in the cervical cancer patients as compared with other groups supports the conclusions of a recent report indicating that antibodies to E6 proteins are markers of HPV-16 associated invasive cancer. However, only 16% of cervical cancer patients were positive to HPV-16 E6 peptides in the peptide ELISA assay described by Muller et al., (1992). Previous analysis of anti-E6 antibody responses using a Western blot assay detected positive responses in one of 23 cervical-cancer patients (Kochel et al., 1991). This low incidence could be due to the use of a E6 β-gal fusion protein which lacks the region containing the major B-cell epitopes (Muller et al., 1992).

The increased frequency of E7 antibody responses observed in cervical-cancer patients compared with normal controls has been described by several other studies

Table 1. Prevalence of antibody to HPV-16 proteins (determined by Western blot) among healthy individuals, patients with pre-malignant cervical lesions, cervical cancer and non-genital cancer.

Study group	Number of patients	Antibody			
		L1	E4	E6	E7
Normal control	123	3(2%)	29(24%)	5(4%)	8(7%)
CIN I	28	5(18%)	10(36%)	4(14%)	4(14%)
CIN II/III	62	6(10%)	24(39%)	8(13%)	4(6%)
CaCx	92	5(5%)	40(43%)	32(35%)	23(25%)
Non-genital cancer	41	3(7%)	17(41%)	5(12%)	10(24%)

(Jochmus-Kudielka et al., 1989; Krchnak et al., 1990; Kochel et al., 1991; Suchankova et al., 1991). A similar incidence of E7-positive sera were found in patients with non-genital cancers (including patients with Hodgkin's disease, lung, oesophageal and breast cancer), which shows a lack of specificity of these responses in cervical disease. Cancer patients are frequently immunocompromised and it is possible that this may facilitate not only primary HPV infection, but also reactivation of latent HPV. Further studies are required to determine the significance of these antibody responses to HPV-16 E7.

Western blot analysis with bacterially expressed fusion proteins has several disadvantages for serological analysis. Antibodies directed against conformational epitopes, or epitopes that are altered by denaturation, will not be detected. Fusion proteins do not undergo post-translational modification in bacteria, and would therefore not detect antibodies directed against epitopes that are dependent upon post-translational modification. In addition, it is labour intensive and non-quantitative. To overcome these problems, recombinant baculovirus vectors expressing the HPV-16 E6 and E7 ORFs were constructed and used to detect the presence of antibodies in human sera.

Radioimmunoprecipitation assays

A eukaryotic expression system based on an insect baculovirus was employed to generate improved target antigens for use in serological assays. The construction and characterisation of recombinant baculovirus vectors expressing HPV-16 E6 and E7 ORFs (bE6 and bE7) are described in Stacey et al.,(1992, 1993).

Cells infected with the vector containing E6 gene sequences expressed a stable protein doublet comprising 18.5K and 19.1K bands. This protein reacted in Western blots with an antiserum raised against a purified E6 fusion protein produced in *E.coli*. This antiserum and others raised against *E.coli*-derived E6 fusion proteins were unable to immunoprecipitate the native bE6. However, serum from a cervical carcinoma patient readily immunoprecipitated the bE6 protein, suggesting that the baculovirus-derived protein represented a realistic antigenic target. The bE7 produced two major forms of the protein; a 16K and an 18K form. The 16K component was shown to be synthesised independently of the 18K form and was truncated at the N-terminus.

A baculovirus based RIPA was developed for the detection of anti-E6 and anti-E7 protein antibodies in patient sera. This assay was chosen because immunoprecipitation is a method that does not involve a denaturing step prior to the antigen-antibody reaction; therefore allowing the detection of antibodies to conformational epitopes. Sera were selected for analysis by RIPA based on their performance in the Western blot assay described above. The aim was to investigate whether similar seronegative and seropositive results would be obtained using the more authentic bE6 and bE7 target antigens and, in particular, whether the RIPA would detect responses which had scored seronegative by Western blot. Samples were encoded and blind-tested at 1:50 dilution. The results of the bE6 and bE7 RIPAs are summarised in tables 2 and 3.

Table 2. Comparison of anti-HPV-16 E6 antibody status determined by Western blot to MS2 fusion proteins and by baculovirus E6 RIPA.

sample	anti-MS2-E6	bE6 RIPA		
		+	+/-	-
CaCx	10+	10	0	0
	10-	3	2	5
Normal control	10-	1	1	8

In the case of E6 antibody responses, all of the cervical carcinoma patients' sera that were positive by Western blot were also positive by bE6 RIPA. In contrast, of the 10 negative carcinoma patients, only five scored negative by bE6 RIPA. Of the 10 normal sera, 8 were negative by both methods, whereas one was positive and one was equivocal by bE6 RIPA. The normal sample that scored positive by bE6 RIPA had previously shown strong antibody responses to the MS2-HPV-16 E4 fusion protein in the Western blot assay.

Table 3. Comparison of anti-HPV-16 E7 antibody status determined by Western blot to MS2 fusion proteins and by baculovirus E7 RIPA.

sample	anti-MS2-E7	bE7 RIPA		
		+	+/-	-
CaCx	10+	9	1	0
	10-	3	2	5
Normal control	10-	0	0	10

An increased rate of detection of anti-E7 antibodies were observed in the bE7 RIPA. Of the 10 carcinoma patient samples previously negative by the Western blot assay, 3 were positive , 2 were equivocal and only 5 were negative by the bE7 RIPA. 4/5 of the samples which scored anti-E7 positive in the RIPA but negative by Western blot had demonstrable antibodies to other HPV-16 proteins.

The increase in detection rate of anti-E6 and E7 antibodies using the bE6 and bE7 RIPAs is likely due to increased sensitivity of these assays relative to Western blot, due to the use of more authentic target epitopes. This result is similar to the increased sensitivity of the TT-RIPA reported by Muller et al., (1992), who compared a RIPA with *in vitro* transcribed and translated HPV-16 E7 protein with an ELISA using E7 peptides. The data suggest that anti-E6 and anti-E7 responses may be more common than previously detected and that serological surveys which rely solely on the use of linear target antigens may be subject to substantial misclassification errors, particularly amongst seronegative carcinoma patients.

129

Development of non-radioactive assays

The bE6 and bE7 RIPA are not easily adaptable to large scale seroepidemiological surveys and the development of higher capacity assays that employ native proteins as serological targets are required. Initially we are concentrating on developing assays using bE7 but new bE6 assays will also be developed. A derivative of the original bE7 recombinant was produced in which the levels of E7 were enhanced. This was achieved by placing the E7 ORF start codon in a favourable Kozak translational initiation context. The resulting baculovirus produced markedly increased levels of the 18K E7 protein, while the production of the 16K, N-terminally truncated form was suppressed (Stacey, unpublished observations). This improved vector is being used to develop: a) a non-radioactive immunoprecipitation assay; and b) an ELISA for E7 serology.

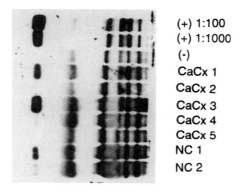

(+) 1:100
(+) 1:1000
(-)
CaCx 1
CaCx 2
CaCx 3
CaCx 4
CaCx 5
NC 1
NC 2

Figure 1. Screening of cervical carcinoma (CaCX) and normal (NC) sera by bE7-IP/Western blot/ECL. Negative control (-), positive control (+).

A non-radioactive immunoprecipitation assay was developed in which the initial immunoprecipitation step was followed by Western blotting of immunoprecipitated E7 protein and developed by ECL using a monoclonal anti-E7 antibody (Triton anti-HPV-16-E7). Several cervical carcinoma and normal sera were tested by bE7-IP/Western/ECL and this is illustrated in Figure 1.

Those samples showing a stronger signal than the 1:1000 positive control were scored positive; those with a stronger signal than the negative, but weaker than the 1:1000 positive, were scored as weak positive; all samples with either a similar or weaker signal than the negative control were scored negative. This assay is being evaluated for disease association using a panel of sera from cervical carcinoma patients, non-genital carcinoma patients and age-matched controls. The results will be compared with those obtained by the Western blot method.

The bE7 is being purified by immunoaffinity for use in an ELISA. This method of purification will enable conformational epitopes to be measured and data obtained from this assay will be compared with Western blot and IP/Western/ECL.

CONCLUSIONS

The Western blot protocol with HPV-16 MS2 fusion protein targets and the baculovirus RIPA have enabled the detection of anti-E6 and anti-E7 serological responses. Anti-E6 antibody responses were significantly associated with cervical cancer. The RIPA was substantially more sensitive and specific than Western blotting, probably due to the detection of conformational epitopes. Non-radioactive serological assays amenable to large scale screening that use native protein as target antigens, are being developed. The use of several different recombinant expression systems for the production of HPV-16 E6 and E7 proteins will allow the detection of antibodies recognising a variety of epitopes. A combination of assay systems may facilitate the monitoring of HPV infection and the development of cervical cancer.

ACKNOWLEDGEMENTS

We would like to thank D. Jordan for technical assistance. This work was supported by the Cancer Research Campaign.

REFERENCES

Connor, M.E., and Stern, P.L., 1990, Loss of MHC-class-I expression in cervical carcinomas, *Int J Cancer* 46:1029

DiMaio, D., 1991, Transforming activity of bovine and human papillomaviruses in cultured cells, *Adv Cancer Res.* 56:133

Dyson, N., Howley, P.M., Munger, K., and Harlow, E.,1989, The human papillomavirus-16 E7 oncoprotein is able to bind to the retinoblastoma gene product, *Science* 243:934

Ghosh, A.K., Smith, N.K., Stacey S.N., Glew,S.S., Connor, M.E., Arrand, J.R., and Stern P.L., 1993, Serological responses to HPV 16 in cervical dysplasia and neoplasia: correlation of antibodies to E6 with cervical cancer, *Int J Cancer* 53:591

Jochmus-Kudielka, I., Schneider, A., Braun, R., Kimmig, R., Koldovsky, U., Schneweis, K.E., Seedorf, K., and Gissman, L., 1989, Antibodies against the human-papillomavirus-type-16 early proteins in human sera; correlation of anti-E7 reactivity with cervical cancer, *Int J Cancer* 81:1698

Kochel, H.G., Monazahian, M., Sievert, K., Hohne, M., Thomssen, C., Teichmann, A., Arendt, P., and Thomssen, R., 1991, Occurrence of antibodies of L1, L2, E4 and E7 gene products of human papillomavirus types 6b, 16 and 18 among cervical-cancer patients and controls, *Int J Cancer* 48:682

Krchnak, U., Vagner, J., Suchankova. A., Kremar, M., Ritterova, L., and Vonka, V., 1990, Synthetic peptides derived from E7 region of human papillomavirus type 16 used as antigens in ELISA, *J Gen Virol.* 71:2719

Mann, V. M., Loo de Lao, S., Brenes, M., Brinton, L.A., Rawls, J.A., Green, M., Reeves, W.C., and Rawls, W.E., 1990, Occurrence of IgA and IgG antibodies to select peptides representing human papillomavirus type 16 among cervical-cancer cases and controls, *Cancer Res.,* 50:7815.

Muller, M., Viscidi, R.P., Sun, Y., Guerrero, E., Hill, P.M., Shah, F., Bosch, X., Munoz, N., Gissman, L., and Shah, K.V.,1992, Antibodies to HPV-16 E6 and E7 proteins as markers for HPV-16-associated invasive cancer, *Virology*, 187:508

Seedorf, K., Oltersdorf, T., Krammer, G., and Rowekamp, W.,1987, Identification of early proteins of the human papillomaviruses type 16 (HPV 16) and type 18 (HPV 18) in cervical-carcinoma cells, *EMBO J.* 6:139

Smotkin, D., and Wettstein, F.O., 1986, Transcription of human papillomavirus type 16 early genes in a cervical cancer and a cancer derived cell line and identification of the E7 protein, *Proc Nat Acad Sci U.S.A.* 83:4680

Stacey, S.N., Bartholomew, J.S., Ghosh, A., Stern, P.L., Mackett, M., and Arrand, J.R., 1992, Expression of human papillomavirus type 16 E6 protein by recombinant baculovirus and use for detection of anti-E6 antibodies in human sera, *J Gen Virol.* 73:2337

Stacey, S.N., Ghosh, A., Bartholomew, J.S., Tindle, R.W., Stern, P.L., Mackett, M., and Arrand, J.R., 1993, Expression of human papillomavirus type 16 E7 protein by recombinant baculovirus and use for the detection of E7 antibodies in sera from cervical carcinoma patients, *J Med Virol.,* 40:14

Suchankova, A., Ritterova,L., Krchmar, M., Krchnak,V., Vagner, J., Jochmus, I., Gissman, L., Kanka, J., and Vonka, V., 1991, Comparison of ELISA and Western blotting for human papillomavirus type-16 E7 antibody determination, *J Gen Virol.* 72:2577

Werness, B.A., Levine, A.J., and Howley, P.M., 1990, Association of human papillomaviruses types 16 and 18 E6 proteins with p53, *Science* 248:76

DETECTION BY ELISA TEST OF ANTIBODIES TO HUMAN PAPILLOMAVIRUS (HPV) TYPE 16 E7 ONCOPROTEIN IN PATIENTS WITH BENIGN OR MALIGNANT PAPILLOMAS FROM SKIN OR MUCOSA

Y. Chardonnet[1], A. Janiaud[1,2], J.J. Chomel[2], J. Viac[1], S. Euvrard[3],
D. Schmitt[1], M. Aymard[2]

[1]INSERM U 346
Affiliée CNRS
Pavillon R
Hôpital E. Herriot
Lyon
France
[2]Laboratoire de Bactériologie, Virologie
Faculté de Médecine
Lyon I
France
[3]Clinique Dermatologique
 Pavillon R
Hôpital E. Herriot
Lyon
France

INTRODUCTION

HPV infections are induced by a wide range of HPV types affecting squamous stratified epithelia. The possible role of HPV types and the prevalence of antibodies to early HPV oncoproteins may be of major importance as markers for invasive cancer. However, antibody response to HPV is still poorly documented. Recently, seroepidemiologic studies have reported the incidence of antibodies against HPV 16 E4

Immunology of Human Papillomaviruses
Edited by M.A. Stanley, Plenum Press, New York, 1994

and E7 proteins in healthy control population and in patients with cervical cancer, using either fusion protein or synthetic peptides as antigens and a solid phase enzyme linked immunosorbent assay (ELISA) or Western blot (Jochmus-Kudielka et al, 1989, 1992, Mann et al, 1990, Reeves et al, 1990, Jenison et al, 1990, 1991 Müller et al, 1990, 1992, Krchnak et al, 1990, Köchel et al, 1991, Suchankova et al, 1991, 1992, Kanda et al, 1992, Gallaway, 1992).The aim of our study was to detect and quantitate anti-HPV 16 E7 IgG in sera of patients with HPV-induced lesions using an ELISA test developed with a peptide chosen in E7 region (aa 41-aa 60), which cross reacts with HPV types 6 and 18 (Krchnak et al, 1990,) in order to determine the incidence of these antibodies in natural infection of the normal population and immunosuppressed patients as compared to women with genital lesions.

MATERIAL AND METHODS

A series of 209 sera was obtained from 188 donors who attended the clinics of Dermatology, Gynecology or Otorhinolaryngology. This included a control group of sera from 27 children of less than 2 years without history of papilloma lesions. Other sera were taken from patients (4-68 years of age) with well-documented HPV infections presenting clinical types of non regressing cutaneous or mucosal papillomas. Sera from 21 transplant recipients (14 renal and 7 cardiac grafted patients) were obtained before or at time of their graft and about a year later.

A synthetic peptide PAGQAEPDRAHYNIVTFCCK from HPV 16 E7 region (aa 41-aa 60) described by Krchnak et al (1990) was used as antigen in the ELISA reaction performed as previously described (Viac et al, 1990). Plates were coated with 2µg per well of peptide to which were added 100 µl of serial dilutions of sera starting at 1:100. After 2 hrs at 37 °C, the reaction was revealed with alkaline phosphatase conjugated goat antihuman IgG (Zymed, 1:3000) and paranitrophenyl phosphate in diethanol amine buffer and stopped by NaOH. The absorbance was measured spectrophotometrically at 405 nm on a multiscan spectrophotometer (Flow). Negative controls were similarly performed on plates without antigen. The differences of optical density between wells with and without peptide were recorded. IgG titre of each serum was determined using the regression curve.

A competition test was performed on a serum with high antibody titer (Krchnak et al, 1990). For adsorption of the reactive antibody with the peptide, 100 µl of serum diluted 1:5 was mixed with 20 µl of peptide in ELISA buffer containing 10 % bovine serum; the mixture was incubated for 2 hrs at 37 °C and overnight at +4°C. The reaction mixtures with or without peptide were centrifuged at 10 000g for 10 min and the supernatants were tested for antibody content.

RESULTS

To determine the cut off, twenty seven sera from children aged 6-22 months without history of warts, were tested in an ELISA test in the absence or presence of the peptide, diluted 1:100. None of these sera fixed aspecifically the plates without antigen. The absorbance ranged from 0 to 0.086 (m= 0.023±0.023). The cut off was taken within m+3SD (m=0.092). Sera were further considered as positive when the absorbance was > 0.1.The specificity of the ELISA test was determined using positive and negative control sera.

Two positive sera from women who had an HPV 16 in cervical intraepithelial neoplasia were selected, reacting with the peptide at 1:800 and 1:300 respectively. They gave consistently similar titers in 21 different ELISA reactions; the mean dilutions in log 2 were m=9.70±0.72 and 8.28±0.78 respectively. Another serum from a young adult without skin or mucosal lesions was used as negative control. Furthermore, these human sera were negative in the ELISA test with HPV type 1 virions previously used (Viac et al, 1990). Preimmune sera from rabbit or mice and a mouse monoclonal antibody containing antibodies directed to HPV 1, gave an absorbance <0.1.

To test the specificity of the reactions, adsorption experiments were done with one human serum strongly reactive with the peptide; specific adsorbed and control samples were tested in parallel. After adsorption, the reactivity of the serum dropped (<1:100).

The sensitivity of the ELISA test was determined by varying the dilutions of positive control antibodies. Human sera were considered as positive when serum dilution 1:200 reacted positively.

In general population (Table 1), antibodies were not detectable in a high proportion of healthy students (85 %) or healthy women (82 %); antibody titers ranged from 1: 200 to 1: 300 in healthy students (15 %) or healthy women (18 %). In women having cervical neoplasia, the proportion of patients (42 %) with antibodies was higher than in controls (18 %) whereas similar proportion was observed in control women and in patients with condylomas (17 %); antibody titers ranged from 1:200 to 1:800 and 1:200 to 1:300, respectively.

Among patients who had typical skin warts corresponding to HPV type 1 or 2, 47 % did not have any detectable antibodies and 53 % had a titer 1:200-1:800. Most adults with condyloma acuminata in which HPV types 6 or 11 have been identified, had antibody titers 1:300-1:600. In the group of children with laryngeal papillomas infected with HPV 6 or 11, only 23 % had low antibody titers 1:200-1:300.

In transplant recipients (Table 1), among 14 patients who had had a renal graft, none of them had IgG antibody just before or at the time of their graft. A year after their graft, two patients acquired antibody titers at 1: 400. Among cardiac transplant recipients, 1/7 had antibodies before graft and another one acquired antibodies at 1:200 after his graft.

Table 1. IgG antibodies to HPV 16 E7 in sera from patients with cutaneous and mucosal lesions from general population, women with genital lesions or from transplant recipients

Donors	Age	Total Number	Absence of antibody	Presence of antibody
General population				
Children	6-24 m	27	27 (100%)	0
Students	21-25 yr	54	46 (85%)	8 (15 %)
Skin warts	15-40 yr	32	15 (47 %)	17 (53 %)
Condyloma acuminata	20-45 yr	6	2 (33%)	4 (67 %)
Laryngeal Papillomas	4-13 yr	13	10 (77 %)	3 (23 %)
Women with genital lesions				
Control women	25-40 yr	11	9 (82%)	2 (18 %)
Women with CIN	27-45 yr	12	7 (58%)	5 (42 %)
Women with condylomas	26-43 yr	12	10 (83 %)	2 (17%)
Transplant recipients				
Renal transplant patients	40-60 yr			
Before graft		14	14 (100%)	0
After graft		14	12 (86 %)	2 (14%)
Cardiac transplant patients	38-65 yr			
Before graft		7	6 (86 %)	1 (14 %)
After graft		7	5 (71 %)	2 (29%)

CIN : Cervical intraepithelial neoplasia

DISCUSSION

In this preliminary study, we found by ELISA test a moderate incidence of IgG antibodies to HPV type 16 E7 oncoprotein (aa 41-aa 60) in the general population with or without papilloma lesions and a low incidence in grafted patients. The ELISA system was specific and sensitive using appropriate negative and positive controls (negative sera from children under two years of age, positive sera from women infected with HPV 16). The cut-off was taken in the same range as in other studies (Krchnak et al, 1990, Mann et al, 1990, Suchankova et al, 1991, Müller et al, 1992) In the general population, we observed the presence of antiE7 IgG antibodies in healthy young adults (15 %) and in control women (18 %) in the same range as reported by others but its significance is not known (Jenison et al, 1990). Using the same peptide, Suchankova et al, (1992) found also that sera from healthy donors may also react with the peptide. The low response in patients with cervical intraepithelial neoplasia may suggest that in the lesions harboring HPV 16 DNA, the low production of E7 oncoprotein is not sufficient to stimulate IgG production.

The incidence of anti-E7 antibodies was high in patients with warts or condyloma acuminatum (53 and 67 %) respectively. This indicate antigenic similarities in various HPV types or unexpected infections. Such cross reactions have been reported for HPV 16 and 18 (Krchnak et al, 1990) but not for HPV 1 or 2. It is still unknown whether any epitope common to the different HPV virions play a role in the immune response in natural infection. The low titers usually observed confirm that HPV proteins are not very immunogenic or that it is difficult to detect the antibody response against a linear epitope.

In transplant recipients who frequently develop benign and malignant lesions harboring HPV 1, 2, 5, 6/11, 16 or 18, the low prevalence of IgG antibodies to E7 oncoprotein may be the result of the immunosuppressive treatment. Our data are very similar to those reported with fusion protein from HPV 16 E7 protein (Jochmus-Kuldielka et al, 1992). A higher number of patients is necessary to confirm the low percentages. It is possible that in such patients, an absence of class switch from IgM to IgG antibodies occurs as already reported for L1 of HPV type 8 (Steger et al, 1990).

In conclusion, in our study there is no evidence for an association between malignant HPV derived lesions and the occurrence of antibodies to HPV 16 E7 oncoprotein. Though the humoral immunity in HPV infection does not seem to play a major role in the defense mechanism, it may reflect the host response to the HPV type and/or any modified antigen during the infection.

Acknowledgments

The authors thank Dr M.J. Carew who reviewed the English manuscript.This work was supported by Fondation de France founds, 1992.

REFERENCES

I. Jochmus-Kudielka, A. Schneider, R. Braun, R. Kimmig, U. Koldovsky, K.E. Schneweis, K.Seedorf and L. Gissmann, Antibodies against the human papillomavirus type 16 early proteins in human sera : correlation of anti-E7 reactivity with cervical cancer, *J Nat Cancer Inst.,* 81: 1698, (1989).

I. Jochmus-Kudielka, J.N. Bouwes-Bavinck, F.J.H.. Class, A. Schneider, F.J. Van Der Woude and L. Gissmann, Seroreactivity against HPV 16 E4 and E7 proteins in renal transplant recipients and pregnant women, *J. Invest Dermatol.* 98:389, (1992).

V. Mann, S. Loo de Lao, M. Brenes, L.A. Brinton, J.A. Rawls, M. Green, W.C. Reeves and W.E. Rawls, Occurence of IgA and IgG antibodies to select peptides representing human papillomavirus type 16 among cervical cancer cases and controls, *Cancer Res,* 50: 7815, (1990).

W.C. Reeves, J.A. Rawls, M. Green and W.E. Rawls, Antibodies to human papillomavirus type 16 in patients with cervical neoplasia, *Lancet.* i: 551, (1990).

S.A. Jenison, X.P. Yu, J.M. Valentine, L.A. Koutsky, A.E. Christiansen, A.M. Beckmann and D.A. Galloway, Evidence of prevalent genital-type human papillomavirus infections in adults and children, *J. Inf. Dis.* 162:60, (1990).

S.A. Jenison, X.P. Yu, J.M. Valentine and D.A. Galloway, Characterization of human antibody-reactive epitopes encoded by human papillomavirus types 16 and 18, *J Virol.* 65: 1208, (1991).

V. Krchnak, J. Vagner, A. Suchankova, M. Krcmar, L. Ritterova and V. Vonka, Synthetic peptides derived from E7 region of human papillomavirus type 16 used as antigens in ELISA, *J Gen Virol.* 71: 2719, (1990).

H.G. Köchel, K. Sievert, M. Monazahian, A. Mittelstäddt-deterding, A. Teichmann and R. Thomssen, Antibodies to human papillomavirus type 16 in human sera as revealed by the use of prokaryotically expressed viral gene products, *Virology,* 182: 644, (1991).

A. Suchankova, L. Ritterova, M. Krcmar, V. Krchnak, J. Vagner, I.L. Jochmus, L. Gissmann, J. Kanka and V. Vonka, Comparison of ELISA and Western blotting for human papillomavirus type 16 E7 antibody determination, *J Gen Virol.,* 72:2572, (1991).

A. Suchankova, M. Krcmar, V. Krchnak, E. Hamsikova, J. Vagner and V. Vonka, Range of HPV 16 E7 antibodies in cervical cancer patients and healthy subjects, *Int. J. Cancer,* 51:837, (1992).

T. Kanda, T. Onda, S. Zanma, T. Yasugi, A. Furuno, S. Wanatabe, T. Kawana, M. Sugase, K. Ueda, T. Sonoda, S. Suzuki, T. Yamashiro, H. Yoshikawa and K. Yoshiike, Independent association of antibodies against human papillomavirus type 16 E1/E4 and E7 protein with cervical cancer. *Virology,* 190: 724, (1992).

M. Müller, I. Jochmus-Kudielka, H. Gausepohl, R. Frank and L. Gissmann, Detection of antibodies against early proteins of human papillomavirus type 16 in human sera, *Contrib. Oncol.,* 39: 193, (1990).

.M. Müller, R.P. Viscidi, Y. Sun, E. Guerrero, P.M. Hill, F. Shah, X. Bosch, N. Munoz, L. Gissmann and K.V. Shah, Antibodies to HPV-16 E6 and E7 proteins as markers for HPV-16 associated invasive cervical cancer, *Virology,* 187:508, (1992).

D.A. Galloway, Serological assays for the detection of HPV antibodies, *in* : The Epidemiology of cervical cancer and human papillomavirus. Ed. N. Munoz, F.X. Bosch, K.V. Shah, A. Meheus, Lyon, 147-161, (1992) .

J. Viac, J.J. Chomel, Y. Chardonnet and M.Aymard, Incidence of antibodies to human papillomavirus type 1 in patients with cutaneous and mucosal papillomas, *J. Med. Virol.,* 32: 18, (1990).

G. Steger, M. Olszewsky, E. Stockfleth and H. Pfister, Prevalence of antibodies to human papillomavirus type 8 in human sera, *J. Virol.,* 64: 4399, (1990).

SEROREACTIVITY TO A L2-DERIVED SYNTHETIC PEPTIDE CORRELATES WITH THE NUMBER OF SURGERY-NECESSITATING RECURRENCES IN PATIENTS WITH LARYNGEAL PAPILLOMATOSIS

Ruth Tachezy,[1,2] Eva Hamsikova,[1] Jaroslav Valvoda,[3] Jan Betka,[3] Robert D. Burk,[2] Vladimir Vonka,[1] and Marc A. Van Ranst[2]

[1]Department of Experimental Virology
Institute of Hematology and Blood Transfusion
Prague 110 00
Czech Republic
[2]Department of Microbiology and Immunology
Albert Einstein College of Medicine
Bronx
New York, NY 10461
U S A
[3]Department of Otorhinolaryngology
Charles University
Prague 128 08
Czech Republic

INTRODUCTION

More than 70 phylogenetically related human papillomaviruses (HPV) have been isolated.[1,2] Numerous HPV types have recently been implicated in the etiology of carcinomatous lesions.[3] Several benign epithelial tumors in the upper aerodigestive tract are associated with the presence of HPVs.[4,5] Recurrent respiratory papillomatosis (RRP), associated with the presence of HPV-6 or -11, is the most common benign tumor of the larynx, affecting both children and adults.[6] Juvenile papillomatosis occurs between the ages of 1 and 5 years, whereas adult onset papillomatosis occurs between the ages of 20 and 50.[7-9] It commonly affects the true vocal cords, the commissures, and/or the epiglottis and occasionally extends into the trachea and bronchial tree. RRP frequently runs a protracted course that necessitates repeated surgical endolaryngeal procedures to remove the papillomas in order to maintain a patent airway.[10]

The immune response is thought to be a determining factor in the natural history of HPV infections, yet is poorly understood. In RRP patients, host immune factors predisposing for papillomavirus infections may be involved since the incidence of cutaneous warts was reported to be higher in these patients than in the general population.[11] Immunoassays capable of measuring type-specific anti-HPV antibodies in patient sera could be useful in the diagnosis and follow-up of HPV-associated diseases. In this study, we have analyzed the presence of HPV-reactive antibodies in a series of patients with RRP lesions.

MATERIALS AND METHODS

Subject Population

Biopsy material was obtained from 10 female and 15 male patients who underwent endolaryngeal treatment for RRP (10 juvenile, 7 adult multiple, and 8 adult solitary papillomas). Most patients had lesions on the vocal cords (n = 20), other lesions were located on the commisures (n = 10) and the epiglottis (n = 4). Part of the surgically removed material was used for histopathological identification and the remainder was immediately frozen at -80°C for virological work-up.

Blood samples were obtained from each patient and age- and sex- matched controls. The control subjects did not have a history of respiratory papillomatosis, and were without visible laryngeal lesions when they underwent tonsillectomy at the same department.

HPV Genotyping

All RRP-biopsies were tested for the presence of HPV DNA by Southern blot hybridization and polymerase chain reaction (PCR). Genomic DNA was extracted from the tissue by a non-phenol extraction procedure.[12]

Southern blot Hybridization. Ten µg of DNA was digested overnight with *Pst* I and electrophoresed through a 1% agarose gel. After depurination and denaturation, the DNA was Southern-transferred to a Nytran membrane (Schleicher & Schuell, Keene, NH).[13] Hybridization was performed with ^{32}P-labelled random primer extended HPV 11, 16 and 18 probes (specific activity >1 x 10^8 cpm/µg). A low stringent wash was performed in solution I (1M NaCl, 50 mM Tris-HCl pH 8.6, 2 mM EDTA pH 8.0 and 1% SDS), solution II (0.5 M NaCl, 25 mM NaPO₄ and 0.5% SDS) and solution III (0.5 M NaCl, 50 mM Tris-HCl pH 8.6, and 0.5% SDS) for 30 minutes each at 55°C. Washing under high stringency conditions was done twice in 0.1 x SSC and 0.5% SDS for 20 minutes at 65°C. Autoradiography was performed using Kodak X-OMAT AR films (Eastman Kodak, Rochester, NY).

PCR. A DNA aliquot was taken from each sample in a PCR-amplicon-free environment. Amplification with HPV-L1 consensus primers MY 11 and MY 09 (0.5 pmol each) was performed in a DNA Thermal Cycler 480 (Perkin Elmer Cetus, Norwalk, CT) in 100 μl reaction mixtures containing 10 mM Tris-HCl, pH 8.5, 50 mM KCl, 4.0 mM MgCl₂, 0.2 mM of each dNTP, and 2.5 U Taq polymerase reaction, and were overlaid with 40 μl of light mineral oil.[14] A control primer set (PC04 and GH20, 0.05 pmol each) which amplified a 268-bp β-globin gene fragment was included to affirm the presence of an adequate amount of amplifiable DNA. After the amplification, 10 μl PCR product was electrophoresed on a 3% agarose gel (2% NuSieve GTG and 1% SeaKem GTG). The gel was depurinated in 0.25 N HCl, and immersed in alkaline transfer solution (0.6 M NaCl, 0.4 N NaOH) for 10 minutes, before transfer to a Nytran membrane.[15] The membrane was neutralized in 1M Tris-HCl pH 7.4 and 1.2 M NaCl for 15 minutes. After a 3 hour prehybridization, the membranes were hybridized overnight at 42°C with a mixture of type-specific ³²P-labelled probes for HPV-6, -16, -18, -51 and the β-globin gene. The membranes were washed under low stringency conditions in 2 x SSC, 0.1% SDS twice for 30 minutes at 50°C. HPV-typing on the amplicons was done using a modification of the method described by Ting and Manos.[16] Briefly, 10 μl PCR product was digested with *Rsa* I and the resulting fragments were resolved by electrophoresis through a 3% agarose gel.

ELISA Screening. A synthetic heptadekapeptide derived from the 3' part of the HPV-6/11 L2 open reading frame (MGTPFSPVTPALPTGPV; amino acids 411 to 427 in HPV 6),[17] was constructed according to a modification of the Merrifield solid phase protocol.[18,19] The peptide was purified by reverse phase liquid chromatography, and was conjugated to bovine serum albumine (BSA) by glutaraldehyde prior to use in the serological assays. The 96-well microplates were coated with 0.2 g of peptide-BSA conjugate in 100 μl of buffer I (50 mmol/l carbonate-bicarbonate buffer pH 9.6, 0.02% NaN₃), incubated for two hours at 37°C and stored overnight at 4°C. Unoccupied sites were blocked with 1% BSA in buffer I for one hour at 37°C. After three times washing with buffer II (0.35 M NaCl, 2.7 mM KCl, 1.5 mM KH₂PO₄, 6.4 mM Na₂HPO₄, 0.1% Triton X-100, pH 7.2), 100 μl of a 1:20 serum dilution was added per well. After one hour incubation at 37°C, the plates were washed five times, and 100 μl of a 1:2000 dilution of peroxidase conjugated swine anti-human IgG (Sevac, Prague) was added for one hour at 37°C. The plates were washed several times with buffer II and once with buffer III (35 mM citrate buffer pH 5.0). The color reaction was elicited with 3.7 mM ortophenylenediamine in buffer III containing 0.006% H_2O_2. The enzymatic reaction was stopped by adding 2 M H_2SO_4, and the optical density was measured in a Titertec Multiscan MCC 340 optical densitometer at 492 nm. Negative and positive serum samples were included in each test. Glutaraldehyde-treated BSA served as a control antigen. To obtain a cut-off value, sera from 39 asymptomatic children aged 1 to 6 years were screened. The cut-off value represents the averaged absorbance value plus 3 SD (standard deviation) (mean OD = 0.134, SD = 0.062, cut-off value = 0.320). Student's t test (two-tailed) was used to compare the mean of different groups. A P-value equal to or less than 0.05 was considered significant.

RESULTS AND DISCUSSION

HPV DNA was detected by Southern hybridization and/or PCR in all tested RRP samples. There was complete agreement between the HPV genotyping by *Pst* I fingerprint on Southern blot and by *Rsa* I digest on PCR L1-amplicons. Fourteen RRP lesions contained HPV-6 DNA, ten cases contained HPV-11 DNA, and one sample was double infected with both HPV-6 and -11. This confirms results reported by Levi et al.[20] and Brandsma et al.,[21] but differs from other reports that found a lower HPV-positivity using less sensitive detection techniques.[22,23]

ELISA screening with a synthetic peptide from the carboxyterminal part of HPV-6/11 L2 did not reveal a difference in antibody response between the RRP-cases and their age- and sex-matched controls (Figure 1). There were 9 cases and 10 controls positive for IgG antibodies against the synthetic peptide. A recent study using complete HPV-11 virions instead of a linear epitope described a difference in antibody titer between juvenile-onset RRP patients and controls. The higher complexity of the antigen used in above-mentioned study might account for the difference.[24]

In our study, female cases and controls (n = 20; mean OD = 0.578) had significantly higher antibody titers than male cases and controls (n = 30; mean OD = 0.312; P < 0.05). For the cases, this can be attributed in part to the fact that juvenile multiple RRP (associated with more severe disease and higher antibody titers) was more prevalent in women than in men. This can however not explain the same observation in the RRP-free controls. In the controls, a higher incidence of (sub)-clinical genital HPV infection in women may account for the difference in antibody levels. We recently reported that the synthetic peptide used in this study showed a higher sero-reactivity in patients with condyloma acuminata than in controls.[17] Condyloma acuminata is a benign disease which is like RRP almost exclusively associated with HPV-6/11.

There was a significant correlation between the number of surgery-necessitating recurrences (a measure for the severity and therapy resistance of the papillomatosis), and the antibody response to the HPV-6/11 derived heptadekapeptide. RRP-patients with a history of more than twenty endolaryngeal surgical interventions (n=4) all had high antibody levels (mean OD = 0.832), whereas patients with one or low surgery-sessions

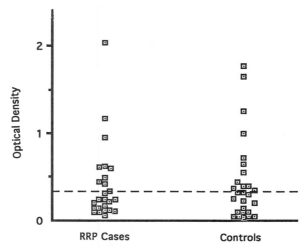

Figure 1. Seroreactivity of a HPV-6/11 L2-synthetic peptide in RRP-patients versus controls.

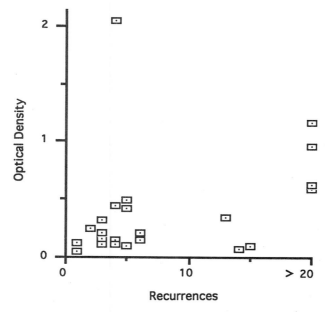

Figure 2. Correlation between seroreactivity against a HPV-6/11 synthetic peptide and number of surgery-necessitating RRP-recurrences.

(n = 5) were likely to be negative on serology (mean OD = 0.181; P < 0.01) (Figure 2). The majority of the former group were women (n = 3; mean OD = 0.913) who suffered from chronic juvenile multiple RRP, a condition associated with long-term maintenance of high quantities of virus. The persistent interaction of these papillomavirus antigens with the immune system, as well as the release of viral particles in the circulation during surgical removal of the papillomas, may be causally linked to the high antibody titers in RRP patients. This observation also indicates that a high anti-HPV-6/11 antibody level does not guarantee resolution or improvement of the RRP. It rather suggests that the seroreactivity is a measure for disease activity. A similar observation was recently made in a study that followed the evolution of the antibody response to HPV-11 in condyloma acuminatum patients treated with interferon . The seroreactivity declined steadily in patients whose papillomas regressed during the course of the interferon trial, whereas the seroreactivity in the interferon-α resistant group increased.[25] It would be of interest to study the evolution of the anti-HPV seroreactivity over prolonged periods of time. A more sensitive immunoassay capable of detecting type-specific anti-HPV antibodies in patient sera would not only be helpful in the diagnosis of HPV associated diseases, but could also be used to follow disease activity and treatment response in certain papillomavirus-related diseases.

REFERENCES

1. E.M. de Villiers, Heterogeneity of the human papillomavirus group, *J Virol.* 63: 4898 (1989).
2. M. Van Ranst, J.B. Kaplan, and R.D. Burk, Phylogenetic classification of human papillomaviruses: correlation with clinical manifestations, *J Gen Virol.* 73:2653 (1992).
3. H. zur Hausen, Human papillomaviruses in the pathogenesis of anogenital cancer, *Virology* 184: 9 (1991).
4. T.L. Green, L.R. Eversole, and A.S. Leider, Oral and labial verruca vulgaris: clinical, histologic and immunohistochemical evaluation, *Oral Surg Oral Med Oral Pathol.* 62: 410 (1986).
5. S.M. Syrjanen, Human papillomavirus infections in the oral cavity, *In*: "Papillomaviruses and human disease," K. Syrjanen, L. Gissman, L.G. Koss, eds., Springer, Berlin (1987).
6. S.R. Jones, E.N. Myers, and L. Barnes, Benign neoplasms of the larynx, *Otolaryngologic Clinics of North America* 17: 151 (1984).
7. A.L. Abramson, B.M. Steinberg, and B. Winkler, Laryngeal papillomatosis: clinical, histopathologic and molecular studies, *Laryngoscope* 97: 678 (1987).
8. H. Lindeberg, S. Øster, I. Oxlund, and O. Elbrønd, Laryngeal papillomas: classification and course, *Clin Otolaryngol.* 11: 423 (1986).
9. B.M. Steinberg, and A.L. Abramson Laryngeal papillomas, *Clin Dermatol.* 3: 130 (1985).
10. M.S. Strong, Recurrent respiratory papillomatosis, *in:* "Scott Brown's Otolaryngology," N.G. Evans, ed, Butterworths, London (1987).
11. H. Björk and C. Weber, Papilloma of the larynx, *Acta Otolaryngol.* 46: 499 (1956).
12. S.A. Miller, D.D. Dykes, and H.F. Polesky, A simple salting out procedure for extracting DNA from human nucleated cells, *Nucleic Acid Research* 16: 1215 (1988).

13. E.M. Southern, Detection of specific sequences among DNA fragments separated by gel electrophoresis, J Mol. Biol. 98: 503 (1975).

14. M.M. Manos, Y. Ting, D.K. Wright, A.J. Lewis, T.R. Broker, and S.M. Wolinsky, Use of PCR amplification for the detection of genital human papillomaviruses, *Cancer Cells* 7: 209 (1989).

15. J. Sambrook, E.F. Fritsch, and T. Maniatis, *in*: "Molecular Cloning: A Laboratory Manual," New York: Cold Spring Harbor Laboratory Press, Cold Spring Harbor (1989).

16. Y. Ting, and M.M. Manos, Detection and typing of genital human papillomaviruses, *in* : "PCR Protocols: A Guide to Methods and Applications," M. Innis, J. Gelfand, J. Sninsky, T. White, eds, Academic Press, San Diego (1990).

17. A. Suchankova, O. Ritter, I. Hirsch, V. Krchnak, Z. Kalos, E. Hamsikova, B. Brichacek, and V. Vonka, Presence of antibody reactive with synthetic peptide derived from L2 open reading frame of human papillomavirus types 6b and 11 in human sera, *Acta Virol.* 34: 433 (1990).

18. G. Barany, and R.B. Merrifield, *in*: "The Peptide Analysis, Synthesis, Biology, Vol. 2.", E. Gross, R. B. Meienhofer,eds, Academic Press, New York, (1980).

19. V. Krchnak, J. Vagner, and I. Hirsch, Simultaneous synthesis of sequence unrelated peptides derived from protein aminoacid sequence, *Anal Biochem.* 165: 200 (1988).

20. J.E. Levi, R. Delcelo, V.N. Alberti, H. Torloni, and L.L. Villa, HPV DNA in respiratory papillomatosis detected by in situ hybridization and the polymerase chain reaction, *Am J Pathol.* 135: 1179 (1989).

21. J.L. Brandsma, A.J. Lewis, A.L. Abramson, and M.M. Manos, Detection and typing of papillomavirus DNA in formaldehyde-fixed paraffin-embedded tissue, *Arch Otolaryngol.* 116: 844 (1990).

22. R.M. Terry, F.A. Lewis, S. Robertson, D. Blythe, and M. Wells, Juvenile and adult laryngeal papillomata: classification by in situ hybridization for human papillomavirus, *Clin Otolaryngol.* 14: 135 (1989).

23. K. Tsutsum, T. Nakajima, M. Gotoh, Y.Shimosato, Y. Tsunokawa, M. Terada, S. Ebikara, and I. Ono, In situ hybridization and immunohistochemical study of human papillomavirus infection in adult laryngeal papillomas, *Laryngoscope* 99: 80 (1989).

24. W. Bonnez, H.K. Kashima, B. Leventhal, P. Mounts, R.C. Rose, R.C. Reichman, and K.V. Shah, Antibody response to human papillomavirus (HPV) type 11 in children with juvenile-onset recurrent respiratory papillomatosis, *Virology* 188:384 (1992).

25. W. Bonnez, C. Da Rin, R.C. Rose, S.K. Tyring, and R.C. Reichman, Evolution of the antibody response to human papillomavirus type 11 (HPV-11) in patients with condyloma acuminatum according to treatment response, *J Med Virol.* 39:340 (1993).

COMPARISON OF PV CONFORMATIONAL EPITOPES EXPRESSED BY L1 PROTEINS IN MAMMALIAN (COS) AND INSECT (SF9) CELLS

Shin-je Ghim[1], Richard Schlegel[1,2], Jeffrey F. Hines[2], Neil D. Christensen[3], John Kreider[3,4] and A. Bennett Jenson[1]

[1]Department of Pathology and [2]Obstetrics and Gynecology
School of Medicine
Georgetown University,
Washington DC 20007
[3]Department of Pathology
[4]Microbiology and Immunology
The Milton S. Hershey Medical Center
Hershey
PA 17033

INTRODUCTION

Papillomavirus (PV) vaccines are currently used to prevent infection by bovine papillomavirus (BPV), canine oral papillomavirus (COPV) and cottontail rabbit papillomavirus (CRPV). Most of these vaccines are derived from either live or formalin-fixed homogenates of productively-infected warts. The humoral immune response that results from prophylactic vaccination has been difficult to study because of a paucity of virions available from most natural PV infections. However, the use of the athymic mouse model developed by Kreider and colleagues[1] for neutralization studies of HPV-11, CRPV, and BPV-1, particularly when the latter

Immunology of Human Papillomaviruses
Edited by M.A. Stanley, Plenum Press, New York, 1994

correlated precisely with neutralization of focus-formation (FF) of C127 cultured cells by BPV-1[4], suggested that conformational epitopes on the surface of PV virions are the primary target of neutralizing antibodies. These epitopes are also type-specific and immunodominant. Recent studies of recombinant PV L1 proteins expressed in eucaryotic cells produced L1 proteins with antigenicity mimicking that of intact PV virions[5]. The BPV-1 L1 protein expressed in Sf9 insect cells self-assembled into empty capsids and induced high-titered neutralizing antibodies[6]. Thus, the use of virion subunits such as the L1 protein as prophylactic vaccines are likely to be successful because they are antigenic and protective in animal models and lack viral DNA that might be carcinogenic to the host.

There appears to be significant variation in the amount of capsid protein produced in lesions caused by different PV types. Cutaneotropic viruses such as HPV-1 and BPV-1 generally produce the greatest quantity of recoverable virions. The mucosotropic viruses, particularly carcinogenic types such as HPV-16, produce low numbers of productively infected cells in the lesion, each of which contains relatively few virions. Viral type, site of infection, and genetic susceptibility of the host have all been invoked as possible explanations for variability of the clinical appearance, pathological features, and viral capsid protein expression in cutaneous warts and mucosal condylomas. Different vectors that encode the exact same PV L1 ORF can now be examined in different expression systems to determine if there is a molecular basis at the level of the viral genome for variability in expression of viral capsid proteins.

Table 1. Antibodies used in study.

Antibodies	Immunogen	Specificity	Source of antibodies
R int.	intact BPV-1	intact BPV1	Georgetown Univ.(Jenson)
R dis. (DAKO)	disrupted BPV-1	most PV	Georgetown Univ.(Jenson)
1H8	disrupted BPV-1	most PV	Georgetown Univ.(Cowsert)
R 639	intact HPV-11	HPV-6/11	Penn.St.Univ. (Christensen)
H11.B2	intact HPV-11	HPV-6/11	Penn.St.Univ. (Christensen)
Camvir 1	HPV-16 fusion prot.	HPV-16/33	Cambridge (McClean)

The major capsid (L1) proteins of BPV-1 and HPV-6, -11 and -16 were expressed in transfected mammalian cells (cos) and infected insect cells (Sf9) to compare the antigenicity and the level of expressed L1 in the two vector systems. The antibodies used for the comparative study are shown in table 1. Hyperimmune rabbit and bovine polyclonal antibodies produced against BPV-1 recognized either conformational or linear surface epitopes on the intact BPV-1 capsid. Polyclonal antibodies and MAbs generated against intact HPV-11 recognized

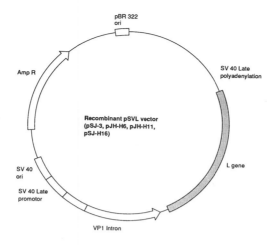

Type		Primers
BPV1	P1	5'-TTA CAT CTC GAG GCC ACC ATG GCG TTG TGG CAA GGC T-3'
	P2	5'-GAT CCA CCC GGG CTT ATA GAA ACT TAG CTT TTA T -3'
HPV6	P1	5'- TTA CAT CTC GAG GCC ACC ATG TGG CGG CCT AG-3'
	P2	5'-GAC ATG AAG CTT TGT AAC AGG ACA CAC-3'
HPV11	P1	5'-TTA CAT CTC GAG GCC ACC ATG TGG CGG CCT AG-3'
	P2	5'-GAT CCA GAG CTC CAC ACT GAC GCG CAT-3'
HPV16	P1(1M)	5'-TTA CAT CTC GAG GCC ACC ATG CAG GTG ACT TTT ATT TCA-3'
	P1(2M)	5'-TTA CAT CTC GAG GCC ACC ATG TCT CTT TGG CTG-3'
	P2	5'-GAT CCA CCC GGG CTT CAA CAT ACA TAC AAT-3'

Figure 1a. Recombinant pSVL constructs and primers used for the L1 ORF amplification

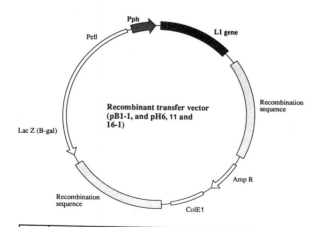

Type		Primers	RE sites
BPV1	P1	5'-GAC ATG GGA TCC GCC ACC ATG GCG TTG TGG CAA-3'	Bam H1
	P2	5'-GAC CTC CTG CAG TTT ATT AGG TGC AGT TGA-3'	Pst 1
HPV6	P1	5'-GAC ATG AGA TCT GCC ACC ATG TGG CGG CCT AGC-3'	Bgl II
	P2	5'-GAC ATG AAG CTT GTG TAA CAA GAG GTA-3'	Hin dIII
HPV11	P1	5'- GAC ATG AGA TCT GCC ACC ATG TGG CGG CCT AGC-3'	Bgl II
	P2	5'-GAC ATG AAG CTT TGT AAC AGG ACA CAC-3'	Hin dIII
HPV16	P1	5'-GAC CGG AGA TCT GCC ACC ATG TCT CTT TGG CTG-3'	Bgl II
	P2	5'-GAC ATG CCA TGG ACA ATT AGT AGG TGT TGA-3'	Nco 1

1b. Constructs used for the recombinant baculovirus and primers of L1 genes

149

conformationally-dependent[2], neutralizing epitopes of HPV-11 and HPV-6 expressed L1 proteins (in press). The camvir MAb that is cross-reactive for HPV-16 and -33[7] defines an in vitro surface linear epitope on the expressed HPV-16 L1. MAb 1H8 recognizes the cryptic epitope[3], FGA, which is present in the linearized L1 of BPV-1, HPV-6 and -11 and HPV-16. This epitope is located internal to intact PV virions. Antigenicity of the expressed L1 protein was considered to mimic that of the intact virion if there was reactivity with either conformationally-dependent antibodies, or, if there was reactivity by immunofluorescence (IF) with a nonconformationally-dependent antibody (ie. camvir for HPV-16) that was significantly different from the IF pattern of MAb 1H8, which only stained the cytoplasm of infected Sf9 cell.

Cos cells were transfected with the recombinant pSVL vector (Fig.1a) encoding the appropriate L1 open reading frame (ORF) by calcium phosphate precipitation and glycerol shock and examined by IF using antibodies depicted in Table 1 to determine the efficiency of transfection, intranuclear localization and the conformation of the L1 protein. The same antibodies used for IF were then utilized in immunoprecipitation (IP) tests to confirm the conformation and molecular weight of the expressed L1.

Sf9 cells were infected by recombinant baculovirus (Fig.1b) containing the L1 ORF downstream of the polyhedrin promoter. At 72 hours post-infection the cells were treated with RIPA buffer, and the unsoluble fractions, which contains the most L1 protein, were examined by SDS-PAGE to compare the quantity of expressed L1 protein among the different PV's tested.

Table 2. Comparison of expression of PV L1 in mammalian (cos) and insect (Sf9) cells.

| | COS | | Sf9 | |
| | Antibody | | Antibody | |
L1 Protein	αIntact	IH8	αIntact	IH8
BPV-1	++++	+	++++	++
HPV-6	+++	±	+++	+
HPV-11	+++	±	+++	+
HPV-16	+	±	+++	++

Transfection/Expression Assayed by IF of L1   Infection/Expression Assayed by IF of L1

BPV-1, HPV-6 and -11 and HPV-16 L1 proteins expressed in cos and Sf9 cells mimicked the antigenicity of the intact virion (Table 2). In cos cells, all of the expressed L1 proteins appeared to assume the same conformation as those of the intact virion. However, this was not true for L1 protein expression in Sf9 cells. Expressed L1 appeared to accumulate as denatured L1 protein in the cytoplasm and, to a lesser extent, in the nucleus of some cells. This distinction was made by IF using MAb 1H8, which only stained denatured L1. Antibodies that recognize denatured L1 proteins, such as Dako and 1H8, are routinely used for the successful detection of productive infections in naturally occurring warts and condylomas. These findings suggest that there are differences in expression and processing of the L1 in the two expression systems. In cos cells, most of the L1 is translocated to the nucleus. Whereas, in the Sf9 cells, although most of the expressed L1 appears to assume a native conformation in the nucleus, a significant amount of the L1 is denatured, either accumulating in the cytoplasm or, to a lesser extent, in the nucleus. The differences in expression of conformational and nonconformational L1-protein epitopes may be related to the expression system.

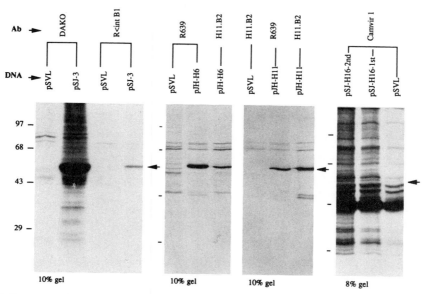

Figure 2. Immunoprecipitation of L1 protein expressed in cos cells with antibodies to corresponding types; L1 proteins are indicated by arrows.

The efficiency of transfection and/or expression of L1 proteins of different PV types in cos cells (Fig.2) appeared to parallel the amount of expressed L1 protein in the Sf9 cells (Fig.3), except for HPV-16 which was highly expressed in the latter. Transfection efficiency determined by the number of cells expressing BPV1 L1 proteins (as determined by IF) was approximately 5-10%, whereas the transfection efficiency of HPV-16 L1 was less than 1%. Up to 90% of Sf9 cells appear to be simultaneous infected with baculovirus, and the amount of L1 protein expressed in Sf9 cells (determined by Coomassie blue staining of 10% SDS-gels) was highest for BPV-1 L1 expression and approximately the same for all 3 HPV (Fig.3). This parallels the amount of L1 protein detected in natural infections by BPV1, but not for the variability seen with mucosotropic PVs. The reasons for the low transfection efficiency of HPV-16 L1 in cos cells is unknown. By IP of proteins from transfected cos cells (Fig.2) and Coomassie blue staining and Western blotting of proteins extracted from infected Sf9 cells (Fig. 3 and 4, respectively), the molecular weight of the capsid protein was always the predicted 55-63kD. Therefore, the expression, translocation and size of the L1 proteins were the same in both expression systems.

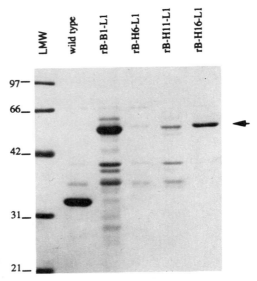

Figure 3. Coomassie blue staining of unsoluble fractions obtained from recombinant baculovirus infected Sf9 cells; L1 proteins are indicated by arrow.

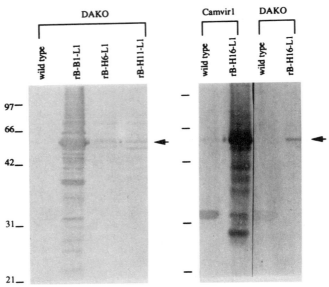

Figure 4. Western blot of recombinant baculovirus infected Sf9 cells with rabbit polyclonal antibody to disrupted BPV1(DAKO) and monoclonal antibody to HPV16 (Camvir); L1 proteins are indicated by arrows.

It is clear from these studies that the Sf9 cells produce more L1 than cos cells. However, there appears to be much more denatured L1 protein in Sf9 cells than cos cells. This means that a vaccine will have to be prepared from purified capsomeres or capsids which will contain the neutralizing conformational epitopes. A preparation containing denatured L1 will produce nonneutralizing antibodies that target linear surface as well as cryptic epitopes. This would cause difficulty in interpreting serological assays used for detecting a protective immunological response.

ACKOWLEDGEMENTS

This research was supported by grants ROICA 4624 (RS) , ROICA 53371 (RS), ROICA50182 (ABJ) and ROICA42011 (JWK) from the National Cancer Institute, NIH, and Jake Gittlen Memorial Golf Tournament (JWK).

REFERENCES

1. N.D. Christensen, and J.W. Kreider, Antibody-mediated neutralization in vivo of infectious papillomaviruses, *J Virol.* 64: 3151 (1990).

2. N.D. Christensen, J.W. Kreider, N.M. Cladel, S.D. Patrick, and P.A. Welch, Monoclonal antibody-mediated neutralization of infectious human papillomavirus type 11, *J Virol.* 64: 5678 (1990).

3. L.M. Cowsert, P. Lake, and A.B. Jenson, Topographical and conformational epitopes of bovine papillomavirus type 1 defined by monoclonal antibodies, *J Natl Cancer Inst.* 79:1053 (1987).

4. S. Ghim, N.D. Christensen, J.W. Kreider, and A.B. Jenson, Comparison of   neutralization of BPV-1 infection of C127 cells and bovine fetal skin xenografts, *Int J Cancer* 49: 285 (1991).

5. S. Ghim, A.B. Jenson, and R. Schlegel, HPV-1 L1 protein espressed in cos cells displays conformational epitopes found on intact virions, *Virology.* 190:548 (1992).

6. R. Kirnbauer, F. Booy, N. Cheng, D.R. Lowy, and J.T. Schiller, Papillomavirus L1   major capsid protein self-assembles into virus-like particles that are highly immunogenic, *Proc Natl Acad Sci USA.* 89: 12180 (1992).

7. C.S. McLean, M.J. Churcher, J. Meinke, G.L. Smith, G. Higgins, M. Stanley, and A. C. Minson, Production and characterisation of a monoclonal antibody to human papillomavirus type 16 using recombinant vaccinia virus. *J Clin Pathol.* 43:488 (1990).

DETECTION OF CLASS-SPECIFIC ANTIBODIES TO BACULOVIRUS-DERIVED HUMAN PAPILLOMAVIRUS TYPE 16 (HPV-16) CAPSID PROTEINS

John Cason, Parminder K. Kambo, Bhavneet Shergill, John Bible, Barbara Kell, Richard J. Jewers and Jennifer M. Best

The Richard Dimbleby Laboratory of Cancer Virology
The Rayne Institute
The United Medical and Dental Schools of Guys and St Thomas's
Hospitals St Thomas' Campus
Lambeth Palace Road
London SE1 7EH
UK

INTRODUCTION

Seroepidemiological studies on the prevalence of HPV16 infections are not possible as HPVs cannot be grown in conventional cell cultures and premalignant and malignant cervical lesions contain few intact HPV-16 particles and only low levels of native viral proteins. Whilst HPV-31b has been propagated *in vitro*[1] and HPV-16 virions have been produced in nude mice[2], virus yields are low. Peptides and prokaryotic fusion proteins have therefore been used as antigens for serological studies[3,4]. As such constructs probably represent poor imitations of native viral proteins[5], we have expressed the L1 and L2 proteins of HPV-16 in insect cells (via recombinant *Autographa californica* nuclear polyhedrosis virus: AcMNPV) for serological studies.

Immunology of Human Papillomaviruses
Edited by M.A. Stanley, Plenum Press, New York, 1994

MATERIALS AND METHODS

AcMNPV-derived HPV-16 proteins

HPV-16 DNA (*Ase*I to *Sph*I, nucleotides 5512 to 7463) containing the entire L1 ORF was ligated into pVl-1392. The complete L2 ORF between *Bam*HI and *Xca*I (nucleotides 6150 to 4138) was inserted into pVl-1393. Recombinant pVl constructs were transfected into *Sf*-21 cells with wild type AcMNPV and recombinants isolated by plaque purification. *Sf*-21 cells were pelleted by centrifugation, lysed by freeze-thawing and homogenised in NP-40. AcMNPV-derived HPV-16 proteins were partially purified by electrophoresis through a 12% SDS-PAGE gel, sections containing recombinant proteins were excised and proteins recovered by electroelution, followed by 5 repeat steps of precipitation in acetone/methanol and resolubilization in distilled water (to remove bound SDS).

Sera

Monoclonal antibody (mAb) 5A4 to a B-gal/HPV-16 L1 protein[6] and rabbit antiserum against B-gal/HPV-16 L2 were used.

Sera from 229 children (C: age range 1-17 yrs), 102 patients with genital warts (GW), 51 patients with cervical intraepithelial neoplasia (CIN) and 46 patients with cervical carcinoma (CA) were tested. Negative control sera consisted of 21 umbilical cord sera (UC: which contain no maternal IgM or IgA as this does not cross the placenta) which had been adsorbed with latex beads coated with anti-human IgG (Behringwerke AG) to remove any maternal IgG antibodies. All human sera were tested at a dilution of 1/50 in EIAs.

Enzyme immunoassays (EIAs)

AcMNPV-derived HPV-16 proteins (or equivalent quantities of coelectrophoresing proteins from *Sf*-21 cells infected with wild-type AcMNPV) were used to coat assay plates. Wells were blocked with 1 mg/ml bovine serum albumin (BSA) for 45 min at room temperature. Test sera in PBS/BSA/Tween were incubated in wells for 17 h at 4°C. Wells were washed with PBS/Tween and then exposed to an appropriate HRP-conjugated anti-species Ig (1/250 in PBS) for 45 min at RT. Plates were washed again then developed with orthophenylene diamine substrate. Reactions were terminated after 5 min with 2 M/l H_2SO_4 and absorbance values at 492 nm (A_{492}) were determined. Results are expressed as A_{492} readings or, as delta A_{492} values (A_{492} of wells coated with HPV-16 protein minus A_{492} of wells coated with co-electrophoresing proteins from wild-type AcMNPV).

RESULTS

Protein preparation

Expression of L1 and L2 proteins in *Sf*-21 was maximal at 72 hours producing proteins of the anticipated molecular weights of 65 and 72 kDa respectively (data not shown). Immunoelectron microscopy studies on thin sections of *Sf*-21 cells infected with AcMNPV/HPV-16 L1, AcMNPV/HPV-16 L2 or both constructs, failed to reveal virus-like particles in *Sf*-21 cells expressing L1 and/or L2 proteins (data not shown). Purification of HPV-16 L1 and L2 proteins by PAGE, electroelution and precipitation/resolubilization resulted in a 90% increase in EIA reactivity and a selective increase in the soluble form of L1 (*e.g.* Table 1).

Optimization of EIAs

Highest absorbance values (A_{492}) were obtained for L1 and L2 EIAs (using mAb 5A4 or rabbit antiserum to B-gal/HPV-16 L2) when Falcon plates were used in conjunction with a carbonate-bicarbonate coating buffer (pH 9.6) (Table 2). Optimal coating concentration of protein was determined for all batches of protein. Optimal time and temperature for coating EIA plates were also determined (Figure 1). Subsequent EIAs were performed in Falcon plates with carbonate-bicarbonate buffer and a coating concentration of 2 mg/l for 2 hours at 24°C was used for L1 and L2 proteins.

Recognition of AcMNPV-derived HPV-16 L1 and L2 proteins by human sera

When sera were tested for antibodies of all classes (IgG, IgA and IgM) to L1, there was no difference ($p>0.05$) between mean delta A_{492} values for UC sera or sera from C or patients with GW, CIN or CA. In contrast, using L2 protein, all four groups of sera (C, GW, CIN & CA) had mean delta A_{492} values which were significantly ($p<0.05$) greater than the mean A_{492} for UC sera (data not shown).

Investigation of the Ig class of antibodies was performed using a cut-off of the mean A_{492} plus 3 standard deviations for UC sera. Using this criterion IgM antibodies to L1 were detected in 14-18% of all groups, while the prevalence of IgG antibodies was 6% among children and patients with GW, 10% among CIN patients and 13% among CA patients (Figure 2). IgA antibodies were detected in 2-8% of patients with GW and CIN, 13% among children and 17% among CA patients. IgM antibodies to L2 were detected in 27-48% of all groups, while IgG antibodies were more frequent amongst children (32%) than among other patients (6-8%). IgA antibodies to L2 were detected in 24% CA patients and 8-10% for other groups.

Table 1. Partial purification of AcMNPV-derived HPV-16 L1 protein.

Preparation[1]	Protein[2] μg	Soluble[3] %	Volume μl	EIA[4] A$_{492}$	Concentration[5] (fold)
Freeze-thaw	1750 (255)	14.5	350 (340)	0.105 (0.098)	1 (1)
Homogenate	1328 (800)	60.2	630 (620)	0.199 (0.105)	1.9 (1.1)
Eluate from PAGE	113 (57)	50.4	610 (600)	1.099 (0.375)	10.4 (3.8)

1. Total protein recovered at each stage from three 25 cm² flasks of confluent AcMNPV/HPV-16 L1 infected Sf-21 cells (i.e. approximately 3x10⁷ cells).
2. Total protein recovered.
   Numbers in parentheses refer to the respective values for supernatants.
3. Percentage of total protein in solution.
4. Mean absorbance at 492 nm/well of duplicate wells coated with 100 ng total protein/well of AcMNPV/HPV-16 L1 protein after subtraction of the A$_{492}$ values for wells coated with equivalent preparations from wild-type AcMNPV infected cells when tested with the monoclonal antibody (mAb) 5A4 in an EIA.
5. Calculated from EIA A$_{492}$ values.

Table 2. Effect of coating buffers and EIA plate types on the binding of AcMNPV-derived HPV-16 L1 and L2 proteins to solid phase.

Plate	Solution (pH)		EIA Antigen				
			L1	Wt$_1$	L2		Wt$_2$
Falcon	C-b	(9.6)	0.56 ±0.02	0.00 -	0.99 ±0.07	0.05 ±0.04	
Falcon	Tris	(7.2)	0.48 ±0.02	0.00 -	0.82 ±0.07	0.09 ±0.00	
Falcon	PBS/T	(7.2)	0.23 ±0.00	0.00 -	0.75 ±0.01	0.03 ±0.02	
Falcon	dH$_2$0	(7.0)	0.27 ±0.00	0.00 -	0.23 ±0.01	0.00 -	
Nunc	C-b	(9.6)	0.34 ±0.01	0.00 -	0.50 ±0.08	0.03 ±0.01	
Nunc	Tric	(7.2)	0.38 ±0.01	0.00 -	0.49 ±0.07	0.02 ±0.01	
Nunc	PBS/T	(7.2)	0.37 ±0.00	0.00 -	0.45 ±0.07	0.05 ±0.01	
Nunc	dH$_2$0	(7.0)	0.23 ±0.00	0.00 -	0.25 ±0.02	0.00 -	

Wt$_1$: proteins from Sf-21 cells infected with wild type AcMNPV which co-electrophorese with L1 protein;
Wt$_2$: proteins from Sf-21 cells infected with wild type AcMNPV which co-electrophorese with L2 protein;
Data as the mean and SD of triplicate A$_{492}$ values for a typical assay of wells coated with L1 or Wt$_1$ at 2mg/1 exposed to mAb 5A4 (diluted 1/10) or, coated with L2 or Wt$_2$ at 2mg/1 exposed to polyclonal antiserum to B-gal/HPV-16 L2 (diluted 1/100). C-b: carbonate-bicarbonate buffer; PBS/T: PBS/Tween; d -: SD not applicable as mean value was zero.

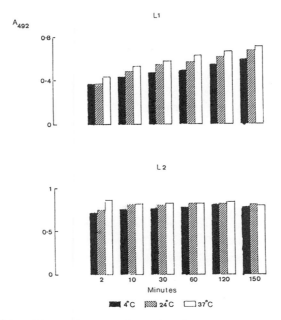

Figure 1. Effect of time and temperature upon the coating of recombinant proteins onto EIA plates.

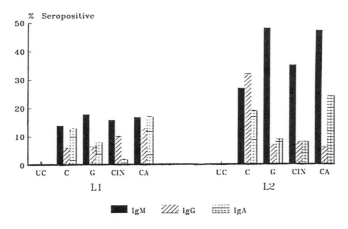

Figure 2. Percentage of sera positive for IgM, IgG, IgA antibodies to HPV-16 L1 or L2 proteins for sera from umbilical cords (UC), children (C), patients with genital warts (GW), cervical intraepithelial neoplasia (CIN) and cervical cancer (CA).

REFERENCES

1. Meyers, C., Frattini, M.G., Hudson, J.B., and Laimins, L.A. 1992, Biosynthesis of human papillomavirus type 31b from a continuous cell line upon epithelial differentiation. *Science* 257:971-973.
2. Sterling, J., Stanley, M., Gatward, G., and Minson, T. 1990, Production of human papillomavirus type 16 virions in a keratinocyte cell line. *J. Virol.* 64:6305-6307.
3. Jenison, S.A., Xiu-ping, Y., Valentine, J.M., Koutsky, L.A., Christiansen, A.E., Beckmann, A.M. and Galloway, D.A. 1990, Evidence of prevalent genital-type human papillomavirus infections in adults and children. *J. Infect. Dis.* 162:60-69.
4. Cason, J., Kambo, P.K., Best, J.M., and McCance, D.J. 1992, Detection of antibodies to a linear epitope on the major coat protein (L1) of human papillomavirus tyep 16 sera from patients with cervical intraepithelial neoplasia and children. *Int. J. Cancer* 50:349-355.
5. Cason, J., and Best, J.M. 1991, Antibody responses to human papillomavirus type-16 infections. *Rev. Med. Virol.* 1:201-209.
6. Cason, J., Patel, D., Naylor, J., Lunney, D., Shepherd, P.S., Best, J.M., and McCance, D.J. 1989, Identification of immunogenic regions of the major coat protein of human papillomavirus type 16 that contain type-restricted epitopes. *J. Gen. Virol.* 70:2973-2987.
7. Pakarian, F., Kaye, J., Cason, J., Jewers, R.J., Kell, B., and Best, J.M. Perinatal transmission and persistence of human papillomavirus types 16 and 18. Submitted for publication.

EVOLUTION OF CLASS I HLA ANTIGEN PRESENTING MOLECULES

Peter Parham

Department of Cell Biology

Sherman Fairchild Building

Stanford Universtiy

Stanford

CA 94305-5400

USA

EVOLUTION OF CLASS I MOLECULES

Two types of cytolytic cells are believed to offer protection against viral infections. Both cell types, the cytolytic T cell (CTL) and the natural killer (NK) cell, function through interaction with class I HLA antigen presenting molecules [1,2]. On viral infection, human cells synthesize viral proteins. Some fractions of these proteins are degraded by a large intracellular protease - the proteasome - and short peptides thus formed are pumped into the endosplamic reticulum (ER). In the ER, peptides of 8-12 amino acids in length associate with class I heavy chains and β_2-microglobulin to form functional class I antigen presenting molecules, which are then targeted to the plasma membrane via the Golgi apparatus and the normal secretory pathway. Once at the cell surface, the viral peptides bound by class I molecules can interact with the antigen receptors of circulating CD8[+] T cell thereby stimulating a CTL response which will kill the infected cell (Figure 1).

In contrast to CTL, which derive a positive signal from the class I molecule, the NK cell appears to be negatively regulated. Thus lysis of a target by NK cells can be inversely correlated with the levels of expression of class I molecules.[2,3]

The class I heavy chains are encoded by genes within a region of 2 megabases within the HLA region on the short arm of chromosome 6.[ref.4] Although some 20 genes pseudogenes and gene fragments have been identified, only the HLA-A,B and C heavy chain genes have been demonstrated to encode antigen presenting functions (Figure 2). Comparison of different mammalian species reveals widely differing numbers of class I genes and only in the most closely related species, for example humans, chimpanzees and gorillas, is similar organization preserved and orthologous genes readily identified.[5]

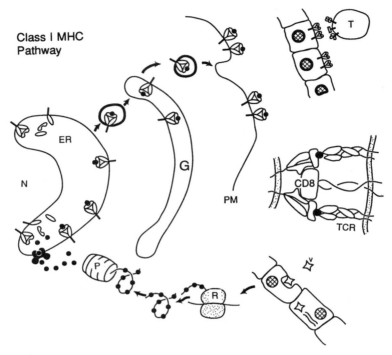

Class I MHC
Pathway

Figure 1 Scheme for the pathway of antigen presentation used by class I Major Histocompatibility Complex (MHC) molecules. Start in the bottom right corner and move clockwise through the figure. A virus (V) infects an epithelial cell and virally encoded proteins begin to be made on host cytoplasmic ribosomes (R). Incorrectly folded proteins are broken down into short peptide fragments by large intracellular proteases called proteasomes (P), two subunits of which are encoded within the MHC. Peptides (¤) are then transported into the endoplasmic reticulum (ER) by a heterodimeric transporter made up of the MHC-encoded TAP 1 and TAP 2 proteins. Peptides are assembled into class I MHC molecules with class I heavy chains and β_2-microglobulin and then routed via the Golgi apparatus (G) to the plasma membrane (PM). At the surface of the virally infected epithelial cell the complexes of peptide and class I MHC molecules can engage the receptors of circulating CD8+ Tcells. The antigen receptor (TCR) interacts with peptide bound to the α_1 and α_2 domains of the class I molecule, while the CD8 co-receptor interacts with the α_3 domain.

Genetic polymorphism, a characteristic of class I genes, correlates directly with antigen presenting function. Thus HLA-A,B and C are highly polymorphic genes whereas the pseudogenes HLA-H and HLA-J have little polymorphism.[6] The HLA-B locus appears to be the most polymorphic of the human class I genes so far defined. The species differences in the numbers of class I genes and the polymorphisms of class I genes within a species attest to the evolutionary instability of antigen presentation by class I molecules. This dynamic nature, perhaps best illustrated by the finding that no single class I allele is shared by humans, and either chimpanzees or gorillas, is believed to result from an ever-changing pressures exerted upon the immune system by viruses and other intracellular parasites.[7]

The Class I HLA Region

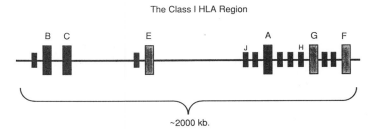

~2000 kb.

Figure 2 Simplified map of the class I region of the HLA region. Vertically oriented rectangles denote the positions of individual genes, pseudogenes or gene fragments. Larger rectangles are used for those genes which produce ß2-m-associated heavy chains: HLA-A,B,C,E,F and G, smaller rectangles denote pseudogenes, for example, HLA-H and J, and gene fragments. Adapted from the map described in Trowsdale and Campbell[4].

The three dimensional structures of various human and mouse class I molecules have been determined by X ray crystallography and shown to be very similar.[8-10] The peptide binding site formed by the α_1 and α_2 domains is where most amino acid substitutions between alleles are found. Moreover, these substititutions are found primarily at positions whose side chains contact peptide directly indicating that the role of the polymorphism is to change the specificity of peptide binding. Comparison of the α carbon backbones of an HLA-A molecule and an HLA-B molecule reveals the CD8 binding loop of the α_3 domain to be the site of greatest difference between the two structures.[11] It is not known if this correlates with any functional difference in the interactions between HLA-A and B molecules and the CD8 coreceptor.

Despite conservation at the level of three dimensional structure tremendous variation exists in the primary structures of class I heavy chains. Sequences from the major classes of vertebrate have been obtained and their comparison reveals absolute conservation of sequence at very few positions. For example, in the α_1 and α_2 domains only 8 of 182 positions are conserved. Seven of these comprise two symmetrically disposed groups of residues involved in interdomain contacts which are essential for the basic structure of the class I molecule (Figure 3). None of these residues are involved in direct contacts with either bound peptide of the T cell receptor. Another feature conserved in the class I structure is the site of N-linked glycosylation at position 86, close to the peptide binding groove.[12] A function for the carbohydrate has yet to be found. Recently a family of proteins expressed by NK cells have been found to have homology with well characterized animal lectins.[13] Thus binding of the glycan of the class I heavy chain by these NK cells. Another possibility is that the carbohydrate affects the binding of peptides.

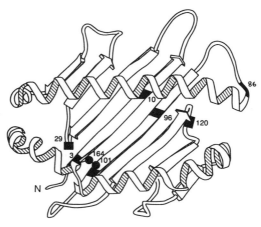

Figure 3 Ribbon diagram of the strcuture of the α1 and α2 domains of the class I molecule showing residues that are conserved in the amino acid sequence of functional class I heavy chains. From Grossberger and Parham[12].

HLA-A,B,C polymorphism is of clinical importance in matching tissues for transplantation and in determining susceptibility to disease. Since its beginning in the early 1960s, typing for HLA-A,B,C alleles has used serological methods employing panels of alloantisera obtained from multiparous women. With this approach some 27 HLA-A, 59 HLA-B and 10 HLA-C antigens have been defined.[14] In the last 15 years, the use of CTL to study class I molecules has revealed heterogeneity in alleles typed as identical by serology. Following up on these observations, direct analysis of the nucleotide sequence has shown that the serological types represent families of related alleles which differ by small numbers of substitutions, often clustered within the primary structure.[15] Although small in numbers, the differences almost always involve peptide binding residues of the antigen recognition site. This property explains why the differences can be detected by T cells and conversely it must be expected that they will also affect antigen presentation and stimulate potent alloreactive T cell responses.

The sensitivity of T cell recognition is illustrated by the finding that the single amino acid differences between the two common subtypes of HLA-B44 can be sufficient to stimulate alloreactive T cells to cause graft rejection.[16] The most extensively studied class I HLA antigens are HLA-A2 and HLA-B27 which have so far been subdivided into 12 and 7 subtypes respectively.[17] As attention turns to other antigens they too are being split in a similar fashion. For example, HLA-B35 has been found to comprise at least 9 distinctive alleles. The rate at which this is happening makes it difficult to estimate the total numbers of HLA-A,B,C alleles in the human population. For instance over 100 HLA-B alleles have been defined at the level of DNA sequence and the number continues to grow. To illustrate the imprecision in serological HLA-A,B,C typing, we shall briefly discuss some recently discovered alleles.

TABLE I

A*8001▲

	TOTAL	5'	3'
A3	7	0	7
A9	10	3	7
A2	19	11	8
A10	15	7	8
A19	18	7	11

Differences in 33 family positions.

From analysis of the HLA-A sequences, Lawlor et al.[36] identified 33 positions within the nucleotide sequence which exhibited family-specific patterns of substitution. Thus the combination of nucleotides at these 33 positions defined unique motifs for the A3,A9,A2,A10 and A19 families into one of which all HLA-A alleles fell. The motif at these 33 positions in the A*8001 sequence is compared to the 5 family motifs and the number of differences ▲ is tabulated. Differences for position in the entire coding region (Total), for the 5' region (exons 1-3) and the 3' region (exons 4-8) are shown.

For many years the HLA-A antigens have been divided into 5 serologically cross reacting groups.[18] When nucleotide sequences of HLA-A alleles were determined they were found to form 5 distinctive families which correlate with the serological grouping.[19] Although the 5 crossreacting groups can account for all the HLA-A antigens in the caucasoid population that is not the case for African and American Black populations in which up to 20% of the alleles have been untypeable i.e. are serologically blank. The segregation of such blank alleles can be demonstrated in families, as revealed when the families of patients needing bone marrow transplantation are tissue typed in order to search for an HLA identical donor. In collaboration with Dr Wilma Bias at the Johns Hopkins

University, we have sequenced HLA-A blank alleles from 3 such families and found them to represent an identical and unusual HLA-A allele.[20] Two other groups have found the same allele independently.[21,22] The sequence is highly distinctive and does not fit the pattern for any of the 5 families defined previously. This allele, now called A*8001, defines a 6th family which appears to be present only in populations of African origin (Table I). The predicted sequence for the A*8001 heavy chain differs from its closest relative, A*0101, by 24 amino acid substitutions, many of which are at exterior positions in the three dimensional structure and potentially capable of stimulating a good alloantibody response. With hindsight one would expect it to have been quite feasible to define the A*8001 molecule serologically. This has now been demonstrated. That it did not happen earlier is probably because caucasoid women have been the source of most typing alloantisera. Knowledge of the structure of this allele should facilitate its typing, either by serology or a DNA-based method, and improve matching for transplantation in black populations, especially between unrelated donors.

Association with arthritic disease has led to extensive study of the HLA-B27 antigen.[23] Analysis using T cells and allelic sequencing has identified 7 serologically identical subtypes of B27 which differ from the most common subtype, B*2705, by small numbers of substitutions.[15] For one subtype, B*2703, the difference is a point substitution, for the others localized clusters of substitutions. This latter pattern is typical of the differences amongst sets of subtypes and is the result of double recombination, or of a mechanism analogous to gene conversion, between alleles.[24] The differences between the subtypes localize to one area of the antigen recognition site while the remainder, including the B pocket, is conserved. It is the B pocket that determines the characteristic presence of basic residues at position 2 of B27-binding peptides[11] a property that has been speculated to relate to disease susceptibility.[25]

Recently, Darke and colleagues have identified a serological variant of the HLA-B7 antigen in the Welsh population.[26,27] Sequencing of the allele encoding this B7Qui antigen reveals it to be structurally more related to HLA-B27 than to HLA-B7.[ref.28] In fact it is a subtype of B27 in which the sequence DLRTLLR at residues 77-83 in B*2705 is replaced with the motif SLRNLRG, found in B*0702 (Figure 4). This region of sequence plays a dominant role in the serology of HLA-B molecules as it encodes the public epitopes Bw4 and Bw6.[ref.29] The B7Qui has the Bw6 public epitope, not normally associated with the B27 antigen and it is probably on this basis that it was assigned serologically as a B7 variant. The sequence indicates that it would be undesirable to match B7Qui with B7 in transplantation and that B27 might provide a more favorable match. Moreover, the similarity with B*2705 and preservation of B pocket suggest B27Qui might also confer susceptibility to disease. This is an issue that we hope to investigate in the future.

From comparison of HLA-A,B,C sequences, a catalogue of recombination events that have moved small segments of sequence from one allele to another, shows a concentration between residues 60 to 116. The most frequent region to undergo exchange involves residues 77-83 which form the Bw4 and Bw6 epitopes. Six pairs of HLA-B alleles which differ solely at residues 77-83 forming the Bw4 and Bw6 epitopes have so far been found. The potential functional importance of the difference is illustrated by the B35/B53 pair of alleles. Both alleles are prevalent in the West African population but only B53 is associated with resistance to severe malaria.[30] Furthermore, Hill et al.[31] have shown that B53 is capable of presenting malarial antigens.

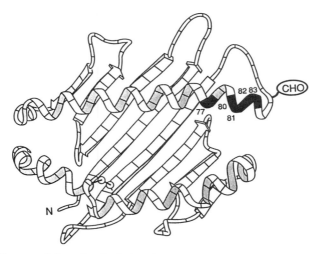

Figure 4 Ribbon diagram of the α1 and α2 domains showing the positions of amino acid substitution (residues 77,80,81,82 and 83) between the B7Qui antigen and the common form of the B27 antigen.

When individual allelic sequences are compared to the consensus derived from all HLA-B alleles, HLA-B27 subtypes emerge as the most divergent, a feature that again may not be unrelated to the disease susceptibility. In contrast, alleles of the HLA-B15 family include those most closely related to the consensus sequence. This lack of individuality is correlated with difficulty in the serological definition of individual B15 alleles and the considerable heterogeneity within the B15 family, 18 alleles of which have been sequenced. These findings have prompted HLA serologists to further examine the nuances of B15 typing, leading to the discovery of further potential variants that await sequencing analysis. As in the case of B27 and other families of subtypes there are distinctive population specificities to many of the subtypes, with alleles characteristic of Africans, Asian Indians, Orientals, American Indians and Caucasians being found. For all the subtypes the differences are placed at functional positions of the antigen recognition site and are expected to alter the nature of peptides bound and the specificity of the T cells to which they present.

Using the distribution of subtypes in human populations it becomes possible to correlate the evolution of a set of subtypes with the historical migration of humans. For example, it is generally believed that the American continent was first colonized by people migrating from Eastern Asia across the Behring Strait during the last ice age. After entering Northern America there followed a relatively rapid colonization of both North and South America. The B*4002 allele, which encodes the B61 antigen, is common in Eastern Asia and can be found in various North and South American Indian tribes. In addition, subtypes of this allele are specific to particular Amerindian groups and appear to have evolved from

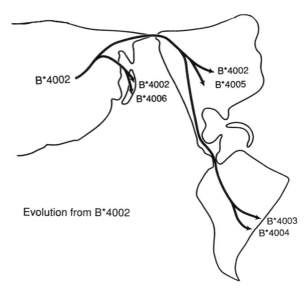

Figure 5 Sketch map showing the dispersal of B*4002 and the evolution of new subtypes in the Americas and Japan.

B*4002 in American populations (Figure 5). The B*4005 allele has been found in the Piman Indians of Arizona[32] while B*4003 and B*4004 have been found in the Guarani tribe of Southern Brazil.[33] Indeed the original B*4002 allele cannot be found in either the Guarani or the Kaingang, another tribe of Southern Brazil. A further subtype, B*4006, has also been found in the Japanese population.[34] The theme seen in the B27 and B15 families is reiterated in the alleles derived from B*4002: all the "new" alleles having been formed by exchange of small segments of sequence between pre-existing alleles which change peptide binding positions of the antigen recognition site.

In our studies and those of David Watkins at the University of Wisconsin[35] molecular analysis of HLA-A and B alleles has been carried out on three tribes of North American Indians and three tribes of South American Indians. The results reveal a contrast in the evolution of the HLA-A and B loci. In North America the majority of HLA-A and B alleles are identical to ones found in Asia and other parts of the world. In South America only the

HLA-A alleles are familiar whereas the majority of HLA-B alleles are new subtypes which can be derived by recombination from those found in North America.[33,35] This shows that in the South American population at least, the HLA-B locus has evolved more rapidly that the HLA-A locus. A similar conclusion is revealed from comparison of HLA-A and B with their homologues in the chimpanzee and the gorilla: the A alleles of the three species are more closely related than the B alleles.[36]

One interpretation of these findings is that the HLA-B locus can adapt more rapidly to changes in the antigenic environment or population structure and thus could be considered the more important class I HLA locus for dealing with new problems of antigen presentation. The example of HLA-B53 and malaria[30,31] shows how a single disease may select for a particular HLA-B allele and it is therefore reasonable to consider that the presence of other geographically localized HLA-B alleles is the result of specific disease selection.

Alternatively, the presence of novel alleles in South American Indians might result from a more general selective force, namely that of heterozygote advantage.[37] Survival to reproductive age necessitates mounting of effective immune responses against an extensive range of potential pathogens. The number of peptides that any single class I molecule can present is limited: of the order of one or two from any given viral protein, and it therefore seems plausible that two allelic products, with distinct peptide binding specificities, are generally better than one. Consistent with this hypothesis is the finding that the frequency of homozygotes in some populations is less than expected from a Hardy-Weinberg equilibrium.[38] It should be emphasized that in this scheme individual alleles are selected for complementarity of their peptide binding specificities not for presentation of a particular peptide or small group of peptides.

The expression of multiple class I loci by many species: HLA-A,B and C in humans, may also act to increase the repertoire of peptide binding specificity in a similar manner to heterozygosity at an indivdual locus. There appears, however, to be selective forces that limit the numbers of antigen presenting class I genes expressed, as all species so far studied express between one and three genes.[5] One hypothesis is that increasing reduction of the T cell receptor repertoire by each additional class I molecule expressed is the limiting factor.

Although the molecular description of HLA-A,B,C polymorphism in human populations is far from complete, the basic principles of their structure and function are now understood. Polymorphism is mostly effected by coding substitutions that change the sequences of peptides bound, indicating that variation is the result of selection by microorganisms. Whether selection alone explains the distinctive frequencies of HLA-A,B,C alleles which distinguish human populations is unclear and the relative contributions of selection and drift are the subject for debate. Assessment of the relative advantage of different HLA-A,B,C alleles requires an understanding of the peptides they bind and of the T cell responses they initiate. This endeavour is in its infancy. Only for a handful of the "well-studied" HLA-A,B,C alleles have viral epitopes been identified and even in those cases the numbers of different epitopes described is small. Thus for the majority HLA-A,B,C alleles nothing is known either of their role in the immune response or the types of peptides they bind. Their ubiquity and role in malignant disease make the papillomaviruses amongst a growing number of human pathogens in which these questions will begin to be addressed.

REFERENCES

1. A. Townsend and H. Bodmer. Antigen recognition by class I restricted T lymphocytes. *Ann. Rev. Immunol.* 7:601 (1989).

2. W.J. Storkus and J.R. Dawson. Target structures involved in natural killing (NK): characteristics, distribution, and candidate molecules. *Crit. Rev. Immunol.* 10:393 (1991).

3. H.G Ljunggren and K. Karre. In search of the 'missing self': MHC molecules and NK cell recognition [see comments]. *Immunol. Today* 11:237 (1990).

4. J. Trowsdale and R.D. Campbell. Physical map of the human HLA region. *Immunol. Today* 9:34 (1988).

5. D.A. Lawlor, J. Zemmour, P.D. Ennis and P. Parham. Evolution of class I MHC genes and proteins: from natural selection to thymic selection. *Annu. Rev. Immunol.* 8:23 (1990).

6. G. Messer, J. Zemmour, H.T. Orr, P. Parham et al. HLA-J: A second inactivated Class I HLA Gene related to HLA-G and HLA-A: Implications for the evolution of the HLA-A related genes. *J. Immunol.* 148:4043 (1992).

7. J.C. Howard. Disease and evolution. *Nature* 352: 565 (1991).

8. P.J. Bjorkman, M.A. Saper, B. Samraoui, W.S. Bennett, J.L. Strominger and D.C. Wiley. Structure of the human class I histocompatibility antigen, HLA-2. *Nature* 329:506 (1987).

9. D.H. Fremont, M. Matsumura, E.A. Stura, P.A. Peterson et al. Crystal structures of two viral peptides in complex with murine MHC class I H-2Kb. *Science* 257:919 (1992).

10. M. Matsumara, D.H. Fremont, P.A. Peterson and I.A. Wilson. Emerging principles for the recognition of peptide antigens by MHC class I molecules. *Science* 267:927 (1992).

11. D.R. Madden, J.C. Gorga, J.L. Strominger and D.C. Wiley. The structure of HLA-B27 reveals nonamer self-peptides bound in an extended conformation. *Nature* 353:321 (1991).

12. D. Grossberger and P. Parham. Reptilian class I major histocompatibility complex genes reveal conserved elements in class I structure. *Immunogenetics* 36:116 (1992).

13. F.M. Karlhofer, R.K. Ribaudo and W.M. Yokoyama. MHC class I alloantigen specificity of Ly-49+ IL-2 activated natural killer cells. *Nature* 358:66 (1992).

14. J.G. Bodmer, S.G.E. Marsh. E.D. Albert, W.F. Bodmer et al. Nomenclature for factors of the HLA system, 1991. in: HLA 1991: Proceedings of the Eleventh International Histocompatiblity Workshop and Conference, Vol. 1, K. Tsuji, M. Aizawa and T. Sasazuki, eds., Oxford Science Publications, Oxford, New York, Tokyo, pp.17 (1992).

15. J.A. López de Castro. HLA-B27 and HLA-A2 subtypes: structure, evolution and function. *Immunol. Today* 10:239 (1989).

16. K. Fleischhauer, N.A. Kernan, R.J. O'Reilly, B. Dupont et al. Bone marrow allograft rejection by T lymphocytes recognising a single amino acid difference in HLA-B44. *New. Engl. J. Med.* 323:1818 (1990).

17. J. Zemmour and P. Parham. HLA Class I nucleotide sequences 1992. *Immunogenetics* 37:239 (1993).

18. G.E. Rodey and T.C. Fuller. Public epitopes and the antigenic structure of the HLA molecules. *CRC Crit. Rev. Immunol.* 7:229 (1987).

19. K. Kato, J.A. Trapani, J. Allopenna, B. Dupont, et al. Molecular analysis of the serologically defined HLA-Aw19 antigens: A genetically distinct family of HLA-A antigens comprising A29, A31 and Aw33 but probably not A30. *J. Immunol.* 143:3371 (1989).

20. J.D. Domena, W.H. Hildebrand, W.B. Bias and P. Parham. A sixth family of HLA-A alleles defined by HLA-A*8001. *Tissue Antigens 42:156* (1993).

21. G.C. Starling, J.A. Wikowski, L.S. Speerbrecher, S.K. McKinney, et al. A novel HLA-A*8001 allele identified in African American population. *Hum. Immunol.*, in press (1993).

22. S. Rosen-Bronson, A.G. Wagner, D. Stewart, S. Herbert, et al. DNA sequencing of a new HLA-A allele using locus specific PCR amplification. Human Immunol., 34: suppl. 1, 18th Annual ASHI Meeting Abstracts, Abstract B2.2.17, pp 15 (1992).

23. M.A. Khan. An overview of clinical spectrum and heterogeneity of spondyloarthropathies. In: Rheumatic Disease Clinics of North America. M.A. Khan, Guest editor, p1, (1992).

24. P.J. Bjorkman and P. Parham. Strucutre, function and diversity of class I major histocompatibility molecules. *Ann. Rev. Biochem.* 59:253 (1990).

25. R. Benjamin and P. Parham. Guilt by association: HLA-B27 and ankylosing spondylitis. Immunol. Today 11:137 (1990).

26. H. Fussell, M. Thomas, J. Street and C. Darke. Serological identification of a new HLA-B7 variant antigen - HLA-B7Qui. Submitted. (1993).

27. P. Reekers, A. Tiilikainen, C. Darke, A. Van der Horst, et al. Antigen Society No. 111, part 2: HLA-B7-like antigen (B703(BPOT), B7Qui, BDT, B7SL, B7x40, BRI, B41V). In: HLA 1991: Proceedings of the Eleventh International Histocompatibility Workshop and Conference, Vol. I (Ed. K. Tsuji, M. Aizawa, T. Sasazuki). p 327. Oxford University Press, New York (1992).

28. W.H. Hildebrand, J.D. Domena, S.Y. Shen, S.G. Marsh, et al. The HLA-B7Qui antigen Is encoded by a subtype of HLA-B27. In preparation.

29. A.M. Wan, P. Ennis, P. Parham and N. Holmes. The primary structure of HLA-A32 suggests a region Involved in formation of the Bw4/Bw6 epitopes. *J. Immunol.* 137:3671 (1986).

30. A.V.S. Hill, C.E.M. Allsopp, D. Kwiatkowski, N.M. Anstey, et al. Common West African HLA antigens are associated with protection from severe malaria. *Nature* 352:595 (1991).

31. A.V.S Hill, J. Elvin, A.C. Willis, M. Aidoo, et al. Molecular analysis of the association of HLA-B53 and resistance to severe malaria. *Nature* 360:434 (1992).

32. W.H. Hildebrand, J.A. Madrigal, M.P. Belich, J. Zemmour, et al. Serologic cross-reactivities poorly reflect allelic relationships in the HLA-B12 and HLA-B21 groups: Dominant epitopes of the α2 helix. *J. Immunol.* 149:3563 (1992).

33. M.P. Belich, J.A. Madrigal, W.H. Hildebrand, J. Zemmour, et al. Unusual HLA-B alleles in two tribes of Brazilian Indians. *Nature* 357:326 (1992).

34. G. Kawaguchi, N. Kato, K. Kashiwase, S. Karaki, et al. Structural analysis of HLA-B40 epitopes. *Hum. Immunol.* 36:193 (1993).

35. D.I. Watkins, S.N. McAdam, X. Liu, C.R. Strang, et al. New recombinant HLA-B alleles in a tribe of South American Amerindians indicate rapid evolution of major histocompatibility complex class I loci. *Nature* 357:329 (1992).

36. D.A. Lawlor, E. Warren, P. Taylor and P. Parham. Gorilla class I MHC alleles: comparison to human and chimpanzee class I. *J. Exp. Med.* 174:1491 (1991).

37. A.L. Hughes and M. Nei. Pattern of nucleotide substitution at major histocompatibility complex class I loci reveals overdominant selection. *Nature* 335:167 (1988).

38. F.L. Black. Interrelationships betwen Amerindian tribes of lower Amazonia as manifest by HLA haplotype disequilibria. *Am. J. Hum. Genet.* 36:1318 (1984).

MAJOR HISTOCOMPATIBILITY COMPLEX (MHC) EXPRESSION AND ANTIGEN PRESENTATION IN CERVICAL CANCER

Jennifer S. Bartholomew[1], Simon N. Stacey[2], Brian Coles[3], Margaret Duggan-Keen[1], Philip A. Dyer[4], Susan S. Glew[1], Patrick J. Keating[1], John R. Arrand[2] and Peter L. Stern[1]

[1]Cancer Research Campaign Department of Immunology
[2]Cancer Research Campaign Department of Molecular Biology
Paterson Institute for Cancer Research
Christie Hospital NHS Trust
Manchester
[3]Department of Molecular Toxicology
University College
London
[4]North West Regional Tissue Typing Laboratory
St. Mary's Hospital
Manchester
U.K.

INTRODUCTION

The strong association between the presence of certain oncogenic types of papillomavirus and the development of cervical cancer has implicated these viruses in the progression of this disease. Human papillomavirus (HPV) types 16 and 18 are most frequently found associated with high grade cervical intraepithelial neoplasia (CIN) lesions and invasive carcinomas of the cervix. The expression of specific viral proteins through the various stages of the natural history of cervical cancer may evoke immunological consequences of relevance to the progression or regression of this disease. Evidence in support of an active role for the immune system in preventing the development of HPV associated malignancies has come from immunocompromised individuals including allograft recipients, cancer and AIDS patients who often exhibit an increased incidence of HPV associated lesions (eg. Halpert et al., 1985). The recognition of antigen by T cells is restricted by the polymorphic products of the MHC whose function is to present short peptides at the cell surface for T cell surveillance. Therefore the expression of HLA and the normal functioning of the peptide processing and transport machinery are crucial factors in the potential recognition of virally infected cells (Neefjes and Ploegh, 1992; Monaco, 1992). This article reviews our work on the expression of polymorphic MHC class I and II antigens in premalignant and malignant lesions of the cervix. To discover whether HPV derived antigens can be presented for immune recognition, specific MHC-bound peptides have been identified, isolated and sequenced from cells expressing HPV 16 transforming proteins. This approach offers an alternative route towards identifying putative T cell epitopes. There is the potential for identification of tumour specific antigens of any origin if a cytotoxic T lymphocyte (CTL) line and a corresponding tumour target are available. Fractionated peptides derived from a tumour cell line can be presented on autologous lymphoblastoid cells as targets for the tumour specific CTL, (derived for example from associated infiltrating T lymphocytes; see Ghosh et al., this volume) and the specific peptide sequenced.

MHC EXPRESSION AND MALIGNANT CERVICAL DISEASE

The following studies have examined the expression of MHC class I and II molecules in cervical lesions and any possible relationship between the presence of HPV and changes in MHC expression. The expression of MHC products in tumours has been investigated primarily by immunohistochemical methods (Connor and Stern, 1990; Glew et al., 1992a, 1993a and P. Keating, unpublished) in cryostat and paraffin embedded sections. The reagents used recognise monomorphic determinants of the heterodimer HLA class I (W6/32) and class II (CR3/43) locus products and additionally monoclonal antibodies (mAbs) recognising chain specific, locus specific and polymorphic determinants have been studied in cervical lesions at various stages of disease.

Studies so far have shown that 11% (17/155) of the squamous cell carcinomas (SCC) of the cervix have a loss of HLA-A, -B, -C and β_2-microglobulin complexed molecules in part or all of the tumour. However using allele specific mAbs, a further proportion of these biopsies have been shown to exhibit downregulation of one or more allelic products (Connor and Stern, 1990). Overall altered HLA class I expression is present in at least 40% of the carcinomas. Patients with early stage cancers with HLA class I down regulation were associated with a significantly poorer clinical outcome (Connor et al., 1993).

Aberrant class II expression has been described in various carcinomas originating from HLA class II negative tissue, however its relevance to clinical outcome is variable

(Garrido and Estaban, 1991). Although normal cervical squamous epithelium is HLA class II negative, the majority of squamous carcinomas (to date, 137/169, 81%) express MHC class II antigens. No apparent correlation between the class II phenotype and the presence of HPV 16 DNA in the cervical cancer specimens was seen (Glew et al., 1992a), suggesting that HPV does not directly influence MHC expression. However, the pathogenesis of cervical cancer is a multifactorial and multistage process and a relationship between MHC class I and/or class II expression and HPV infection may be more evident in the evolution of premalignant lesions.

MHC EXPRESSION IN PREMALIGNANT CERVICAL DISEASE

Virtually all benign and premalignant lesions of cervical epithelia analysed are HLA class I positive; a single exception was a full thickness loss in a CIN II lesion (Glew et al., 1993a). It is possible that this low frequency of HLA class I down regulation compared to the invasive tumours reflects important events that occur at the step that breaches the threshold of invasion and would be supported by data from other premalignant and malignant epithelial lesions (Garrido et al., 1993).

High risk HPV types (16, 18, 31, 33) were not detected in normal or metaplastic epithelia with or without warty changes, but there was an increase in the detection in CIN I (27%), CIN II (54%) and CIN III (79%) paralleling the change in HLA class II expression (Glew et al., 1993a). Local cytokine production does not appear to be the sole cause of the epithelial cell class II expression since there is a sharp demarcation of class II expression at the interface of CIN III/normal squamous epithelium in some specimens. No correlation between class II expression and heavy sub-epithelial leucocyte infiltration (eg. in 'chronic active cervicitis') was seen in normal epithelium, CIN or HPV infection, nor was any correlation seen between class II phenotype and the presence or absence of high risk HPV DNA. These observations imply that HLA class II expression is neither a consequence nor a requirement of HPV infection in the cervix.

Finally the function of MHC to present short peptides at the cell surface for T cell recognition requires the correct operation of the peptide processing and transport pathway. Recently, studies have established a correlation between HLA class I down regulation and the absence of a peptide transporter protein (TAP 1) in cervical disease (Cromme et al., 1993) emphasising the role of the peptide transport machinery in the functional expression of HLA class I molecules. The polymorphic nature of MHC glycoproteins is reflected in their peptide binding repertoire, different alleles presenting different peptides for cell mediated recognition. Thus down regulation of particular MHC alleles may be a critical factor in the development of cervical tumours. If this were the case, there should be a difference in the HLA frequencies in patients with cervical disease compared with the normal population.

HLA POLYMORPHISM AND CERVICAL CANCER

An association of HLA-DQ3 with SCC of the cervix has been reported by groups in Germany and Norway (Wank and Thomssen, 1991; Helland et al., 1992). In contrast, our preliminary report (Glew et al., 1992b) failed to show any signficant differences in patients and controls from North-West England. We have now examined in detail the HLA polymorphism in cervical carcinoma patients, with respect to HPV infection, MHC class II expression within the tumour, serological response to HPV and other relevant clinical variables such as disease stage (Glew et al., 1993b). No significant association of any HLA-A, -B, -C, -DR or -DQ antigen with SCC patients was found in this study of 65 patients. Molecular typing for HLA-DQ allowed for the definition of 14 HLA-DQ alleles, but no differences between patients and controls were apparent. While a possible explanation of the differences between this and the other studies could be disease heterogeneity, the various tumour and clinical factors examined do not account for the observed differences. However, the extensive polymorphism of HLA antigens limits the interpretation of this and other studies, due to relatively small patient subgroups. A much larger study is required to understand fully the interaction between HPV, HLA and cervical disease. Appropriately selected control populations must be typed at the same level of discrimination as patient groups and in view of the linkage disequilibrium between loci within the MHC, it is important not to consider polymorphism of individual loci in isolation.

IDENTIFICATION OF NATURALLY PROCESSED PEPTIDES PRESENTED BY HLA CLASS I MOLECULES

Self peptides eluted from isolated MHC molecules are normally 8-9 amino acids in length and usually contain allele specific structural motifs. MHC peptide elution studies in cells infected with vesicular stomatitis virus or influenza virus have shown that virally derived peptides become associated with MHC class I following infection and are recgonised by viral specific CTL (Rotzschke et al., 1990; Van Bleek and Nathenson, 1990). This approach is being used as a means to identify not only viral peptides but any alteration in self peptides which may be relevant for potential immune recognition of cervical cancer cells.

In preliminary studies, endogeneously processed peptides bound to MHC class I molecules have been isolated from JY lymphoblastoid cells (homozygous HLA-A2.1, -B7) infected either with recombinant vaccinia virus expressing the HPV 16 E6 open reading frame (ORF) or the non-recombinant (WR) virus at 10 pfu/cell. By comparison of the peptide profiles from these cells, unique peaks have been identified, further fractionated and sequenced. HLA-A2 proteins were isolated with the mAb HB82 followed by the mAb W6/32 to obtain the remaining MHC class I molecules. The MHC-bound peptides were purified based on the procedures of Rotzschke et al (1990), using Protein A Sepharose, 10% acetic acid elution and the peptide fraction obtained as a Centricon 10 filtrate. The analysis of the isolated peptides was performed by reverse phase chromatography in a 0.1% trifluoroacetic acid (TFA)/water and 0.1% TFA/acetonitrile gradient using SMART (Pharmacia) technology.

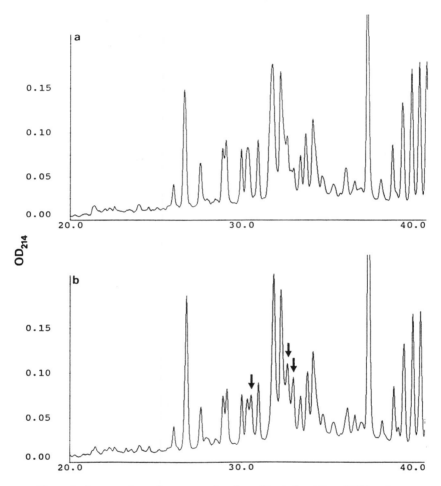

Figure 1. Reverse phase chromatography of peptides isolated from MHC molecules immunopurified with the mAb HB82. (a). Peptide fraction isolated from JY cells infected with wild type (WR) vaccinia virus. (b). Peptide fraction isolated from JY cells infected with vaccinia virus expressing HPV 16-E6. Peak differences between the peptide profiles are marked with an arrow.

The expression of E6 protein in cells infected with recombinant vaccinia expressing the E6 ORF was confirmed using immunoprecipitation of ^{35}S-cysteine labelled proteins with serum from an E6 seropositive cervical carcinoma patient. There was no alteration in the level of MHC class I synthesis at 8h post infection. Analysis of the peptides eluted from HLA class I complexes by reverse phase chromatography produced multiple absorbance peaks at 214 nm. Comparison of these peptide profiles from cells infected with WR and recombinant vaccinia expressing HPV 16 E6 for HB82 is shown in Figure 1.

The peptide profiles were reproducible for each mAb used within each experiment and between separate infections. This allowed comparison of profiles obtained from control and HPV 16 E6 expressing cells and unique peaks were identifiable which eluted at differing times to the control runs, depending on the antibody used. The short peptides of interest eluted in the gradient between 20 and 40% acetonitrile. Profiles obtained with W6/32 showed greater complexity than those isolated with HB82. Peaks have been selected on the basis of comparison of WR control and vaccinia expressing HPV 16 E6 and these have been rechromatographed and subjected to sequential Edmann degradation. Preliminary analysis has identified sequences of known self proteins but also an HPV derived E6 sequence. These results indicate the potential of this approach for the identification of endogenously processed peptides for any putative target antigen. It will of course be of great interest to discover whether the antigen processing and presentation machinery of the keratinocyte can perform the same feats as the lymphocyte.

ACKNOWLEDGEMENT

This work was supported by the Cancer Research Campaign and North-West Regional Health Authority. PJK and SSG were Joseph Starkey Clinical Research Fellows.

REFERENCES

Connor, M.E., and Stern, P.L., 1990, Loss of MHC class I expression in cervical carcinomas, *Int J Cancer* 46:1029.

Connor, M.E., Davidson, S.E., Stern, P.L., Arrand, J.R., and West, C.M.L., 1993, Evaluation of multiple biological parameters in cervical carcinoma: high macrophage infiltration in HPV-associated tumours, *Int J Gynecol Cancer* 3:103.

Cromme, F.V., Airey, J., Heemels, M.T., Ploegh, H.L., Keating, P.J., Stern, P.L., Meijer, C.J.L.M., and Walboomers, J.M.M., 1993, Loss of transporter protein encoded by the TAP-1 gene is highly correlated with loss of HLA expression in cervical carcinomas. In press *J Exp Med.*

Garrido, F., Cabrera, T., Concha, A., Glew, S.S., Ruiz-Cabello, F., and Stern, P.L., 1993, Natural history of HLA expression during tumour development, *Immunol Today* 14:491.

Garrido, F., and Ruiz-Cabello, F., 1991, *in*: Seminars in Cancer Biology, E. Klein, and F. Garrido, ed., Saunders, 2:3.

Glew, S.S., Duggan-Keen, M., Cabrera, T., and Stern, P.L., 1992a, HLA class II antigen expression in human papillomavirus-associated cervical cancer, *Cancer Res.* 52:4009.

Glew, S.S., Stern, P.L., Davidson, J.A., and Dyer, P.A., 1992b, HLA antigens and cervical carcinoma, *Nature* 356:22.

Glew, S.S., Connor, M.E., Snijders, P.J.F., Stanbridge, C.M., Buckley, C.H., Walboomers, J.M.M. *et al*, 1993a, HLA expression in preinvasive cervical neoplasia in relationship to human papillomavirus infection, *Eur J Cancer* In press.

Glew, S.S., Duggan-Keen, M., Ghosh, A.K., Ivinson, A., Sinnott, P., Davidson, J. *et al*, 1993b, Lack of association of HLA polymorphisms with HPV-related cervical cancer, *Human Immunol.* 37:15.

Halpert, R., Fruchter, R.G., Seclus, A., Butt, K., Boyce, J.G., and Sillman, F.H., 1985, HPV and lower genital tract neoplasia in renal transplant patients, *Obstet Gynecol.* 68:251.

Helland, A., Borresen, A.L., Kaern, J., Ronningen, K.S., and Thorsby, E., 1992, HLA antigens and cervical carcinoma, *Nature* 356:23.

Monaco, J.J., 1992, A molecular model of MHC class I-restricted antigen processing, *Immunol Today* 13:173.

Neefjes, J.J., and Ploegh, H., 1992, Intracellular transport of MHC class II molecules, *Immunol Today* 13:179.

Rotzschke, O., Falk, K., Deres, K., Schild, H., Norda, M., Metzger, J., Jung, G., and Rammensee, H., 1990, Isolation and analysis of naturally processed viral peptides as recognised by cytotoxic T cells, *Nature* 348:252.

Van Bleek, G.M., and Nathenson, S.G., 1990, Isolation of an endogenously processed immunodominant viral peptide from the class I H-2K^b molecule, *Nature* 348:213.

Wank, R., and Thomssen, C., 1991, High risk of squamous cell carcinoma of the cervix for women with HLA-DQw3, *Nature* 352:723.

Wank, R., Schendel, D.J., and Thomssen, C, 1992, HLA antigens and cervical carcinoma, *Nature* 356:22.

ANALYSIS OF MHC CLASS I EXPRESSION IN HPV 16 POSITIVE CERVICAL CARCINOMAS, IN RELATION TO C-*MYC* OVEREXPRESSION

F.V. Cromme[1], P.J.F. Snijders[1], A.J.C. van den Brule[1], M.J. Stukart[1], P. Kenemans[2], C.J.L.M. Meijer[1] and J.M.M. Walboomers[1]

[1] Department of Pathology, Section of Molecular Pathology
[2] Department of Gynaecology and Obstetrics
Free University Hospital
De Boelelaan 1117
1081 HV Amsterdam
The Netherlands

INTRODUCTION

Certain human papillomavirus (HPV) genotypes are considered to play a crucial role in the development of cervical neoplasia, in particular HPV 16. However there are several indications that additional events besides HPV infection are involved in the pathogenesis of cervical cancer[1]. A hint that failure of the immune response might play a role is given by the reduced expression of major histocompatibility complex class I (MHC-I), frequently observed in cervical carcinomas[2,3]. This could facilitate escape of neoplastic cells from killing by cytotoxic T-cells (CTLs), since cell surface expression of MHC-I molecules is necessary for recognition and subsequent killing of antigen bearing cells by CTLs[4]. It is tempting to speculate on a role of HPV in MHC-I down-regulation, in analogy with other viruses[5]. In a previous study we focused on the E7 gene of HPV 16, since this gene is consistently expressed in cervical carcinomas[6]. The HPV 16-E7 protein shows functional homology with the Adenovirus E1A gene product[7], which is responsible for MHC-I down-regulation[8]. However, the observed reduction of class I expression was not found in all HPV 16-E7 expressing carcinomas[3], indicating no direct effect of E7 on down-regulation of MHC-I expression.

Immunology of Human Papillomaviruses
Edited by M.A. Stanley, Plenum Press, New York, 1994

Alternatively, an indirect effect of HPV on MHC-I expression could involve the c-*myc* oncogene product, which has been implicated in modulating MHC-I expression in melanomas[9]. Cis-activation of c-*myc* gene expression has been suggested as a result of integration of HPV 16 and 18 DNA nearby the c-*myc* gene[10,11]. In addition, complex formation between the retinoblastoma tumour suppressor protein (pRB) and HPV 16-E7 could cause increased levels of c-*myc*, either by abrogating the inhibitory effect of transforming growth factor β1 (TGF-β1)/pRB complex on c-*myc* transcription[12], or by preventing binding of the c-*myc* protein by pRB[13].

In either way HPV 16/18 could effectuate increased levels of c-*myc*, which would lead to MHC-I down-regulation. Therefore we investigated in this study whether overexpression of c-*myc* leads to down-regulation of MHC-I expression in cervical carcinomas. In addition carcinomas were examined on the presence of class I coding transcripts, since it has been suggested that c-*myc* exerts its effect on MHC-I expression at the transcriptional level[14]. The majority of the c-*myc*/MHC-I expression studies performed thus far have used tumour cell line extracts *in vitro* and did not allow to correlate both parameters *in vivo*. Therefore immunohistochemistry and RNA *in situ* hybridisation were applied for analysing the relationship between HPV 16-E7 transcription, c-*myc* overexpression and MHC-I down-regulation in cervical carcinomas with preservation of morphology.

MATERIALS AND METHODS

Details of the methods used for HPV detection[15], MHC-I/c-*myc* immunohistochemistry[3] and RNA *in situ* hybridisation[6] have been published[16], and are briefly summarized under the figure.

RESULTS AND DISCUSSION

HPV DNA detection and E7 transcription

After applying PCR with general primers for HPV detection and type-specific primers for HPV typing[15], 23 squamous cell carcinomas of the uterine cervix containing only HPV 16 DNA were selected for this study. RNA *in situ* hybridisation revealed presence of E7-coding transcripts in all carcinomas with proper RNA quality (n=15), as determined with the human β-actin probe, which is in accordance with previous findings[6]. Signals were restricted to neoplastic cervical cells, while stroma and infiltrating cells of the immune system were negative.

MHC-I expression

The percentage of neoplastic cells that show staining for MHC-I heavy chains or β2-microglobulin was estimated by two independent observers, with normal epithelium and cells of the immune system serving as positive internal controls. Carcinomas showing more than 25% of the neoplastic cells with strongly reduced to negative staining were classified as reduced.

In Figure 1 a typical example of carcinoma cells showing negative staining is shown (Fig. 1B) while adjacent normal epithelium in the same section stained positive (Fig. 1A). When reduction of class I heavy chains was observed, both heavy chain specific antibodies showed comparable staining patterns. Reduced expression of MHC-I was observed in 18/23 carcinomas. In all carcinomas that showed reduction of staining for heavy chain expression, a coordinate loss of staining for β2-microglobulin was observed.

C-*myc* overexpression in relation to MHC-I expression

C-*myc* expression was analysed with a monoclonal antibody 6E10, which is generated against a mixture of oligopeptides spanning the exons 2 and 3 of the c-*myc* gene and recognizes the p62 c-*myc* protein[17]. Overexpression of c-*myc* in neoplastic cells was scored, when groups of neoplastic cells (in total more than 5% of the neoplastic cells in a section) showed positive nuclear staining, while normal epithelium and infiltrating immune cells were negative. C-*myc* overexpression was found in 12 out of 23 cervical carcinomas studied (52%). This frequency is comparable with the frequency (44%) found by others using Northern blot analysis[18].

In order to correlate c-*myc* and MHC-I expression at the single cell level, immunohistochemical double stainings were performed, and a typical example is shown in Figure 1. In normal epithelium, adjacent to one of the carcinomas, no detectable levels of c-*myc* expression can be observed (Fig. 1A), whereas staining for MHC-I (brown) is clearly positive. Invasive neoplastic cells exhibit varying levels of nuclear staining for c-*myc* (black), and are also positively stained at the membrane for MHC-I (brown) (Fig. 1C). In total 4 c-*myc* overexpressing carcinomas showed positive staining for MHC-I, while 8 c-*myc* overexpressing carcinomas were found with reduced MHC-I expression. Therefore no absolute correlation could be established between overexpression of c-*myc* and down-regulation of MHC class I. Immunohistochemical staining results for MHC-I and c-*myc* are summarized in Table 1.

An additional argument against a role for c-*myc* in MHC-I down-regulation in cervical neoplasia is the observation that c-*myc* specifically down-regulates expression of the HLA-B locus at the transcriptional level in melanomas[19], while expression of the A-locus and β2-microglobulin is unaffected. In contrast down-regulation of MHC-I in cervical carcinomas generally involves both A- and B-locus products[3,22], and is consistently accompanied by the simultaneous loss of ß2 microglobulin expression. Therefore a B-locus locus specific effect of c-myc in cervical carcinomas is probably not involved.

Furthermore, reduction of expression of MHC Class I antigens can occur independent from c-myc in neuroectodermal tumors, non-small cell lung cancer and colon carcinomas (reviewed in 9). These data indicate that a possible down-regulatory effect of c-myc on HMC-I expression occurs in a tissue-specific manner, and probably involves addition cell- or tissue-specific factors. However also a dose-dependent effect of c-myc on MHC-I expression could explain the different findings.

Table 1 MHC-I polypeptides, transcripts and c-myc overexpression

	positive MHC-I	reduced MHC-I
c-myc -	1 (4%)	10 (43%)
HLA-B RISH +	**1/1**	**6/6**
c-myc +	4 (17%)	8 (35%)
HLA-B RISH +	**2/2**	**6/6**

MHC class I expression (MHC-I) and c-myc expression are summarized for 23 cervical carcinomas, as determined with immunohistochemistry. Reduced MHC-I was scored when 25% or more of the neoplastic cells show strongly reduced to negative staining for MHC-I. c-myc + was scored when 5% or more of the neoplastic cells show positive staining for c-myc. The figures given in bold are the number of lesions, positive by RNA in situ hybridisation (RISH) with the HLA-B probe, out of the number of lesions analysed of each result group.

$$\longrightarrow$$

Figure 1 Immunohistochemical double staining for c-myc and MHC class I heavy chain expression (1A,C), monostaining for MHC-I (1B) and RNA in situ hybridisation (RISH) with an HLA-B specific RNA probe (1D). A: Normal squamous epithelium is positive for MHC-I on basal and parabasal cells (brown), and show no detectable levels of c-myc. B: MHC class I negative carcinoma cells, with infiltrating immune cells staining positive. C: cervical carcinoma cells show positive membranous staining for MHC-I (brown). In the same cells varying levels of positive staining are observable for c-myc (black). D: Reflection signals of the antisense HLA-B specific RNA-probe reveals B-locus specific transcripts in neoplastic cells that show lack of heavy chain polypeptides in the consecutive tissue section (1B).

Antibodies 6E10 (c-myc) and HC10 (HLA-B/C) were detected in a three step immunohistochemical detection system using peroxidase. HC10 signals were visualised with diaminobenzidine (DAB), while c-myc signals were visualised with DAB-Nickel and silver intensification[16]. RNA in situ hybridisation was performed non-radioactively with biotinylated RNA-probes[6], which were detected immunohistochemically with immunogold staining, enhanced with silver. Signals were visualised with confocal laserscan microscopy. Control HLA transgenic mouse tissues only showed positive signals for the HLA-B expressing mice, indicating that the HLA-B RNA-probe is B-locus specific[16].cervical carcinomas generally involves both A- and B-locus products[3,22], and is consistently accompanied by the simultaneous loss of β2-microglobulin expression. Therefore a B-locus specific effect of c-myc in cervical carcinomas is probably not involved. Reproduced by kind permission from The MacMillan Press Ltd, see Reference 16 Cromme et al 1993.

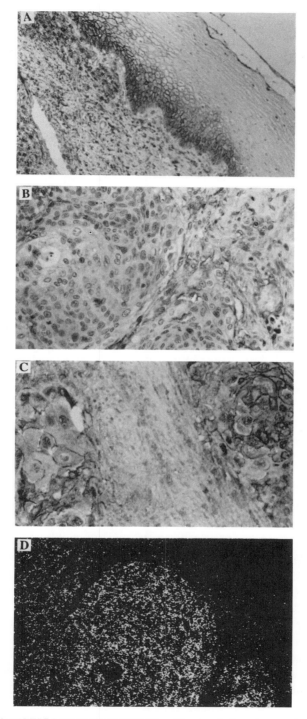

Figure 1. Analysis of MHC-I expression in HPV 16 positive cervical carcinomas, in relation to C-MYC overexpression.

MHC-I RNA *in situ* hybridisation

Fifteen carcinomas with different patterns of MHC-I and c-*myc* expression were subjected to RISH with HLA-B specific RNA-probes. No differences in RISH signals could be detected between neoplastic cells with positive and with reduced staining for heavy chain polypeptides. As shown in Figure 1D HLA-B transcripts can be detected in an neoplastic area in which staining for class I polypeptides is negative (Fig. 1B). Similar results were obtained on the other carcinomas with and without detectable levels of c-*myc* overexpression.

In conclusion these data indicate that the reduced steady state levels of class I polypeptides are not due to c-*myc* mediated inhibition of MHC-I transcription, and are the result of a post-transcriptional regulation defect. A candidate mechanism is the lack of stabilization of the heavy chain/light chain dimer in the endoplasmic reticulum (ER) due to loss of peptide binding. This could be related to the lack of peptide translocation over the ER membrane by the presumed peptide transporter, encoded by the TAP-1 and -2 genes[20,21]. Indeed analysis of the cervical carcinomas described in this paper concerning Tap gene expression reveals a coordinate loss of class I heavy chain and Tap gene expression as determined by immunohistochemical double staining procedures[22]. All these findings justify further research of the regulation of class I intracellular transport and assembly in cervical cancer.

ACKNOWLEDGMENTS

Authors would like to thank Ms. M de Wit and Mr. W. Vos for excellent technical assistance, E.J. Baas for generously supplying the transgenic mouse tissues, and Guus Hateboer for fruitful discussions. This work was supported by grants from the Prevention Fund (28-1502.2) and the Dutch Cancer Society "Koningin Wilhelmina Fonds" (IKA VU 91-10), The Netherlands.

REFERENCES

1. H. zur Hausen. Human papillomaviruses in the pathogenesis of anogenital cancer. *Virology* 184: 9 (1991).
2. M.E. Connor & P.L Stern. Loss of MHC class-I expression in cervical carcinomas. *Int. J. Cancer* 46:1029 (1990).
3. F.V. Cromme. C.J.L.M. Meijer, P.J.F. Snijders, A. Uyterlinde, P. Kenemans, Th. Helmerhorst, P.L. Stern, A.J.C. van den Brule & J.M.M. Walboomers. Analysis of MHC class I and II expression in relation to presence of HPV genotypes in premalignant and malignant cervical lesions. *Br. J. Cancer* 67:1372 (1993).

4. P. Björkman, P. Saper, B. Samraoui, W. Bennet, J. Strominger & D. Wiley. The foreign antigen binding site and T-cell recogniton regions of class I histoccompatibility antigens. *Nature* 329:512 (1987).

5. D.J. Maudsley & D.J. Pound. Modulation of MHC antigen expression by viruses and oncogenes. *Immol. Today* 12(12):429 (1991).

6. A.J.C. van den Brule, F.V. Cromme, P.J.F. Snijders, L. Smit, C.B.M. Oudejans, J.P.A. Baak, C.J.L.M. Meijer & J.M.M. Walboomers. Non radioactive RNA *in situ* hybridisation detection of HPV-16 E7 transcripts in squamous cell carcinomas of the uterine cervix using confocal laserscan microscopy. *Am. J. Pathol.* 139(5):1037 (1991).

7. W.C. Phelps, C.L. Yee, K. Münger & P.M. Howley. The human papillomavirus type 16 E7 gene encodes transactivation and transformation functions similar to those of Adenovirus E1A. *Cell* 53:539 (1988).

8. P.I. Schrier, R. Bernards, R.T.M.J. Vaessen, A. Houweling & A.J. van der Eb. Expression of class I Major Histocompatibility antigens switched off by highly oncogenic adenovirus 12 in transformed rat cells. *Nature* 305:771 (1983).

9. P.I. Schrier & L.T.C. Peltenburg. Relationship between myc oncogene activation and MHC class I expression. *Adv. Cancer Res.* 60:181 (1992).

10. M. Dürst, C.M. Croce, L. Gissmann, E. Schwartz & K. Hübner. Papillomavirus sequences integrate near cellular oncogenes in some cervical carcinomas. Proc. *Natl. Acad. Sci. U.S.A.* 84:1070 (1987).

11. J. Couturier, X. Sastre-Garau, S. Scheider-Manoury, A. Labib & G. Orth. Integration of papillomavirus DNA near *myc* genes in genital carcinomas and its consequence for proto-oncogene expression. *J. Virol.* 65(8):4534 (1991).

12. J.A. Pietenpol, R.W. Stein, E. Moran, P. Yaciuk, R. Schlegel, R.M. Lyons, M.R. Pittelkow, K. Münger, P.M. Howley & H.L. Moses. TGF-β1 inhibition of c-myc transcription and growth in keratinocytes is abrogated by viral transforming poteins with pRB binding domains. *Cell* 61:777 (1990).

13. A.K. Rustgi, N. Dyson & R. Bernards. Amino-terminal domains of c-*myc* and N-*myc* proteins mediate binding to the retinoblastoma gene product. *Nature* 352:541 (1991).

14. R.K. Versteeg, I.A. Noordermeer, M. Krüse-Wolters, D.J. Ruiter & P.I. Schrier. c-*myc* down-regulates class I HLA expression in human melanomas. *E.M.B.O. J.* 7:1023 (1988).

15. J.M.M. Walboomers, P.W.J. Melkert, A.J.C. van den brule, P.J.F. Snijders & C.J.L.M. Meijer. The polymerase chain reaction for screening in diagnostic cytopathology of the cervix. In: *Diagnostic Molecular Pathology* vol. 2, Herrington, C.S., and McGee, O.D. (eds), p 153-172. IRL press, Oxford, U.K. (1992).

16. F.V. Cromme, P.J.F. Snijders, A.J.C. van den Brule, P.Kenemans, C.J.L.M. Meijer & J.M.M. Walboomers. MHC class I expression in HPV 16 positive cervical carcinomas is post-transcriptionally controlled and independent from c-myc overexpression. *Oncogene*, 8:2969 (1993).

17. G. Ramsay, G.I. Evan & J.M. Bishop. The protein encoded by the human proto-oncogene c-*myc*. *Proc. Natl. Acad. Sci U.S.A.* 81:7742 (1984).

18. T. Iwasaka, M. Yokoyama, M. Oh-Ouchida, K. Matsuo, K. Hara, K. Fukuyama, T. Hachisuga, K. Fukuda & H. Sugimori. Detection of human papillomavirus genome and analysis of expression of c-myc and Ha-ras oncogenes in invasive cervical carcinomas. *Gynaecol. Oncol.* 46:298 (1992).

19. R.K. Versteeg, M. Kruse-Wolters, A.C. Plomp, A. van Leeuwen, N.J. Stam, H.L. Ploegh, D.J. Ruiter and P.J. Schrier. Suppression of class I human histocompatibility leukocyte antigen by c-*myc* is locus-specific. *J. Exp. Med.* 170:621 (1989).

20. T. Spies & R. DeMars. Restored expression of major histocompatibility class I molecules by gene transfer of a putative peptide transporter. *Nature* 351:323 (1991).

21. J. Trowsdale, I. Hanson, I. Mockridge, S. Beck, A. Townsend & A. Kelly. Sequences encoded in the class II region of MHC related to the 'ABC' superfamily of transporters. *Nature* 348:741 (1990).

22. F.V. Cromme, J. Airey, M.-T. Heemels, H.L. Ploegh, P.J. Keating, P.L. Stern, C.J.L.M. Meijer & J.M.M. Walboomers. Loss of transporter protein, encoded by the TAP-1 gene, is highly correlated with loss of HLA expression in cervical carcinomas *J Exp Med.* in press.

IMMUNOGENETIC STUDY OF WOMEN WITH HPV RELATED CANCER OF THE UTERINE CERVIX

Patrizia Tenti, Miryam Martinetti,[1] Solange Romagnoli, Enrico Silini, Cinzia Pizzochero,[1] Rita Zappatore, Luciana Babilonti,[2] Luciano Carnevali, and Mariaclara Cuccia[3]

Department of Pathology of the University of Pavia and IRCCS Pol. San Matteo Pavia
[1]Immunohematology and Transfusion Service of the IRCCS Pol. San Matteo Pavia
[2]Department of Obstetrics and Gynaecology of the University of Pavia and IRCCS Pol. San Matteo Pavia
[3]Department of Genetics and Microbiology of the University of Pavia Pavia
Italy

INTRODUCTION

It has been suggested that women carrying the HLA-DQ3 antigen are at increased risk of developing cervical squamous cell carcinoma (SCC)[1]. Since the association between cervical SCC and human papillomavirus (HPV) types 16 and 18 has been proved by molecular studies[2] and in animal models the tumorigenic effect of HPV may differ according to the immunogenetic background,[3] the presence of a given HLA type might help linking environmental risk factors with individual susceptibility to cervical SCC. Subsequent studies however have reported different findings[4,5] that could be in part explained by differences in HLA phenotype among populations.

The aim of our study was to investigate HLA antigens distribution in Italian patients with HPV-related cervical SCC.

Immunology of Human Papillomaviruses
Edited by M.A. Stanley, Plenum Press, New York, 1994

MATERIAL AND METHODS

Forty five patients with invasive SCC of the uterine cervix (median age 55 years, range 27-78) were investigated for HLA phenotype and 39 of them also for HPV infection. HLA class I and II polymorphism was assessed by NIH microlymphocytotoxicity, on T and B enriched lymphocyte suspensions. The serum set employed for the typing has been standardized during the 11th International Histocompatibility Workshop.[6] B cell enrichment was obtained by rosetting with sheep's red cells. As controls, the HLA phenotype frequencies in 510 healthy individuals from Continental Italy were employed.[7]

Associations between HLA markers and cervical SCC were analyzed by 2 x 2 contingency tables. Chi square with Yate's correction and Fisher's probability values were calculated for all defined specificities. Probability values were corrected for the number

Table 1. Oligonucleotide primers and probes for the Polymerase Chain Reaction (PCR).

HPV type		sequence (5'-3')	Genomic location*	Size of amplified products (base pairs)
16	pr	GAACAGCAATACAACAAACCG	368-388	201
	pr	CCATGCATGATTACAGCTGG	549-569	
	pb	TGTCCAGATGTCTTTGCT		
18	pr	TGCCAGAAACCGTTGAATCC	426-445	197
	pr	CAATGTCTTGCAATGTTGCC	604-623	
	pb	CGTTGGAGTCGTTCCTGT		

pr= primers; pb= probes; *amplified sequences were localized within E6-E7 ORF.

of comparison made. Relative Risk (RR) was calculated according to Woolf's method, reviewed by Svejgaard and colleagues.[8]

The presence of HPV 16 and 18 genomic sequences was investigated by Polymerase Chain Reaction (PCR) with virus type specific primers (table 1) using DNA extracted from formalin-fixed paraffin-embedded sections of the tumors. Human cell lines containing a known number of HPV DNA sequences were used as positive controls in the reactions (SiHa cells for HPV 16 and HeLa cells for HPV 18). Appropriate negative controls were used in each set of reactions and all recommended precautions to avoid PCR product carry over were observed.

Table 2. HLA-A, -B, -Cw, -DR, -DQ and HPV status in 45 patients affected by squamous cell carcinoma of uterine cervix.

Patient	Age (yr)	HLA-A	-B	-Cw	-DR	-DQ	HPV
B.M.L.	40	3,24	7,35	4,7	15,-	6,-	-
B.M.	61	2,3	35,51	4,-	1,13	6,-	16
B.W.	54	1,30	51,57	6,-	11,15	6,7	16,18
B.I.	45	2,23	27,57	2,6	1,11	5,7	16
C.I.	75	3,25	35,44	4,5	2,8	1,4	ND
C.G.	30	2,3	14,51	2,-	3,6	1,2	16,18
C.M.	78	1,28	35,37	6,-	1,11	1,7	-
C.L.	27	2,28	51,57	6,-	2,11	1,7	16,18
C.F.	74	2,3	53,62	3,4	6,7	1,2	18
D.P.	56	1,2	49,57	6,-	7,11	2,7	16,18
F.F.	58	2,26	38,51	1,-	10,11	5,7	-
F.A.	47	2,11	55,60	3,-	3,8	2,4	18
G.A.	62	1,25	18,51	1,-	11,-	7,-	-
G.A.	29	1,3	37,49	6,7	1,14	1,-	16,18
G.N.	57	23,24	18,49	7,-	11,14	5,7	-
G.L.	51	2,3	51,62	4,-	1,8	1,4	16
G.A.	63	1,3	7,35	4,7	1,8	4,5	16
G.P.	59	2,30	14,55	3,-	4,15	4,6	16
L.L.	57	2,26	35,63	7,-	1,11	5,7	16,18
M.E.	35	2,24	7,45	6,7	7,15	2,6	16
M.L.	61	3,11	35,-	4,-	3,11	2,7	18
M.C.	59	1,29	35,-	4,-	11,-	7,-	18
M.B.	49	1,24	7,58	7,-	7,12	2,7	16
M.M.	45	3,25	39,47	6,-	15,-	6,-	16
N.L.	44	2,3	58,62	3,-	6,-	1,-	-
N.R.	33	3,31	44,51	1,2	8,12	7,-	ND
O.M.	67	2,28	51,-	6,-	1,11	5,7	16,18
P.G.	70	1,28	7,51	7,-	ND	ND	ND
P.M.	40	2,3	47,51	2,6	1,6	1,-	ND
P.E.	50	2,11	8,44	5,7	3,11	2,7	ND
P.G.	60	2,24	49,51	5,7	2,7	1,2	16,18
R.G.	46	1,3	8,35	2,-	15,3	2,6	16
R.M.R.	52	2,32	14,61	2,-	1,11	5,7	16,18
R.M.	49	2,32	35,51	4,-	1,4	3,5	16,18
S.S.	54	1,24	8,57	6,7	3,7	2,-	16,18
S.C.	61	2,33	39,51	6,7	3,9	2,7	18
S.S.	64	2,28	35,51	1,2	1,15	6,-	-
T.M.A.	38	2,24	13,50	6,-	7,-	2,-	16,18
T.C.	55	1,-	13,41	6,-	7,10	2,5	-
V.G.	56	2,11	38,57	7,-	4,13	3,6	ND
V.L.	65	2,3	14,51	2,-	3,6	1,2	16
Z.T.	76	2,11	7,37	5,6	2,11	1,7	16
Z.G.	67	2,24	27,44	1,5	4,15	1,3	16
Z.M.	55	2,29	7,18	-,-	7,11	2,7	16,18
Z.M.R.	35	2,29	13,44	6,-	7,-	2,-	16,18

ND: not determined

RESULTS

The complete list of patients and of their HLA phenotype is reported in table 2. With respect to HLA class II polymorphysm the differences between patients and controls antigens are not statistically significant. However some deviations may be observed: HLA DR1, DR8, and DQ1 antigens are weakly overrepresented in patients with cervical SCC: 26.6% vs. 16.5% of controls, 11.1% vs. 6.5% and 68.9% vs. 58% respectively . On the contrary, HLA-DR4 was underrepresented in patients: 8.9% vs. 13.5% of controls (Table 3).

Table 3. HLA deviated frequencies in 45 patients with SCC of the uterine cervix.

	Controls* (N°=510)	Patients (N°=45)	p corrected
HLA-DR1	16.5%	26.6%	>0.05
HLA-DR8	6.5%	11.1%	>0.05
HLA-DR4	13.5%	8.9%	>0.05
HLA-DQ1	58%	68.9%	>0.05
HLA-B51	6.8%	**35.6%**	**0.0021**
HLA-Cw6	19.8%	**37.8%**	**0.0061**

* XI IHW

Deviations have been found also with respect to HLA class I polymorphism. In particular, HLA-B51 and Cw6 antigens show a higher frequency in patients than in controls: 35.6% vs. 16.8% (X2=10.79; p=0.0021; p corr.=O.05; RR=2.88) and 37.8% vs. 19.8% (X2=7.98; p=O.0061; p corr.=0.04; RR=2.46) respectively.

The overall rate of HPV infection in our series is 79.5% (30.8% HPV 16; 12.8 % HPV 18; 35.9% HPV 16 and 18). We did not identify any correlation between HLA class I antigens and HPV infection. Among HLA class II polymorphisms however, HPV negative patients show an increase of DQ1 frequency, 87.5% in HPV negative vs. 64.9% in HPV positive patients (p value not significant) (table 2).

DISCUSSION

It is known that viral antigens are presented to T cells by HLA molecules. Therefore the association of HPV-related cervical SCC with a specific HLA sequence motif like HLA-DQ3, as suggested by Wank and Thomssen,[1] might be important for understanding the susceptibility to cervical SCC on an immunogenetic basis. Subsequent investigations[4,5] have not confirmed the previously proposed association, but many difficulties in replicating results in studies on HLA-associated diseases may be explained by the linking of susceptibility genes with different HLA markers in various ethnic groups, or by different frequences of HLA antigens. Therefore the full understanding of HLA alleles involvement in susceptibility to cervical SCC could be obtained by analyzing the associations between HPV infection and HLA in distinct populations and/or by studying other Major Histocompatibility Complex linked genes.

In our study we did not confirm the results of Wank and Thomssen[1] regarding the HLA- DQ3 association nor the HLA-DR distribution in patients with cervical SCC as reported by Glew and Stern.[4,5] HLA class I polymorphisms instead of HLA class II seem to be involved. In particular HLA-B51 and -Cw6 alleles are significantly more frequent in patients than in controls. We therefore suggest the possible involvement of HLA-class I linked genes in cervical SCC susceptibility.

REFERENCES

1. R. Wank and C. Thomssen. High risk of squamous cell carcinoma of the cervix for women with HLA DQw3. *Nature* 352:723 (1991).
2. H. zur Hausen. Papillomavirus in anogenital cancer as a model to understanding the role of viruses in human cancer. *Cancer Res.* 49:4677 (1989).
3. R. Han, F. Breitburd, P.N. Marche, and O. Orth.Linkage of regression and malignant conversion of rabbit viral papillomas to MHC class II genes. *Nature* 356:66 (1992).
4. S.S. Glew and P.L. Stern. HLA antigens and cervical carcinoma. *Nature* 356:22 (1992).
5. A. Helland and A.L. Borrensen. HLA antigens and cervical carcinoma. *Nature* 356:23 (1992).
6. "HLA 1991" Proceedings of the Eleventh International Histocompatibility Workshop and Conference, K.Tsuji, M. Aizawa, and T. Sasazuki eds., Oxford University Press, Oxford (1992).
7. T. Imanishi, T. Akaza, A. Kimura, K. Tokunaga, and T. Oojoboi. Allele and haplotype frequencies for HLA and complement loci in various ethnic groups. In: "HLA 1991", K.Tsuji, M. Aizawa, and T. Sasazuki eds., Oxford University Press, Oxford (1992).
8. A. Svejgaard, P. Platz, and L.P. Ryder. Insulin-dependent diabetes mellitus. In: "Histocompatibility testing 1980", P.I. Terasaki, ed., UCLA Tissue Typing Laboratory Press, Los Angeles (1980).

RECURRENT RESPIRATORY PAPILLOMATOSIS (RRP): ENRICHED HLA DQw3 PHENOTYPE AND DECREASED CLASS I MHC EXPRESSION

Vincent R. Bonagura,[1] Mary Ellen O'Reilly,[1]
Allan L. Abramson,[2] Bettie M. Steinberg[2]

[1]Department of Pediatrics,
[2]Department of Otolaryngology
Long Island Jewish Medical Center
New Hyde Park
New York 11042
U S A

INTRODUCTION

Human papillomavirus (HPV) infection of the upper respiratory tract and larynx can cause recurrent, life-threatening disease in both adults and children [1]. Type 6 and 11 HPV are the most frequent causes of this disease [2,3]. Latency is the most common and benign outcome of acute HPV infection [6]. However, some HPV infected patients have a chronic course requiring many operative procedures to maintain a patent airway. The immunologic response(s) that should prevent recurrent respiratory papilloma (RRP) development are not well characterized. We recently identified a restricted expression of immune response genes by patients with RRP. This observation indicates that T-cell dysregulation may predispose susceptible individuals to develop RRP. Little is understood about the regulation of cellular immune responses to HPV. These patients show strong humoral and non-MHC restricted cellular responses to HPV [4-13], yet fail to prevent HPV reactivation.

We have identified the restricted expression of an immune response gene associated with immune suppression, DQw3, in RRP patients. We have also identified down-regulation of Class I MHC expression on papillomas. These results implicate immune suppression of MHC restricted T-cell responses in patients with RRP as a possible pathogenic mechanism inducing defective T-cell containment of HPV.

Non-MHC Restricted Immunity In Patients With RRP

To rule out the possibility that reduced general immune function was present in our RRP patients, we first evaluated a number of immunologic parameters by standard methods [14-16]. No statistically significant differences in the absolute number of circulating lymphocytes, or T cell subsets were observed. Lectin-induced mitogenesis, natural cytotoxicity to the myeloid cell line K562, generation of lymphokine-activated killer (LAK) cells against RAJI target cells, and production of IFN-α in response to herpes simplex virus also were intact. LAK cell killing of papilloma target cells was observed with both HLA-unmatched normal controls and papilloma patients' autologous effectors. Therefore, non-MHC restricted immunity in these RRP patients was normal.

MHC Expression By Patients With RRP

HLA restriction for the MHC Class II immune response gene has been identified in patients with cervical carcinoma[17]. We therefore identified the HLA phenotypes of 16 RRP patients to determine if the expression of a specific Class II MHC immune response gene was associated with the susceptibility to RRP, thereby implicating MHC-restricted T-cell function in the development of RRP. Patients included 10 adults and 6 children, 4 females and 12 males.

Table 1. MHC Class II phenotype of papilloma patients, compared to the population as a whole.

	DR5	P Value	DQw3	P Value
Papilloma Patients	50%	0.0044	75%	<0.0001
Total Population	17%		22%	

Patients were phenotyped for Class I and Class II expression by the fluorocytochromasia method [18]. Frequencies of RRP patient allele expression were compared with those reported in the 11th International Histocompatibility Workshop[19]. Patients were derived from all parts of the United States, and therefore should reflect the broad base in this Workshop. Data was analyzed by 1-tailed Fisher's exact test using the approximation of Woolf. Bonferroni's correction was made because of multiple comparisons in the retrospective analysis of Class I MHC expression by the RRP patients; p <0.0125 would be considered equivalent to 0.05 for a single comparison.

The HLA Class II DQw3 phenotype was expressed by most RRP patients (Table 1). Comparing the frequency of DQw3 expression in our population (12/16 or 75%) with that recorded in the 11th International HLA Workshop (controls, 21.7%) (19), the incidence of DQw3 expression in our population was highly significant (p<0.0001). In addition, the DQw3 phenotype in humans is further split into the 7, 8, or 9 subtypes, and 10/12 (83%) of the DQw3 RRP patients show the DQw3(7) split compared with 28.1% in the controls (78). This comparison was also highly significant (p=0.0002). Expression of the Class II major histocompatibility gene DR5 (8/16 or 50.0%) by the RRP patients (controls, 17.0%) was also significant (p=0.0044). In retrospective analysis, we compared Class I, HLA-A and HLA-B expression by these RRP patients. A11 and B14 were also frequently expressed (5/11 or 45% each), p=0.006.

Class I and II expression by papillomas

We then asked whether an alteration in Class I or Class II MHC antigen expression by the papillomas could facilitate HPV evasion of specific T-cell immunity, contributing to RRP pathogenesis. Five micron sections of frozen papilloma tissue and normal squamous vocal cord epithelium were stained with murine monoclonal antibody W6/32 conjugated with fluorescein isothiocyanate (specific for a monomorphic determinant on HLA Class I heavy chains in association with β2 microglobulin)[20], and counterstained with a murine monoclonal anti-Class II antibody (specific for a monomorphic determinant of DR)[21] conjugated with tetramethyl rhodamine isothiocyanate. A similar staining with murine monoclonal anti-DQ antibody (Leu-10) in a separate experiment showed similar results.

Table 2. Papilloma expression of Class I and II MHC molecules compared with normal respiratory epithelium .

Tissue	Class I MHC Expression	Class II MHC Expression
Papilloma	- or +/-	++++
Normal Respiratory Epithelium	++++	++++

Class I MHC expression on papillomas was markedly reduced compared to normal larynx epithelium. A similar observation has been made in cervical cancers associated with HPV expression, due to decreased expression of transporter proteins (the TAP proteins) required for Class I MHC expression on the cell membrane[22]. Alternatively, down-regulation of Class I MHC antigens in papilloma tissue could represent the effect of an HPV-specific protein on movement of Class I molecules to the cell surface, similar to the Adenovirus 12 E3 protein inhibition of Class I MHC surface expression[23]. In contrast, expression of the Class II MHC gene products, DR and DQ, appeared equivalent in normal and papillomas.

DISCUSSION

The association of particular class II MHC gene products with antigen may trigger either stimulatory or suppressive immune responses[24-26]. The DQ gene regulates antigen-specific suppression through CD8+ suppressor T-cells activation by antigen-specific CD4+ suppressor/inducer T-cells [25,26].

The highly enriched Class II DQw3(7) gene expression by RRP patients suggests that select immune response genes, namely DQw3 and perhaps DR5, are important in conferring susceptibility to this disease following HPV infection. Expression of HLA-A11 and B14 may also influence HPV recognition by Class I restricted cytotoxic T-cells. Prosepective experiments specifically designed to identify Class I MHC expression by RRP patients are needed to confirm these observations.

Although we did not detect differences in T cell subsets in peripheral blood of patients, it is conceivable that locally, Ts cells are involved in respiratory papillomatosis. Carson et al[21] found a significant increase in CD8+ T cells in HPV-16 containing genital malignancies. Taken collectively with our results on Class I distribution and specific Class II phenotypes, these observations indicate that susceptibility to HPV represents combined viral and host defense elements. T-suppressor function may have a role in down-regulating immunologic recognition of, and responsiveness to, active HPV infection.

Leprosy as a model of immune suppression

Leprosy serves as a model system for understanding mechanisms of immune suppression. Leprosy is expressed in two forms, tuberculoid (TL) and lepromatous (LL). The first is associated with a strong specific cytotoxic T-cell response. associated with stimulatory lymphokines. In contrast, LL patients show specific immune unresponsiveness. They have absent cytotoxic T-cell responses to *M. leprae*, and activated CD8+,28-suppressor T-cells synthesize immunosuppressive cytokines when lepromin protein is presented by cells expressing the DQw3 Class II genes[25,26].

RRP resembles LL in several ways: 1) They both show evidence of an chronic infectious pathogen with antigen-specific cellular immunologic "tolerance" to that pathogen. 2) There is a paucity of mononuclear cells in the cellular infiltrates found in lesions in both diseases. 3) Regression of lesions can occur following repeated immunization with the respective pathogen, shifting disease susceptibility to resistance (HPV-infected wart lesions have shown this phenomenon). 4) In both diseases high titers of specific antibodies to the pathogen are found without specific CTC responses during the period of immune tolerance when the disease progresses or recurs. 5) They share the same restricted expression of immune response genes. 6) Immunosuppressive cytokines are found within lesions in both diseases[27-32], V. Bonagura et al, unpublished.

Therefore, if the immune mechanisms active in LL are similar to those in RRP, T-cell mediated immune suppression effected by immunosuppressive cytokines may be expected in RRP. This argument finds support in the temporary disappearance of papillomas in some RRP patients treated with interferon-alpha[33]. The clinical and immunologic parallels between these diseases suggest that a strategy to illuminate the suppressive mechanism(s) in RRP may aid in achieving better disease control.

REFERENCES

1. Holinger P.H., Johnson K.C., and G.C. Anison, Papilloma of the larynx: review of 109 cases with preliminary report of aureomycin therapy. *Ann Otol Rhinol Laryngol.* 59:547(1950).
2. Mounts P., Shah K.V., and H. Kashima H, Viral etiology of juvenile and adult-onset squamous papilloma of the larynx. *Proc Natl Acad Sci USA.* 79:5425(1982).
3. Steinberg B.M., Topp W.C., Schneider P.S., and A.L. Abramson, Laryngeal papillomavirus infection during clinical remission. *N Engl J Med.* 308:1261(1983).
4. Perrick D., Wray B.B., Leffel M.S., Harmon J.D., and E.S.Porubsky, Evaluation of immunocompetency in juvenile laryngeal papillomatosis. *Ann Allergy* 65:69(1990).
5. Bonnez W., Kashima H.K., Leventhal B., Mounts P., Rose R.C., Reichman R.C., and K.V. Shah, Antibody response to human papillomavirus (HPV) type 11 in children with juvenile-onset recurrent respiratory papillomatosis (RRP). *Virology* 188:384(1992).
6. Christensen N.D., and J.W. Kreider, Antibody-mediated neutralization in vivo of infectious papillomaviruses. *J Virol.* 64:3151(1990).
7. Naiman H.B., Doyle A.T., Ruben R.J., and A.S. Kadish, Natural cytotoxicity and interferon production in patients with recurrent respiratory papillomatosis. *Ann Otol Rhinol Laryngol.* 93:483(1984).
8. Jakubikova J., Oravec C., and I. Klacansky, Modulation of humoral and cellular resistance in children with laryngeal papillomatosis. *Intl J Pediatr Otorhinolaryngol.* 23:229(1992).
9. Denis M., Chadee K., and G.J. Matlashewski, Macrophage killing of human papillomavirus type 16-transformed cells. *Virology* 170:342(1989).
10. Kirchner H., Immunobiology of human papillomavirus infection. *Prog Med Virol* 33:1(1986).
11. Siegal F.P., Lopez C., Fitzgerald P.A., Shah K., Baron P., Leiderman I.Z., Imperato D., and S. Landesman, Opportunistic infections in acquired immune deficiency syndrome result from synergistic defects of both the natural and adaptive components of cellular immunity. *J Clin Invest.* 78:115(1986).

15. Santiago-Schwarz F., Panagiotopoulos C., Sawitsky A., and K.R. Rai, Distinct characteristics of lymphokine-activated killer (LAK) cells derived from patients with B-cell chronic lymphocytic leukemia (B-CLL). A factor in B-CLL serum promotes natural killer cell-like LAK cell growth. *Blood* 76:1355(1990).

16. Steinberg B.M., Abramson A.L., and R.P. Meade, Culture of human laryngeal papilloma cells in vitro. *Otol Head Neck Surg.* 90:728(1982).

17. Wank R, and C. Thomssen. 1991. High risk of squamous cell carcinoma of the cervix for women with HLA DQw3. *Nature* 352:723-725.

18. Bodmer W.F. and J.C. Bodmer. "NIAID Manual of Tissue Typing Techniques (1979- 1980). NIH, Washington D.C.

19. The central data analysis committee: allele frequencies, Section 6.3 splits combined (five loci). In: The data book of the 11th international histocompatibility workshop. Yokohama, 2:807(1991).

20. Parham P., Barnstable C.J., and W.F. Bodmer, Use of a monoclonal antibody (W6/32) in structural studies of HLA-A,B,C, antigens. *J Immunol.* 123:342(1979).

21. Quaranta V., Walker L.E., Pellegrino M.A., and S. Ferrone S, Purification of immunologically functional subsets of human Ia-like antigens on a monoclonal antibody (Q5/13) immunoadsorbent. *J Immunol.* 125:1421(1980).

22. Townsend A., and J. Trowsdale, The transporters associated with antigen presentation. *Semin Cell Biol.* 4:53(1993).

23. Wold W.S., and L.R. Gooding, Region E3 of adenovirus: a cassette of genes involved in host immunosurveillance and virus-cell interactions. *Virology* 184:1(1991).

24. Benacerraf B., and H.O. McDevitt. Histocompatibility-linked immune response genes. *Science* 175:273(1972).

25. Bloom B.R., Modlin R.L., and P. Salgame, Stigma variations: observations on suppressor T cells and leprosy. *Annu Rev Immunol.* 10:453(1992).

26. Salgame P., Convit J., and B.R. Bloom, Immunological suppression by human CD8+ T cells is receptor dependent and HLA-DQ restricted. *Proc Natl Acad Sci USA* . 88:2598(1991).

27. Thivolet J., Hegazy M.R., Viac J., and Y. Chardonnet, An in vivo study of cell mediated immunity in human warts. Preliminary results. *Acta Derm Venereol Stockh.* 57:317(1977).

28. Viac J., Thivolet J., and Y. Chardonnet, Specific immunity in patients suffering from recurring warts before and after repetitive intradermal tests with human papilloma virus. *Br J Dermatol.* 97:365(1977).

29. Majewski S., and S. Jablonska, Epidermodysplasia verruciformis as a model of human papillomavirus-induced genetic cancers: The role of local immunosurveillance. *Am J Med Sci* 304:174(1992).

30. Modlin R.L., Mehra V., Wong L., Fujimiya Y., Chang W.C., Horwitz D.A., Bloom B.R., Rea T.H., and P.K. Pattengale, Suppressor T lymphocytes from lepromatous leprosy skin lesions. *J Immunol.* 137:2831(1986).

31. Yamamura M., Wang X.H., Ohmen J.D., Uyemura K., Rea T.H., Bloom B.R., and R.L. Modlin, Cytokine patterns of immunologically mediated tissue damage. *J Immunol.* 149:1470(1992).

32. Lin Y.L., Borenstein L.A., Selvakumar R., Ahmed R., and F.O. Wettstein, Progression from papilloma to carcinoma is accompanied by changes in antibody response to papillomavirus proteins. *J Virol.* 67:382(1993).

33. Kashima H., Leventhal B., Clark K., Cohen S., Dedo H., Donovan D., Fearon B., Gardiner L., Goepfert H., Lusk R., McCabe B.F., Mounts P., Muntz H., Richardson M., Singleton G., Weck P., Whisnant J., Wold D., and A. Yonkers, Interferon alfa-n1 (Wellferon) in juvenile onset recurrent respiratory papillomatosis: results of a randomized study in twelve collaborative institutions. *Laryngoscope* 98:334(1988).

HPV 16-DERIVED SYNTHETIC PEPTIDES WITH ABILITY TO UPREGULATE MHC CLASS I EXPRESSION ON RMA-S OR T2 CELLS, AS DETECTED BY ENZYME IMMUNOASSAY

Joakim Dillner

Department of Virology
Karolinska Institute
Stockholm
Sweden

INTRODUCTION

The measurement of the ability of peptides to interact with MHC class I molecules has been greatly facilitated in recent years, by the introduction of mutant cell lines with surface expression of unstable MHC class I molecules lacking endogenously bound peptides[1,2]. The murine lymphoma cell line RMA-S, a mutant of the T cell lymphoma line RMA, was generated by selection for low surface class I expression[1]. RMA-S expresses only about 5% of class I K^b and D^b molecules compared to the wild type cell line RMA[1]. These MHC class I molecules are unstable at physiological temperature, due to lack of normal peptides in the antigen binding groove[1]. However, they can be stabilized by supplementing the culture medium with exogenous peptide with ability to bind to the allele in question[1,2]. The binding ability of a given peptide can thereafter be quantified by measuring the amount of class I molecules by immunoprecipitation or by quantitative immunofluorescence[1,2,3,4,5]. Although the use of immunofluorescence represents a significantly more rapid assay than immunoprecipitation, it still requires a considerable amount of time on a Fluorescence Activated Cell Sorter (FACS), which was not available. In the past 5 years, our laboratory has synthesized a large amount of peptides (>2000), derived from a variety of viruses including HPV. All these peptides are approximately 20 residues long, which is much longer than the optimal size of a MHC class I binding peptide (8-10 residues long)[6]. In the present study, we wished to 1) develop a rapid assay that does not require a FACS for measurement of the ability of synthetic peptides to interact with MHC class I and 2) investigate whether 20-mer peptides could be used for screening for agretopes, in spite of their suboptimal length.

MATERIALS AND METHODS

The enzyme immunoassay used will be described in detail elsewhere[7]. Briefly, 40000 RMA-S or 30000 T2 cells were incubated with synthetic peptides at a 300 uM concentration in 96-well U-bottomed tissue culture plates overnight at 37 degrees, 5% CO_2. Surface MHC class I expression was then measured by incubation with the monoclonal antibodies HB27, HB158 or BB7.2 (specific for D^b, K^b and A2.1, respectively), goat anti-mouse IgG-peroxidase conjugate, 1% formaldehyde and finally the ABTS peroxidase substrate. These incubations were for 30 minutes on ice and in-between incubations the cells were washed extensively with ice-cold PBS. Finally, the absorbances at 405 nm were recorded in a Dynatech microplate reader.

RESULTS

An example of results is shown in the Figure. A set of 78 21-residues long E7 peptides, overlapping each other by 20 residues, was tested for ability to upregulate D^b expression on RMA-S cells. As can be seen, several peptides were able to induce upregulation of D^b expression to levels equal or greater than those of the parental cell line RMA. A summary of the major D^b and K^b-binding peptides found in the E6 and E7 open reading frames after testing of 107 peptides is presented in Table 1.

Comparison of the present data with the 2 previous reports (by Stauss et al[4] and Feltkamp et al[5]) that have screened HPV 16 E6 and E7 peptides in RMA-S-based assays shows that almost all the reactive peptides reported in this work contain an agretope found either by Feltkamp or by Stauss, except for the D^b-binding activity in the E6 carboxyterminal part. It should be emphasized that the overlap between the tested peptides was 20 residues and that several of the reactive peptides are therefore likely to contain the same MHC class I-interacting agretope. As shown in Table 1, seven of the peptides with strong upregulating ability are derived from the same region of E7 and all share the sequence AHYNIVTFCCK. Since the work of Feltkamp et al[5] reported that RAHYNIVTF and AHYNIVTFC were D^b-binders and HYNIVTFCC was a K^b-binder, it is likely that the upregulatory activity of these peptides was indeed induced by agretopes in this overlapping part of the peptides.

For analysis of which peptides were able to interact with the human HLA allele A2.1, we used the human lymphoblastoid cell line T2, which also has a peptide processing defect[1], but otherwise similar assay conditions as for the RMA-S assay. Among the 107 E6 and E7-derived peptides that were tested, 7 were found to be strong binders. The most reactive peptide was YMLDLQPETTDLYCYEQLNDS (from E7) which induced upregulation even at a 9 uM concentration. Interestingly, whereas most of the peptides that induced K^b also induced D^b, and vice versa, the A2.1-inducing peptides were in almost all cases different from the D^b and K^b inducers (not shown).

Table 1. Synthetic peptides from HPV 16 E6 or E7 with ability to restore full H-2 expression on RMA-S. From E7, 78 21-residue peptides, overlapping by 20 residues, and from E6 29 21-residue peptides, overlapping by 16 residues were tested. The peptides that lacked cysteine had an extra cysteine added to the carboxyterminus, since this appeared to enhance upregulatory ability.

Peptide number	Peptide sequence	D^b-induction(%)	K^b-induction(%)
HPV 16 E7:			
4140	GPAGQAEPDRAHYNIVTFCCK	108	184
4141	PAGQAEPDRAHYNIVTFCCKC	69	105
4146	EPDRAHYNIVTFCCKCDSTLR	99	162
4147	PDRAHYNIVTFCCKCDSTLRL	116	154
4148	DRAHYNIVTFCCKCDSTLRLC	104	132
4149	RAHYNIVTFCCKCDSTLRLCV	92	118
4150	AHYNIVTFCCKCDSTLRLCVQ	65	104
4157	FCCKCDSTLRLCVQSTHVDIR	113	96
4158	CCKCDSTLRLCVQSTHVDIRT	124	170
4162	DSTLRLCVQSTHVDIRTLEDL	33	116
4177	RTLEDLLMGTLGIVCPICSQK	133	101
HPV 16 E6:			
41101	YRDGNPYAVCDKCLKFYSKIS	142	102
41111	INCQKPLCPEEKQRHLDKKQR	-8	184
41113	EKQRHLDKKQRFHNIRGRWTC	429	386
41114	LDKKQRFHNIRGRWTGRCMSC	90	187
41115	RFHNIRGRWTGRCMSCCRSSR	260	274
41116	RGRWTGRCMSCCRSSRTRRET	88	130

DISCUSSION

The present study has utilized a simple and efficient enzyme immunoassay for measuring the ability of a large panel of synthetic peptides to interact with different MHC class I alleles. Our use of a small-scale assay enabled the testing of peptides at a high concentration at low cost. The high peptide concentration used resulted in that MHC class I expressions could be upregulated at least 30-fold for several peptides. The assay was therefore very easily interpretable as to which peptides were able to interact with the class

I alleles or not. The low cost and rapidity of the assay were considered to outweigh the assay variability seen, since repeated testing and multiple replicates can easily be used also in large-scale screenings.

In analogy with previous studies[1,2,3], we observed that the ability to bind and induce MHC class I expression on RMA-S cells was not limited to 8-10 residue peptides, although naturally processed peptides presented in MHC class I molecules have a distinct size, usually 8-10 residues[6]. HPLC-separation of synthesized peptide material and testing of all HPLC fractions showed that upregulatory activity was found in the main peak, suggesting that the activity was not due to shorter analogs present as impurities in the synthesized peptides. The reason why the longer peptides also work is likely to be due to

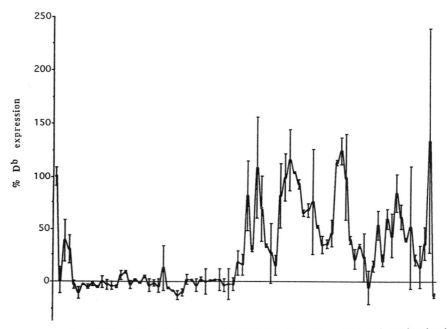

Figure 1. Screening of 78 peptides derived from HPV 16 E7, 21 residues long and overlapping by 20 residues, for ability to upregulate D^b expression on RMA-S. Values are given as percent D^b expression relative to RMA (100%) and RMA-S (0%). Each point represents the mean of duplicate values with standard deviation error bars extending from each point. The first point is RMA, point 2 is RMA-S, point 3 is an influenza virus epitope known to bind to D^b, point 4 is a Sendai virus epitope known to bind to K^b and points 5-82 are the overlapping E7 peptides. The peptides were tested at concentrations of about 300 uM (E7 peptides) or 100 uM (influenza and Sendai virus control peptides). A more detailed presentation of this data will appear elsewhere[7].

that a fraction of the longer peptide is degraded to shorter analogs during the overnight incubation of peptides and cells at 37 degrees.

It will now be most interesting to analyze shorter analogs of the peptides with MHC upregulatory activity, in order to define agretopes with optimal binding affinity. Such peptides could be useful in studies of the CTL response against HPV.

REFERENCES

1. H.G. Ljunggren, C. Öhlén, P. Höglund, L. Franksson, and K. Kärre, The RMA-S lyphoma mutant: Consequences of a peptide loading defect on immunological recognition and graft rejection. *Int J Cancer* suppl 6, 38 (1991).

2. A. Townsend, C. Öhlén, J. Bastin, H.G. Ljunggren, and K. Kärre, Association of class I major histocompatibility heavy and light chains induced by viral peptides. *Nature* 340:443 (1989).

3. G. Stuber, S. Modrow, P. Höglund, L. Franksson, J. Elvin, H. Wolf, E. Klein, K. Kärre, and G. Klein, Assessment of MHC class I interaction with EBV and HIV peptides by elevation of membrane H-2 and HLA in peptide loading deficient cells. *Eur J Immunol.* 22:2697 (1992).

4. H. J. Stauss, H. Davies, E. Sadovnikova, B.M. Chain, N. Horowitz, and C. Sinclair, Induction of cytotoxic T lymphocytes with peptides in vitro: Identification of candidate T-cell epitopes in human papillomavirus. *Proc Natl Acad. Sci USA* 89:7871 (1992).

5. M. Feltkamp, H. Smits, M. Vierboom, R. Minnaar, B. de Jongh, J. Drijfhout, J. ter Schegget, C. Melief, and W.M. Kast, Vaccination with cytotoxic T-lymphocyte epitope-containing peptide protects against a tumor induced by human papillomavirus type 16-transformed cells. *Eur J Immunol.* in press (1993).

6. K. Falk, O. Rötzschke, S. Stevanovic, G. Jung, and H.G. Rammensee, Allele-specific motifs revealed by sequencing of self-peptides eluted from MHC molecules. *Nature* 351:290 (1991).

7. J. Dillner. Synthetic peptides from the E6 and E7 regions of human papillomavirus type 16 that induce MHC class I expression on RMA-S cells, as detected by enzyme immunoassay. *J Immunol Methods* in press (1993).

REGULATION OF MHC CLASS I, CLASS II AND ICAM-1 EXPRESSION BY CYTOKINES AND RETINOIDS IN HPV-HARBORING KERATINOCYTE LINES

Slawomir Majewski[1], Francoise Breitburd[2], Gerard Orth[2], and Stefania Jablonska[1]

[1]Department of Dermatology
Warsaw School of Medicine
Koszykowa 82a
02-008 Warsaw
Poland
[2]Unite des Papillomavirus
Institut Pasteur
25 rue du DR. Roux
75724 Paris, Cedex 15
France

INTRODUCTION

The growth and progression of HPV-associated,potentially malignant anogenital lesions seems to be controlled by local immunosurveillance mechanisms. These mechanisms include tumor antigen presentation, tumor cell recognition and eradication by specific T cytotoxic lymphocytes (Chen et al., 1992) and natural cytotoxic cells (Malejczyk et al., 1989). The immune recognition and cytolysis are dependent, in a part, on the expression on effector/target cells of some adhesion molecules, eg.LFA-l/ICAM-1 and CD2/LFA-3 receptor/ligand pairs, as well as class I and class II MHC-glycoproteins reacting with CD8 and CD4 molecules, respectively.

The aim of the study was to examine, by means of quantitative immunoperoxidase and Northern blot techniques, the expression of ICAM-1, LFA-3, class I and class II MHC molecules in several human keratinocyte lines containing HPV DNA and displaying

Immunology of Human Papillomaviruses
Edited by M.A. Stanley, Plenum Press, New York, 1994

various tumorigenic potential. We have also studied the mechanisms of regulation of the adhesion molecule expression by various immunomodulatory cytokines and retinoids.

MATERIAL AND METHODS

Keratinocyte lines

The study was performed on Skv cell lines, established from vulvar bowenoid papulosis containing HPV16 DNA (Schneidder-Maunoury et al, 1987. In vitro passaging of Skv cells resulted in selection of two nontumorigenic sublines (Skv-e1, Skv-l1) and two tumorigenic counterparts (Skv-e2 and Skv-l2). The latter, when transplanted into nude mice, show a fast growth and reconstitute tumors with histopathological pattern of cancer in situ with Bowen's atypia. The cells were propagated in MEM supplemented with 10% FCS, Hepes buffer, 2mM L-glutamine and antibiotic solution.

Quantitative immunoperoxidase staining (modified ELISA)

For the detection of adhesion molecules on the surface of the keratinocyte lines we used a modified immunohistochemistry with specific monoclonal antibodies against ICAM-1, LFA-3, HLA-A,B,C, and HLA-DR (Immunotech). The second antibody (peroxidase-conjugated rabbit immunoglobulins to mouse IgG) was derived from DAKO GmbH, Hamburg. The cells were seeded into 96-well plates in a number of 2×10^4/well and incubated overnight at 37°C. Then several cytokines (IFNg, TNFa) or other substances (acitretin, B-carotene) at various concentrations were added for 24-48 hours. The cells were washed, incubated for 1 hr with the first antibody followed by second antibody treatment. The staining procedure was performed with the use of 3-amino-9-ethylcarbazol. The intensity of color reaction was determined in an ELISA reader at 450nm.

Northen blot analysis

The cells were grown on 10cm plates and, after cytokine pulse for 24-48 hrs, they were washed and lysed followed by ultracentrifugation. Ten micrograms of total RNA were electrophoresed under denaturing conditions, then blotted onto nitrocellulose membrane. Hybridization with ^{32}P-labeled cDNA probes was performed for 18 hrs followed by washing of the filters twice in 0.1xSSC/0.1%SDS at 50°C (ICAM-1),55^{0}C (class I, class II MHC and c-myc) or 65°C (B-actin).

RESULTS

Using quantitative immunocytochemistry (ELISA) method we found a high ICAM-1 and class I MHC expression on nontumorigenic Skv sublines as compared to the tumorigenic counterparts (Table 1, Fig.1). No significant HLA-DR and LFA-3 molecule expression was detected in both tumorigenic and nontumorigeic Skv cells. ICAM-1, MHC-class I, class II expressions were upregulated by IFNg (1-1000ng/ml), TNFa (1-100ng/ml), and retinoids: all trans retinoic acid, acitretin (both at $10^{-6}M$) and beta carotene ($5 \times 10^{-6}M$). In Fig.1 the upregulation is shown for ICAM-1 but similar results were obtained for other adhesion molecules and compounds studied (not shown).

Table 1. ICAM-1 expression in nontumorigenic and tumorigenic HPV16-harboring Skv keratinocyte sublines measured by ELISA.

Skv cell lines	ICAM-1 Protein (Absorbance x1000)	HLA-A,B,C Protein (Absorbance x1000)
Skv-e1 (nontu)	62.5 ± 9.3	52.5 ± 7.2
Skv-e2 (tu)	22.3 ± 5.5	35.8 ± 3.5
Skv-11 (nontu)	75.3 ± 10.1	66.4 ± 5.7
Skv-12 (tu)	41.5 ± 11.3	24.9 ± 6.9

The values for nontumorigenic SKv lines significantly higer (p<0.05), compared to those for tumorigenic counterparts.

Interestingly both Skv-e1 and Skv-e2 cells responded better to IFNg than Skv-11 and Skv-12 which differed in HPV16 DNA integration pattern. The upregulation of ICAM-1 expresssion by IFNg was not associated with changes in c-myc expression, however, constitutive expression of this oncogene was higher in tumorigenic cells (Fig.2). Cycloheximide blocking experiments revealed that expression of HLA-DR (but not other molecules) required a trans-acting protein (data not shown).

DISCUSSION

Differences in the constitutive expression of ICAM-1 and class I MHC molecules in various HPV-harboring tumor cells and differences in their response to immunomodulatory cytokines may be important factors determining recognition and killing of neoplastic cells by immune mechanisms. Of special interest are retinoids which, in addition to their known inhibitory effect on cell proliferation, were shown also to stimulate ICAM-1 expression in HPV16-harboring keratinocytes.

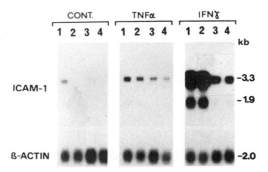

Figure 1. ICAM-1 mRNA expression in nontumorigenic (1, 3) and tumorigenic (2, 4) HPV-harboring Skv keratinocyte sublines.

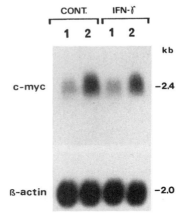

Figure 2. The expression of c-myc in nontumorigenic (1) and tumorigenic (2) Skv cells and the effect of IFNg.

ACKNOWLEDGMENTS

The study was supported by grant from Centre National de la Recherche Scientifique (Fellowship: S.Majewski), and Polish Committee for Scientific Research, KBN, no. 0507/S4/92/03.

REFERENCES

Chen, L., Mizuno, M.T., Singhal, M.C., Hu, S.L., Galloway, D. A., Hellstrom, I., and Hellestrom, K.E., 1992, Induction of cytotoxic T lymphocytes specific for a syngenic tumor expressing E6 oncoprotein of human papillomavirus type 16, *J Immunol.* 148:2617.

Malejczyk, J., Majewski, S., Jablonska, S., Rogozinski, T.T., and Orth, G., 1989, Abrogated NK-cell lysis of human papillomavirus (HPV) -16-bearing keratinocytes in patients with pre-cancerous and cancerous HPV-induced anogenital lesions, *Int J Cancer* 43:209.

Schneider-Maunoury, S., Croissant, O., and Orth, G., 1987, Integration of human papillomavirus type 16 DNA sequences: a possible early event in the progression of genital tumors, *J Virol.* 61:3295.

Springer, T.A., Adhesion receptors of the immune system, 1990, *Nature* 346:425.

MURINE CYTOTOXIC T CELL RESPONSES TO HUMAN PAPILLOMAVIRUS E7 PROTEIN

Elena Sadovnikova, Xiaojiu Zhu, Shona M.Collins, Peter Beverley, Hans J. Stauss

Imperial Cancer Research Fund
Tumour Immunology Unit
Courtauld Institute of Biochemistry
91 Riding House St, London W1P 8BT

INTRODUCTION

HPV type 16 is commonly associated with human cervical carcinomas (Crawford, 1993). It has been demonstrated that cell-mediated immunity plays an important role in human host defence against some viral infections such as herpes viruses and hepatitis B virus (Wildy and Gell, 1985). The link between cellular immunodeficiency and the high incidence of HPV-induced lesions (Kirshner, 1986; Alloub et al., 1989) suggests a possible involvement of lymphocytes in the control of HPV associated diseases. But little is known about CTL response to different virus encoded gene products (Altmann et al.,1992). The expression of virus encoded E7 gene is often observed in biopsies from malignant tissues (Smotkin and Wettstein, 1986; Seedorf et al., 1987) which makes it a good candidate for targeting an immune attack. The aim of the present study was to investigate whether E7 gets access to the MHC class I presentation pathway in H-2^b mice and is able to induce a CTL response.

Immunology of Human Papillomaviruses
Edited by M.A. Stanley, Plenum Press, New York, 1994

RESULTS AND DISCUSSION

Since permissive replication systems for HPV are not available either for human or animal cells we have used recombinant vaccinia virus to express E7 in murine cells. Vaccinia virus recombinants were successfully used for the induction of neutralising antibodies and specific cytotoxic T cell responses to a variety of antigens (Paoletti et al., 1984: Zhou et al., 1991). We used E7 containing recombinant vaccinia virus (Vac-E7) or alternatively cell lines transfected with the E7 coding sequence to immunise H-2[b] mice. Only those immunised with Vac-E7 developed an E7 specific response, which can be explained by higher level of E7 expression in vaccinia infected cells compared to transfectants. Following Vac-E7 *in vivo* immunisation, spleen cells were repeatedly boosted *in vitro* with transfected stimulators. The CTL obtained were able to recognise specifically E7 but not E6 expressing targets (Fig. 1). However even in long-term cultures the recognition of Vac-E7 infected cells never exceeded 35% of specific release in ^{51}Cr release assays, which can be attributed to a relatively inefficient presentation of E7. In order to confirm the specificity of the CTL and to further characterise CTL epitopes we have isolated peptides from Vac-E7 infected cells and separated them by reverse phase HPLC. Individual HPLC fractions were collected and tested for the presence of CTL epitopes. As shown in figure 2 only fractions 27 and 28 were efficiently recognised by anti-E7 CTL.

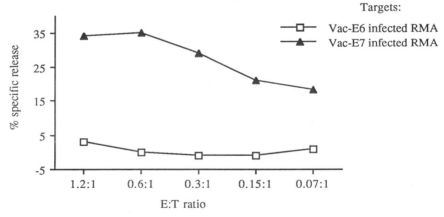

Figure 1. CTL recognition of Vac-E7 infected RMA. The T cells were induced by immunisation of H-2[b] mice with Vac-E7 and *in vitro* restimulation with E7 transfected EL4 cells (reproduced from Sadovnikova et al., Int. Immunology 6, 1994 with kind permission of Oxford University Press).

No cross reactivity was observed with peptide material isolated from Vac-E6 infected or uninfected cells which demonstrates that the CTL are highly specific. The recognition of peptides isolated from Vac-E7 infected cells was significantly more efficient than the recognition of whole cells. This was probably due to the fact that peptide material from approximately 2.5×10^7 infected cells was used to coat 5×10^3 target cells, which probably resulted in higher epitope density and more efficient effector-target interaction. Thus the use of HPLC fractionated material made it possible to increase the sensitivity of the assay system.

To map the CTL epitope we used a set of 10 and 15mer synthetic peptides overlapping by 5 amino acids and corresponding to E7 protein. Two 10 amino acid long peptides E7 46-55 and E7 51-60 and one 15mer E7 51-65 covering the same region of E7 were recognised (Fig. 3). The same set of peptides was analysed previously for binding to MHC class I molecules using RMA-S cells which have a peptide loading defect (Stauss et

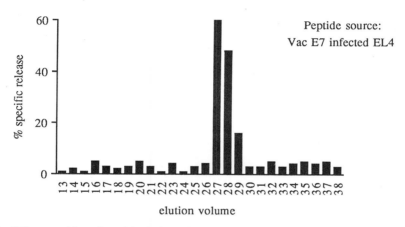

Figure 2. CTL recognition of peptides isolated from Vac-E7 infected EL4 cells. Low molecular weight peptides were isolated from 2.5×10^8 cells and separated by HPLC using a Pharmacia Pep-S column. Individual fractions were resuspended in 300 μl PBS and 30 μl were used to pulse RMA-S target cells. E7-specific effector CTL were generated as described in figure 1 (reproduced from Sadovnikova et al., Int Immunology 6, 1994 with kind permission of Oxford University Press).

al., 1992). The most efficient H-2K^b-binding peptide corresponded to amino acids 21-30 (DLYCYEQLN). E7 21-30 was the only peptide in E7 sequence which contained a strong K^b-binding motif (Falk et al., 1991) and was predicted as a potential CTL epitope. However, E7-specific CTL did not recognise the 10mer E7 21-30 peptide or 9mer and 8mer variants (Fig. 3).

The failure to function as natural CTL epitope prompted a detailed analysis of the E7 21-28 peptide. This peptide readily induced a primary CTL response in cultures of H-2^b splenocytes indicating that the relevant precursors are present in the T cell repertoire. However, T cells generated against synthetic E7 21-28 peptide did not recognise natural peptides isolated from cells expressing E7 endogenously (Fig. 4).

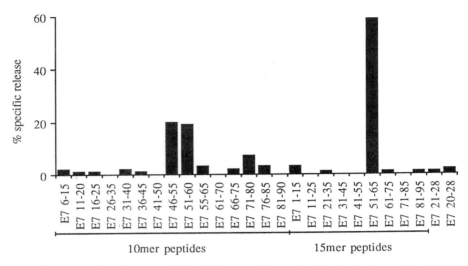

Figure 3. CTL recognition of a panel of 10 and 15mer peptides overlapping by 5 amino acids by E7 specific T cells. Included in the panel was a predicted CTL epitope corresponding to residues 21-28 (8mer and 9mer versions were tested). RMA-S cells pulsed with 100 µM of indicated synthetic peptides were used as targets (reproduced from Sadovnikova et al., Int. Immunology 6, 1994 with kind permission of Oxford University Press).

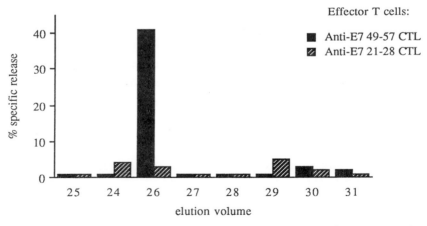

Figure 4. The specificity of CTL induced by E7 21-28 and E7 49-57 synthetic peptides. Anti-peptide E7 49-57 but not anti-peptide E7 21-28 CTL can recognise peptides isolated from Vac-E7 infected EL4 cells. Target cells were prepared as discribed in figure 2 (reproduced from Sadovnikova et al., Int. Immunology 1994 with kind permission of Oxford University Press).

Since we used an incomplete set of peptides overlapping by 5 amino acids several epitopes were missing in our binding assays, including E7 49-57 (RAHYNIVTF) which was shown to bind well to D^b molecules (Feltkamp et al., 1993). E7 49-57 peptide could not be predicted on the basis of MHC class I binding motifs. Surprisingly this peptide was recognised most efficiently by Vac-E7 specific T cells and CTL induced by synthetic E7 49-57 lysed E7 expressing targets (Fig. 4). E7 49-57 co-eluted from HPLC columns with active peptides isolated from Vac-E7 infected cells (not shown).

The data demonstrate the limitations of predictive MHC class I binding motifs. The use of binding motifs for CTL epitope prediction and synthetic peptides for mapping can be misleading. If judged by binding motifs E7 21-28 peptide would be chosen as a potential CTL epitope instead of the natural E7 49-57. Additional complications are introduced by the cross reactivity of synthetic peptides as demonstrated for three E7 derived peptides (E7 46-55, E7 51-60 and E7 51-65) which were recognised by E7 specific T cells but did not contain the complete epitope. CTL mapping with natural peptides can overcome potential problems associated with the synthetic peptide approach.

REFERENCES

Alloub, M.I., Barr, B.B.B., McClaren, K.M., Smith, I.W., Bunney, M.H., and Smart, G.E., 1989, Human papillomavirus infection and cervical intraepithelial neoplasia in women with renal allografts. *Brit. Med. J.* 298:153.

Altmann, A., Jochmus-Kudelka, I., Rainer, F., Gausepohl, H., Moebius, U., Gissmann, L., and Meuer, S.C., 1992, Definition of immunogenic determinants of the human papillomavirus type 16 nucleoprotein E7. *Eur. J. Cancer* 28:326.

Crawford, L., 1993, Prospects of cervical cancer vaccines. *Cancer Surveys* 16:215.

Falk, K., Rötzschke, O., Stevanovic, S., Jung, G., and Rammensee, H-G., 1991, Allele-specific motifs revealed by sequencing of self-peptides eluted from MHC molecules. *Nature.* 351:290.

Feltkamp, M.C.W., Smits, H.L., Vierboom, M.P.M., Minnar, R.P., de Jongh, B.M., Drijfhout, J.W., ter Schegget, J., Melief, C.J.M., and Kast, W.M., 1993, Vaccination with cytotoxic T lymphocyte epitope-containing peptide protects against a tumor induced by human papillomavirus type 16-transformed cells. *Eur.J.Immunol.* in press.

Kirshner, H., 1986, Immunobiology of human papillomavirus infection. *Prog.Med .Virol .*33:1.

Paoletti, E., Lipinskas, B.R., Samsonoff, C., Mercer, S., and Panicali, D.,1984, Construction of life vaccines using genetically engineered poxviruses: Biological activity of vaccinia virus recombinants expressing the hepatitis virus B surface antigen and the herpes simplex virus glycoprotein D. *Proc. Natl. Acad. Sci. USA* 81:193.

Sadovnikova, E., Zhu, X., Collins, S., Zhou, J., Vousden, K., Crawford, L., Chain, B., Beverley, P., and Stauss, H.J., 1993, Limitations of predictive motifs revealed by CTL epitope mapping of the human papillomavirus E7 protein. *Int. Immunol.,* submitted for publication.

Seedorf, K., Ottersdorf, T., Kramer, G., and Rowekamp, W., 1987, Identification of early proteins of human papillomavirus type 16 (HPV 16) and type 18 (HPV 18) in cervical carcinoma cells. *EMBO J.* 6:139.

Smotkin, D., and Wettstein, F.O., 1986, Transcription of human papillomavirus type 16 early genes in cervical cancer and in a carner-derived cell line and identification of the E7 protein. *Proc. Natl. Acad. Sci. USA* 83:4680.

Stauss, H.J., Davies, H., Sadovnikova, E., Chain, B., Horowitz, N., and Sinclair, C., 1992, Induction of ytotoxic T lymphocytes with peptides *in vitro* : identification of candidate T-cell epitopes in human papillomavirus. *Proc. Natl. Acad. Sci. USA* 89:7871.

Wildy, P., and Gell, P.G.H., 1985, The host response to herpes simplex virus. *Brit. Med. Bull.* 41:86.

Zhou, J., McIndoe, A., Davies, H., Sun, X-Y., and Crawford, L., 1991, The induction of cytotoxicT-lymphocyte precursor cells by recombinant vaccinia virus expressing human papillomavirus type 16 L1.*Virol.* 181:203.

IMMUNE RESPONSE TO HUMAN PAPILLOMAVIRUS TYPE 16 E6 ONCOPROTEIN

L. Gao[1], B. Chain[1], C. Sinclair[1], L. Crawford[2], J. Zhou[3], J. Morris[4], X. Xhu[5], H. Stauss[5] and P.C.L. Beverly[5]

[1] ICRF Papillomavirus Group
Department of Biology
University College London
London WC1E 6BT
UK

[2] ICRF Tumour Virus Group
Department of Pathology
University of Cambridge
Cambridge CB2 1QP

[3] Papillomavirus Research Unit
Lions Human Immunology Laboratories
University of Queensland
Woolloongabba 4102,
Australia,

[4] Ludwig Institute for Cancer Research
St. Mary's Hospital Medical School
London W2 1PG

[5] ICRF Human Tumour Immunology Group,
91 Riding House St
London W1P 8PT

INTRODUCTION

Cervical cancer presents a promising model system in which to explore the possibilities of immunologicaly based cancer therapies (Davies *et al*, 1991). The need for such novel therapeutic strategies is reinforced by the epidemiological data suggesting that the incidence of this disease is increasing in many countries, despite the introduction of extensive screening programmes. The association between this cancer and infection with human papilloma viruses identifies clearly certain target antigens which could act as tumour specific markers, and thus as potential targets for immune system recognition. Specifically, there is strong evidence that the expression of the HPV early proteins E6 and E7 is a characteristic feature of neoplastic transformation. A variety of immunisation strategies can potentially be used to generate HPV specific responses for therapy. In this project we used a murine model system to test the immunogenicity of a vaccinia construct, rVV16 E6/360 which can express HPV16 E6 protein in infected cells. These studies have demonstrated that this vector can be used to stimulate antibody, T cell cytotoxic and T cell proliferative responses in mice. Analysis of the epitope specificity of the response have demonstrated that the epitope profiles recognised by these different arms of the immune system are largely non-overlapping, and have illustrated the extreme selectivity of this response in terms of epitope profile. Such selectivity may be a limiting factor in terms of therapeutic potential, since it will provide strong selective pressures for escape mutants. The epitope studies have also provided unexpected new information on the nature of CTL epitopes, and have suggested that predictive motifs may be of limited application in the quest for novel CTL epitopes.

RESULTS

Antibody studies

DBA/2 (H-2d) mice were immunised by scarification at the base of the tail with rVV16 E6/360 (1.6×10^6 units per mice). The vector was constructed and validated according to previously published methods (Zhou et al, 1990). The development of E6 specific antibody was evaluated using sera taken 10 days after the second immunization with rVV16 E6/360 (Fig. 1A). Since sufficiently pure E6 protein was not available, the sera were tested by Western blot analysis using lysates of A20 cells (a murine B cell lymphoma) transfected with the E6 gene. Antibody binding was detected using peroxidase conjugated rabbit anti-mouse or swine anti-rabbit IgG and visualised using enhanced chemiluminescence (ECL). A band of approximately 18 Kd corresponding to the expected molecular weight of the E6 protein was detected in the transfected cells, but not the parent cells using sera from 3 animals immunized with rVV16 E6/360. None of the five animals given the control WR virus developed antibody against E6 (not shown). For comparison, Fig. 1B also shows the reactivity of a polyclonal rabbit antiserum raised against the E6 C-terminal peptide, which recognises the intact E6 protein.

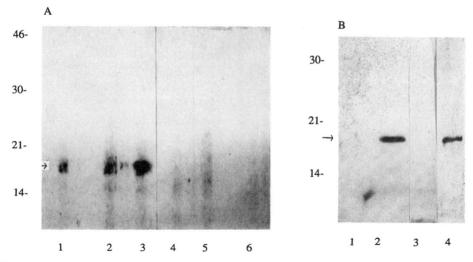

Fig.1 Antibody response to HPV16 E6 protein. Specific antibody was tested by ECL Western blotting Sera (diluted 1/100) taken from 3 mice infected with vaccinia recombinant, rVV16E6/360 recognized a 18 Kd band corresponding to HPV16 E6 in the E6 gene transfected A20 cells (panel A, lane 1-3), but not the parent cells (lane 4-6). Panel B shows the expression of HPV16 E6 protein in E6 gene transfected cells detected by ECL Western blotting using rabbit anti-E6 C terminal peptide polyclonal antibodies. E6 protein (arrowed) is expressed in E6 gene transfected EL4/E6 (lane 2) and P815/ E6 (lane 4) but not in EL4 (lane 1) and P815 (lane 3) parent lines

Cytotoxic T cell responses

In order to provide in vitro stimulators, and targets for cytotoxic cell assays, a PJ4Ω plasmid containing whole HPV16 E6 ORF, PJ4Ω16 E6 (Storey *et al.*, 1988), was introduced into EL4 and RMA cells (expressing H-2^b haplotype MHC class I molecules) by electroporation (using the Biorad Gene Pulser). The cells were cloned by limiting dilution and tested for E6 expression by ECL Western blotting.using rabbit anti-E6 and anti-E6 C'-terminal peptide antibodies.

In order to induce CTL responses, C57Bl (H-2^b) and DBA/2 mouse spleens were harvested 10 days after the animals had been primed with rVV16 E6/360 or WR vaccinia virus. Single cell suspensions at 1 X 10^5/ml were restimulated *in vitro* with 1 X 10^4/ml irradiated (5000 rads) E6 gene transfected syngeneic cells, for 8 days in *vitro* in RPMI 1640 medium containing 10% fetal calf serum and 2-mercaptoethanol (1 X 10^{-5} M). Cytolytic activity of *in vitro* secondary CTL was measured as previously described (Zhou *et al.*, 1990), using a 4-hour ^{51}Cr release assay. After one or more rounds of restimulation, the responding T cells were assayed on the same or different transfectants of the same haplotype (Fig. 2). To exclude the possibility that the lysis of transfected cells was due to their greater fragility than the nontransfected cells, a transfectant line

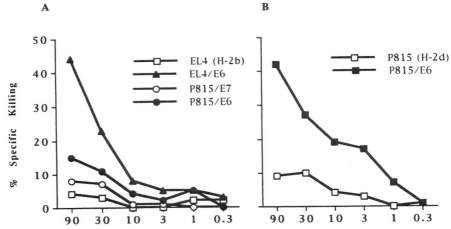

Fig.2 E6 specific cytotoxic T cell responses of spleen cells from mice immunised with rVV16 E6/360. C57 Bl (H-2^b) (panel A) and DBA/2 (H-2^d)(panel B) were inoculated with rVV16 E6/360 and tested for cytotoxic activity. The targets used were transfected or untransfected P815 (class I MHC of H-2^d haplotype) or EL4 (H-2^b haplotype). Spleen cells were restimulated in vitro with autologous transfectants for 8 days before assay of cytotoxic activity.

expressing an irrelevant protein was also used as control targets in some experiments. Fig. 2 shows that rVV16 E6/360 primed immune spleen cells elicited an E6 specific response in C57Bl mice. Similar results were obtained in DBA/2 (H-2^d) mice. Although the response was mainly haplotype specific, some weak cross-reaction on E6-expressing allo-targets was frequently observed perhaps reflecting weak NK or LAK cell reactivity in the cultures. Spleen cells from wild type WR vaccinia infected mice showed no specific killing of the HPV16 E6 transfected cells (not shown).

Epitope analysis of E6 secific antibody and cytotoxic immune responses

Candidate linear B cell epitopes were identified by testing immune sera taken from rVV16 E6/360 inoculated mice against a series of overlapping E6 peptides by ELISA. Fig.3A shows the results from a typical experiment. The pooled sera from five rVV16 E6/360 inoculated mice reacted with six peptides (O.D greater than three times the mean of the control sera from WR virus infected mice) corresponding to candidate linear B-cell epitopes (residues 86-95, 96-100, 111-120, 136-140, 141-146 and 146-150). Three of these peptides were clustered at the C-terminal end of the protein, consistent with the fact that immunisation of rabbits with a C-terminal peptide induced an antibody response recognsing the whole molecule. Sera from five mice infected with another recombinant rVV16 E6/42 (with a 42K promoter instead of 360 synthetic promoter), also recognised the same three peptides (data not shown). Sera from WR virus infected mice identified two weakly cross-reactive peptides . E6 specific CTL populations generated as described above were assayed on RMA cells incubated with individual peptides from a set of overlapping 10-mer peptides which covered the E6 sequence. As shown in Fig 3B, specific cell lysis could be elicited with only one peptide in this haplotype. Wild type WR vaccinia did not prime cells for any of the E6 peptides. The cells from the rVVE6/360 primed H-2^b mice recognised peptide 131-140 only in the context of presenting cells expressing the autologous MHC molecules molecules, and not when the same peptide was presented on cells of the H-2^d haplotype (not shown).

Proliferative responses

E6 protein for use as an *in vitro* antigen was not available in concentrations and purity adequate for in vitro proliferation assays. To study whether rVV16 E6/360 was capable of eliciting a proliferative T-cell response, the ability of a set of synthetic peptides spanning the E6 sequence to induce specific proliferation in vitro of lymph node cells from rVV16 E6/360 vaccinia recombinant primed mice was determined. Such proliferative responses have been very well documented and are known to be largely restricted to the helper T cell (Th) population. Ten days after a second inoculation with rVVE6 or WR the draining inguinal and peri-aortic lymph nodes were taken and passed through a nylon mesh to produce a single cell suspension. Viable cells were counted and resuspended at 2 X 10^6 cells/ml in RPMI 1640 medium supplemented with 1% normal mouse serum and 2-mercaptoethanol (1 X 10^{-5} M). Synthetic HPV16 E6 peptides and a control peptide (corresponding to the HPV16 E7 sequence amino acids 1-10) were diluted in PBS to give final concentrations of 0.016 to 5 μM. Peptide or concanavalin A (Con A, 10μg/ml) were added to flat-bottomed 96 well tissue culture plates containing 2 X 10^5 lymph node cells/well; controls containing medium only were also included. The cells were then incubated for four days and then pulsed with 1μCi (^{3}H)thymidine (Amersham) /well for 16 hours prior to harvesting onto glass filters using an automatic cell harvester. The amounts of thymidine incorporated into the cells were measured by liquid scintillation. Proliferative response of lymph node cells from C57BL mice immunized with rVV16 E6/360 to a series of overlapping E6 peptides are shown in Fig 3C. The results show that peptides 41-50, 91-100 and 146-151 induced specific proliferation, significantly above that of cells without peptide and of that with the same dose of irrelevant peptide, E7 1-10. The rest of the E6 peptides gave no significant proliferation above that of the medium and peptide controls. Concentrations as low as 0.016 μM of E6 peptide 41-50 gave a significant response (data not shown) suggesting this peptide contains a potent proliferative T cell epitope. Cells from mice immunized with wild type (WR) gave no significant response (not shown).

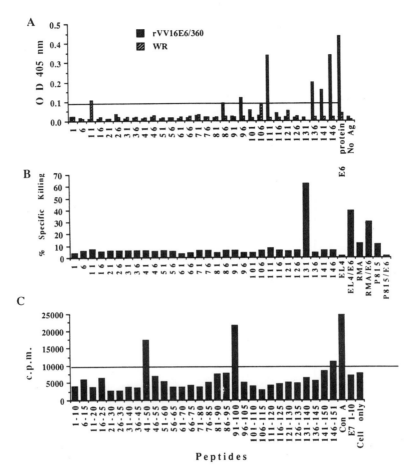

Fig. 3. Comparison of antibody, T cell cytotoxic and T cell proliferative epitopes. Panel A. Pooled sera from 5 DBA/2 mice inoculated with HPV16 E6 rVV or WR were collected. Reactivity (OD 405 nm) of the sera in ELISA with a series of synthetic decamer overlapping peptides and E6 protein expressed in transformed E coli. Peptide numbers corresponding to the HPV16 E6 sequences are indicated e.g. 1=1-10, 6=6-15, etc. The solid line is drawn at an O.D. value corresponding to three times the mean of all the sera from the WR virus infected mice. Sera giving O.D. values above this line were considered to give positive binding. Panel B. CTL epitope recognition by T cells from rVV16 E6/360 immunised C57Bl mice. ^{51}Cr labelled RMA(H-2^b) cells were pulsed with individual HPV16 E6 peptide and used as target. HPV16 E6 gene transfected P815 (H-2^d, P815/E6) and EL4 (H-2^b, EL4/E6), and the parent lines were used as controls. Panel C. Proliferative response of lymph node cells from C57Bl mice (H-2^b) to HPV16 E6 peptides (10 μM). Con A (positive) and a peptide corresponding to the E7 sequence 1-10 (negative) were used as controls. Amino acid residue numbers representing HPV16 E6 sequences are indicated. The line corresponds to the mean + twice standard error of the mean for control cultures.

DISCUSSION

The E6 protein of HPV16 is a good candidate for a target tumour antigen for immunotherapy or immunoprophylaxis of cancer of the cervix, since its distribution is highly specific and mRNA for E6 is found in a high proportion of cervical high grade neoplasias (Higgins *et al.*, 1992). Our results indicate that rVV16 E6/360 immunise mice to produce an antibody, proliferative and cytotoxic response specific for E6. In agreement with our findings, studies in rats have shown that immunisation with E6 vaccinia recombinants can indeed partially protect against tumour challenge (Meneguzzi *et al.*, 1991). In contrast to humoural response, T cells are likely to be the dominant effector cell in effective responses to E6. However, it is still unclear whether optimum protection can be provided by CD8[+] class I restricted cytotoxic T cells, or CD4[+] class II restricted "inflammatory" T cells. There is some evidence in animal models that E6 or E7 expressing tumours can be controlled by cytotoxic T cell responses Chen *et al.*, 1991; Chen *et al.*, 1992). However, inflammatory T cells clearly play an important role in regression of non-malignant HPV warts (Benton *et al.*, 1992).

The detailed analysis of the epitopes recognised within E6 by the three compartments of the immune response revealed a number of interesting features. As described previously in a number of other systems, the repertoire of the response is restriced to a very few epitopes. Interestingly, there was no overlap in the repertoire recognised by antibody, proliferative T cells and cytotoxic T cells. Thus, it should be possible to probe the relative importance of each type of response, and the interaction between the diverse cell types involved, by independently stimulating antibody, proliferative T cells (which are likely to represent the CD4[+] helper cell population) or cytotoxic T cells.

The factors which operate to govern the repertoire of the immune response have not been clearly defined. Because of the likely importance of cytotoxic responses in tumour lysis, we have previously analysed in detail the MHC class I (H-2[b]) binding ability of all the E6 peptides, and the ability of these peptides, on their own, to stimulate a cytotoxic T cell response (Stauss *et al.*, 1992). Unexpectedly, there appears to be no correlation between our ability to measure binding of the peptides to bind H-2K and H-2D molecules in vitro, and to act as epitopes in rVVE6 primed mice. The reasons why the peptide binding assay used in our previous study did not detect the binding of these peptides to class I MHC are not yet clear. In addition, we were unable to identify any of the previously described allele specific motifs (Falk *et al.*, 1991) in the epitope (RWTGRCMSCC) identified inw H-2[b] haplotype.

Our results have a number of important implications in terms of the design of vaccines for HPV16. Firstly, we believe that our results demonstrate that it is unwise to rely solely on either theoretical predictions (based on motifs) or even class I binding assays in identifying potential peptide epitopes for vaccine design. Secondly, our results confirm that the T cell immune response to a protein is limited to a very few epitopes, dictated by the HLA haplotype of the host. This phenomenon imposes severe restraints on the use of synthetic peptides as immunogens in outbred human populations. It raises the possibility that several haplotypes may exist with no E6 epitopes at all, although the expression of six class I MHC molecules in human (outbred) populations make it less likely that an individual would be unable to mount any response to E6. Finally, the restricted nature of the response, particularly to a small protein such as E6, compounds the difficulties due to sequence variability among HPV types, since mutations at single loci may be sufficient to convert an immunogenic protein to a non-immunogenic variant.

REFERENCES

Benton, C., Shahi-Dullah, H. & Hunter, J. A. A. 1992, HPV in the immunosuppressed. In *Papilloma virus report* 3, 23-26 Leeds: Leeds University Press.

Chen, L., Thomas, E. K., Hu, S-L. & Hellstrom, I. 1991, Human papillomavirus type 16 nucleoprotein E7 is a tumour rejection antigen. *Proceedings of the National Academy of Sciences, USA* **88**,110-114.

Chen, L, Miruno, M. T., Singhal, M. C., Hu, S-L., Galloway, D A., Hellstrom, i. & Hellstrom, K. E. 1992, Induction of Cytotoxic T lymphocytesspecific for syngeneic tumor expressing the E6 oncoprotein of human papillomavirus.

Davies, D. H., Mcindoe, G. A. J. & Chain, B. M. 1991, Current status review: Cancer of the cervix: prospects for immunological control. International Journal of Experimental Pathology. **72**, 2691-2698.

Falk, K., Rotzschke, O., Stevannovic, S., Jung, G. & Rammensee, H. G. 1991, Allele-specific motifs revealed by sequencing of self-peptides eluted from MHC molecules. *Nature* **351**, 290-296.

Higgins, G. D., Uzelin, D. M., Phillips, G.E., Marin, R. & Burrell, C. J. 1992, Transcription patterns of human papillomavirus type 16 in genital intraepithelial neoplasia: evidence for promoter usage within the E7 open reading frame during epithelial differentiation. *Journal of General Virology* 73, 2047-57.

Meneguzzi, G., Cerni, C., Kieny, M. P. & Lathe, R. 1991, Immunization against human papillomavirus type 16 tumor cells with recombinant vaccinia viruses expressing E6 and E7. *Virology* **181**, 61-69.

Stauss, H. J., Davies, H., Sadovnikova, E., Chain, B., Horowitz, N. & Sinclair, C. 1992,. Induction of cytotoxic T lymphocytes with peptides *in vitro*: Identification of candidate T-cell epitopes in human papillomavirus. *Proceedings of the National Academy of Sciences, USA* . **89**, 7871-7875.

Storey, A., Pim, D., Murray, A., Osborn, K., Banks L. & Crawford, L. 1988, Comparison of the in vitro transforming activities of human papillomavirus types. *EMBOJournal.* 7,1815-1820.

Zhou, J., Crawford, L., Mclean, L., Sun X. Y., Stanley M., Almond, N. & Smith, G. L. 1990, Increased antibody responses to human papillomavirus type 16 L1 protein expressed by recombinant vaccinia virus lacking serine protease inhibitor genes. *Journal of General Virology.* **71**, 2185-2190.

HUMAN CYTOTOXIC T CELL EPITOPES IN HPV 11: RELATIONSHIPS BETWEEN ALLELE-SPECIFIC MOTIFS, HLA BINDING, AND STIMULATION IN VITRO

Huw Davies,[1] Ian Tarpey,[1] Simon Stacey,[2] Julian Hickling,[3] Jennifer Bartholomew,[2] Humphrey Birley,[4] Adrian Renton,[5] and Angus McIndoe [6]

[1] Division of Life Sciences
King's College
London W8 7AH
[2] CRC Paterson Institute for Cancer Research,
Christie Hospital NHS Trust
Manchester M20 9BX
[3] ICRF, Human Tumour Immunology Group
University College and Middlesex School of Medicine,
London W1P 8BT
Departments of [4] Genitourinary Medicine, [5] Public Health [6] Obstetrics
and Gynaecology
St. Mary's Hospital
London, W2 1PG.

INTRODUCTION

The identification of cytotoxic T lymphocyte (CTL) epitopes in HPV may offer a route to peptide vaccine design. However, the screening of suitable peptides from a virus usually requires CTL that have been elicited during natural infection. The difficulty in obtaining viable HPV (used to infect stimulator cells for in vitro propagation of naturally-occurring CTL) has complicated the issue. One approach to overcome this is to prime CTL in vitro with HPV antigen processed endogenously and presented by dendritic cells (I. Tarpey, S. Stacey, J. Hickling, H. Birley, A. Renton, A. McIndoe and H. Davies; Immunol, in press). This allows the peptides of endogenous processing to be presented to T cells which may mimic the events that occur in vivo. There are other approaches to locating epitopes that are independent of pre-existing CTL. These include screening of candidate peptides for binding to HLA molecules, or to predict epitopes on the basis of possession HLA allele-specific motifs.

In this context we describe the testing of 6 peptides from HPV 11 E6 and E7, which contain published HLA A2 (A*0201) or A3 (A*0301) motifs, for their ability to stimulate CTL in vitro. The A2-motif peptides have also been tested for stabilization of the A2 molecule on .174/T2 cells. We found that both of the A2 motif-containing peptides elicited CTL, whereas only one out of four A3 motif-containing peptides stimulated CTL in vitro. Using vaccinia viruses containing HPV 11 E6 and E7 we show that of these three peptide-specific CTL lines, one (to peptide HPV 11 E7 4-12, which contains an A2 motif) killed targets expressing endogenously-processed E7. This peptide, however, showed negligible binding to the A2 molecule in the T2-binding assay.

MATERIALS AND METHODS

The details of construction of vaccinia virus recombinants will be published elsewhere (Tarpey et al, Immunol, in press). Two viruses were made containing HPV 11 E6 and E7 ORFs (designated vC614 and vC714, respectively).

Peptides were chosen on the basis of allele-specific motifs and synthesized using F-moc chemistry There are 6 peptides in the putative sequences of HPV 11 E6 and E7 that contain the A2 and A3 motifs as described [1,2]. The A2 motif peptides are E7 4-12 (RLVTLKDIV), and E7 82-90 (LLLGTLNIV). The A3 motif peptides are E6 69-77 (ELQGKINQY), E6 97-105 (ILKVLIRCY), E6 110-118 (PLCEIEKLK), and E6 120-128 (ILGKARFIK). In addition, three A2 motif peptides from HPV 6b E7 were made: E7 21-30 (GLHCYEQLV), E7 47-55 (PLKQHFQIV) and E7 82-90 (same as HPV 11).

A2 motif peptides were tested for binding to the A2 molecule using the mutant .174/T2 line [3] by incubation overnight in different concentrations of peptide (100μM to 6.25μM) in the presence of b2-microglobulin. Stabilization of A2 was determined by flow cytometry using the BB7.2 antibody.

Peptide stimulation of CTL was performed according to a method based on that reported elsewhere [4]. Briefly, PBMC were obtained from healthy HLA A2 or A3 laboratory donors and cultured overnight on plastic (T75 flasks). Non-adherent cells were further separated on analytical grade metrizamide (Sigma; grade 1) gradients prepared by adding 14.5g to 100ml RPMI with 10% FCS. Low density cells were incubated in 100μM peptide for 1h prior to returning to the pellet of cells (mostly lymphocytes) at a ratio of around 10:1 lymphocytes per low density cell. This procedure is able to prime CTL in vitro [4]. Cells were cultured for 6 days in 24 well plates in IMDM with 10% autologous serum prior to chromium release assay for cytotoxicity using B-lymphoblastoid cell lines (B-LCL), either matched at A2 or A3 as appropriate, or completely mismatched. B-LCL line KM was supplied by Dr. J. Stewart (CRC Paterson Institute, Manchester).

RESULTS AND DISCUSSION

Figure 1 shows the results of a T2 binding assay of three of the four A2 motif-containing peptides. Peptide 21-30 binds at levels comparable with the positive control peptide from the influenza virus matrix protein [5]. Peptide HPV 11 E7 4-12 exhibits only minimal binding, whereas peptide 47-55 is negative in this assay. Peptide HPV 11 E7 82-90 has not been tested to date; however, the homolog from HPV 16 (LLMGTLGIV), which has two substitutions in non-anchor residues, binds well to A2 on T2 cells (Hickling, unpublished observations).

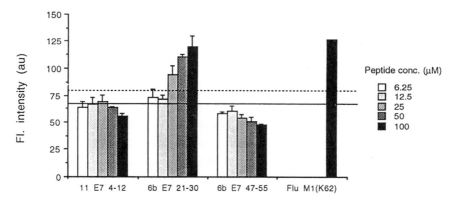

Figure 1. Typical peptide binding assay using .174/T2 cells. The solid line represents the mean fluoresence intensity (in arbitrary units) of control cells incubated for 18h in the absence of peptide. The dotted line represents the control mean plus 3 x SD. Peptide Flu M1 (K62) is the A2 restricted epitope from influenza matrix protein 57-68 (KGILGFVFTLTV; Ref. 5) with a F to K substitution at position 62.

These peptides have not been screened for their ability to bind to A2 molecules using the T2 lysate assay [2] thus it is possible that peptides that appear negative here may be revealed as binding to A2 using different or more sensitive assays.

In parallel with the binding assays, all of the peptides were tested for their ability to stimulate CTL in vitro. Figure 2 shows the results obtained from two different HLA A3 donors stimulated in vitro with autologous low density cells pulsed with the HLA A3 motif-containing peptide 11 E7 69-77. Neither donor responded to any of the other three A3 motif peptides. Although peptide 11 E6 69-77 elicited CTL from both donors, neither of these CTL lines recognized targets expressing endogenously processed HPV 11 E6.

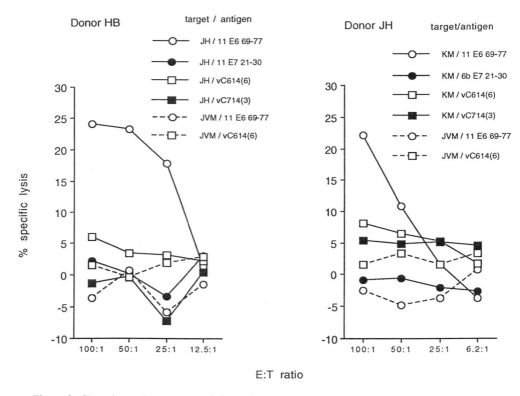

Figure 2. Chromium release assays of CTL stimulated for 6 days with peptide HPV 11 E6 69-77 (containing an A3 motif). PBMC from two different A3 donors (HB and JH) were used. Targets were B-lymphoblastoid cell lines selected to share only HLA A3 (JH for donor HB, KM for donor JH) or to be mismatched (JVM for both) and pulsed with peptide or infected with vaccinia viruses as shown.

Of the four A2 motif-containing peptides, all elicited CTL to varying degrees (Tarpey et al, in press). The hierarchy was 6b E7 21-30 > 6b E7 47-55 > 11 E7 4-12 > 6b/11 E7 82-90. All responses seen were peptide-specific and A2-restricted. In addition to the 11 E6 69-77 specific CTL shown in Figure 2, two of the A2 motif containing peptides (11 E7 4-12 and 11 E7 82-90) were also tested for recognition of endogenously processed protein. The results from these three assays are summarized in Figure 3. Only the percent specific lysis at an E:T ratio of 100:1 is depicted, although the lysis titrated down with lower ratios.

It can be seen from Figure 3 that only peptide 11 E7 4-12 elicits CTL that recognize endogenously processed protein. In reciprocal experiments (not shown) CTL elicited to endogenously processed 11 E7 recognized peptide 4-12 (Tarpey et al; in press). These data suggests that the region 4-12 is the product of natural processing. Suitable vaccinia virus recombinants for testing CTL stimulated to the peptides from HPV 6b E7 are currently being made, thus it is unknown whether these mimic the products of endogenous processing.

It was not our intention to formally test the predictive value of motifs or HLA binding data for locating dominant epitopes since this would require a more thorough set of peptides. Rather, it was our intention to use peptides to establish conditions for CTL priming in vitro. However, on the small number of peptides analyzed, a few observations can be made. Possession of a published A2 motif[1] correlated well with ability to stimulate CTL in vitro, whereas possession of the published A3 motif[2] correlated less well. Results of A2 stabilization on T2 cells did not correlate well with possession of an A2 motif or with the

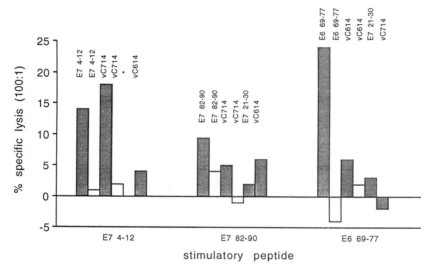

Figure 3. Summary of assays of peptide specific CTL where appropriate vaccinia recombinants were available to determine whether the CTL recognize endogenously processed protein. CTL to peptides 11 E7 4-12 and 11 E7 82-90 (both containing A2 motifs) were obtained from the same A2 donor. A2 matched targets (JVM; solid bars) and mismatched (KM; white bars) were used. CTL from peptide 11 E6 69-77 were obtained from an A3 donor. A3-matched targets (JH, solid bars) and mismatched (JVM; white bars) were used. Lysis at an E:T ratio of 100:1 is shown. * = irrelevant peptide not done.

capacity to induce CTL in vitro; the only peptide to elicit CTL that recognized endogenously processed protein had a poor capacity to stabilize A2 on T2 cells. Nevertheless, the A2 motif has allowed us to locate an epitope that is apparently the product of endogenous processing.

ACKNOWLEDGEMENTS

This work was supported by the CANCER RESEARCH CAMPAIGN.

REFERENCES

1. K. Falk, O. Rötzschke, S. Stevanovic´, G. Jung, and H-G. Rammensee. Allele-specific motifs revealed by sequencing of self-peptides eluted from MHC molecules. *Nature*. 351:290 (1991).

2. M. DiBrino, Parker, K. C., Shiloach, J., Knierman, M., Lukszo, J., Turner, R. V., Biddison, W. E. and Coligan, J. E. Endogenous peptides bound to HLA-A3 possess a specific combination of anchor residues that permit identification of potential antigenic epitopes. *Proc Natl Acad Sci USA*. 90, 1508-12 (1993).

3. V. Cerundolo, J. Alexander, K. Anderson, C. Lamb, P. Cresswell, A. McMichael, F. Gotch, and A. Townsend. Presentation of viral antigen controlled by a gene in the major histocompatibility complex. *Nature*. 345:449 (1990).

4. S. E Macatonia, S. Paterson, and S. C. Knight. Primary proliferative and cytotoxic T cell responses to HIV induced in vitro by human dendritic cells. *Immunol*. 74:399 (1991).

5. F. Gotch, A. McMichael, and J. Rothbard Recognition of influenza A matrix protein by HLA A2-restricted cytotoxic T lymphocytes. Use of analogues to orientate the matrix peptide in the HLA A2 binding site. *J Exp Med*. 168:2045 (1988).

AN IMMUNODOMINANT REGION IN HPV16.L1 IDENTIFIED BY T CELL RESPONSES IN PATIENTS WITH CERVICAL DYSPLASIAS

Philip S. Shepherd, Andrea J. Rowe, Jeremy C. Cridland,
Michael G. Chapman,* Jenny C. Luxton and Lee S. Rayfield

Depts of Immunology and *Obstetrics and Gynaecology
Guy's Hospital Medical School
UMDS
London Bridge, SE1 9RT
UK

INTRODUCTION

Human papillomaviruses are truly epitheliotropic and give rise to skin and mucosal lesions. How the host controls and eliminates HPV infections at these surfaces remains largely unknown. In the genital tract HPV has been shown to cause genital warts, cervical dysplasias and carcinomas of the cervix. Most cases of genital warts and early lesions of cervical dysplasias will spontaneously regress if left untreated suggesting that the host mounts a protective response against the virus. High grade dysplasias and tumours appear not to be controlled despite the fact that high risk HPV types (16,18,31, 33 etc.) are found in both situations. The role of immune mechanisms in HPV infections can now be examined where previously it was impossible through the development of new assay techniques. This has come about following the availability of good antigen sources, namely HPV capsids for B cell (serology) studies and recombinant HPV proteins and synthetic peptides for T cell work. Our present study looks for proliferative T cell responses to HPV16.L1 in patients with cervical dysplasias by generating short term T cell lines from their peripheral blood *in vitro* and using these to map immunodominant T cell epitopes on the molecule with overlapping synthetic peptides.

Immunology of Human Papillomaviruses
Edited by M.A. Stanley, Plenum Press, New York, 1994

REAGENTS

Tissue culture medium

The standard medium used was RPMI 1640 with L-glutamine (041-01875M; Life Technologies Ltd, Paisley, Scotland), supplemented with : 1mM sodium pyruvate (16-820-49; Flow Laboratories, Irvine, Scotland), 2mM L-glutamine (043-05030H; Life Technologies, Paisley, Scotland), 10mM HEPES (44285; BDH, Poole, UK), 100u/ml of penicillin, 25mg/ml of gentamycin (16-762-45; Flow Laboratories, Irvine, Scotland), 50mM 2-mercaptoethanol (M-6250; Sigma, Poole, UK), and 0.25mg/ml Fungizone (16-723-46; Flow Laboratories, Irvine, Scotland). This medium was supplemented with autologous human sera.

HPV Antigens

The β-galactosidase HPV16.L1 fusion protein (β gal-HPV16.L1) was constructed from a 637 bp fragment of DNA (Bam HI and Pst I) from the L1 gene of HPV16 cloned into the pEX1, -2 and -3 vectors (Stanley & Luzio, 1984) and used to transform *E.coli* strain pop. 2316. The resulting fusion protein (Mr of 141 K) was induced by raising the temperature of the bacterial cultures from 28°C to 42°C for 90 min. Isolation of the protein from pelleted bacteria was performed according to the method of Doorbar *et al* (1986). Removal of sodium dodecyl sulphate (SDS) from the final protein preparation was achieved by extensive dialysis against several changes of phosphate buffered saline (PBS, 137mM NaCl 10mM Na_2HPO_4, 18mM KH_2PO_4 and 27mM KCl) and then passing it through a 2ml Extracti-Gel column (Pierce, UK).

Synthetic peptides

A set of overlapping peptides (15 mers overlapping by 5 amino acids) representing the HPV16.L1 fragment between amino acids 199-409 were kindly supplied by Dr H Davies (King's College, London, UK) as shown in Figure 1. In preliminary experiments the peptides were pooled (8 tri-pools and 1 di-pool) and used in the three day specificity assays to define responses to regions of HPV16.L1. Later studies used individual peptides to map more accurately the T cell epitopes recognised.

Patient selection and HPV typing

Ethical Committee approval was obtained to collect peripheral blood samples from patients referred to the colposcopy clinic at Guy's Trust Hospital for investigation of abnormal cervical smears. Clinical diagnoses were made on histological evidence from cervical biopsy material taken at the same visit. A normal control group of women were selected on the basis of no previous history of genital warts or abnormal cervical smears. HPV typing was performed by Dr J. M. Walboomers (Department of Pathology, Free University Hospital, 1081 HV Amsterdam, The Netherlands), on DNA extracted from tissue sections cut from the same paraffin embedded blocks and amplified by polymerase chain reaction using HPV L1 consensus primers and type specific primers (van den Brule, et al. 1992).

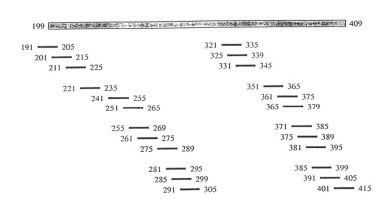

Figure 1. Overlapping peptides representing the HPV16.L1 fragment between amino acids 199-409

Preparation of patient's cell samples

50ml of venous blood was taken from each patient and defibrinated by rotating it in a sterile centrifuge tube containing glass beads for 5 min at room temperature. The serum was collected after centrifugation (780g x 5min) and the cells diluted to 100mls with Hanks balanced salt solution (042-04060H; Life Technologies Ltd, Paisley, Scotland) and then 25mls aliquots layered onto 15mls Lymphoprep (Nycomed, Oslo, Norway) and spun at 942g for 30 min at 23°C. The cells at the interface were collected and washed once by adding an equal volume of Hanks BSS and spinning them at 350g for 10 min. Each patient's cells were resuspended in autologous serum containing 10% (v/v) Dimethylsulphoxide (10323; BDA, Poole, Dorset) and stored as three 1.5ml aliquots in liquid nitrogen until required.

Short term lines

These were set up using one of the three vials of stored patient cells. The cells were rapidly thawed in a 37°C waterbath, diluted to 25ml in culture medium and spun at 350g for 10 min at room temperature. The pelleted cells were then resuspended in 2mls culture medium containing 10% human serum and counted and the cell numbers adjusted to $2x10^6$/ml. The fusion protein of HPV16.L1 (aa 199-409) was diluted in culture medium containing 10% human serum and 100µl (10µg/ml) was dispensed into 30 wells of a 96 well round bottomed microtitre plate (Greiner). 100µl of cell suspension (2×10^5 cells) was added to each well and the plates incubated at 37°C in a humidified 5% CO_2 atmosphere for 14 days. The cell cultures were fed on days 3 and 7 by removing 100µl of supernatant and replacing it with medium containing 5% human serum and recombinant IL2 (25 units/ml, Sandoz) and r IL4 (2 units/ml, Glaxo), and on day 11 with medium containing 5% serum only.

Specificity assays on short term lines

Antigen specificity assays were performed on day 14. Each of the 20 short term lines was tested against β gal-HPV16.L1 fusion protein (1µg/ml); β-galactosidase (G-6008, Sigma, UK) 10µg/ml; HPV16.L1 synthetic peptides and culture medium. Peptides were combined into 9 pools comprising three individual peptides (15 mers) per pool (except for peptide pool 305-329 which was a di-pool) and spanned amino acid residues 191-415 of the HPV16.L1 protein. Peptides within pools were used at 10µM in all assays. Cell counts were performed on 5 pooled cell lines and the mean counts used to estimate the numbers of cells per line ($\pm 2x10^5$ cells). Each cell line was set up in duplicate in 96 well round bottomed microtitre plates against the 11 antigens listed above and one medium control in the presence of autologous antigen presenting cells (APC). The later were from two vials of the patient's cells stored in liquid nitrogen, thawed, washed and irradiated (4000 Rads) within 2 hours of thawing. APC numbers varied between patients ($\pm 2.5x10^7$ cells) and were used in the assays at $2.5x10^5$/ml.

The peptide pools (see Figure 1) were dispensed (100µl/well) together with irradiated APCs ($2.5x10^5$/ml) and line cells (10^5/ml) in 100µl of medium. The plates were incubated for three days at 37°C in 5% CO_2 before adding of [Methyl-^{3}H] thymidine (TRA 120, Amersham; 9.25KBq/well) and incubating for a further 4h. Incorporation of labelled thymidine was measured by counting the harvested wells in a liquid scintillation β-spectrometer (LKB). The data was plotted as dpm for all the antigens and medium controls for each cell line and a positive response was taken as a stimulation index (SI) of > 2.5 that of the medium control for each line and having a Δ dpm of > 500 (see Figure 2).

RESULTS

Response of short term T cell lines to HPV16 fusion protein and synthetic peptides

Peripheral blood mononuclear cells were thawed from the frozen state and cultured with β gal-HPV16.L1 (amino acids 199-409) fusion protein at a concentration of 1-2x10⁵ cells/well. After two weeks, cells from 5 replicate cultures were pooled and counted to establish cell yields and the mean count was usually comparable to the number set up per line and these were used for the specificity assays. The contents of each well were split to provide duplicate cultures assayed against β gal-HPV16.L1 and 9 separate pools of synthetic peptides in the presence of freshly prepared and irradiated autologous mononuclear cells. The composition of the peptide pools and their relationship to the β gal-HPV16.L1 antigen is shown in Figure 1. In addition, controls of medium alone and β-galactosidase were included with each cell line. For each patient 20 separate lines were tested in a single experiment. An example of the responses given by two cell lines from two patients (12T and 7M) are shown in Figure 2. The four lines responded (S.I. > 2.5, Δ dpm > 500) to the β gal-HPV16.L1 used to select and expand them. Patient 12T responded to peptide pool 305 (peptides 305-319 and 315-329) in both lines and to pool 191 (peptides 191-205, 201-215 and 211-225) in line 1 and to pool 385 in line 2. Of the remaining 18 lines from this patient, 11 responded to pool 305 but none reacted against pool 191. In addition, one of these 11 lines proliferated to pool 385 and another recognised pool 255 (peptides 255-269, 261-275 and 275-289) and pool 281 (peptides 281-295, 285-299 and 291-305). To reduce the possibility of uncovering random proliferative

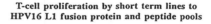

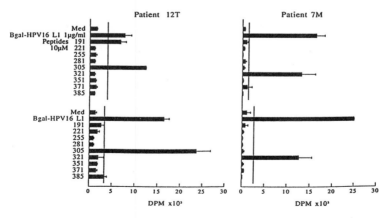

Figure 2. ——— = Stimulation index (SI) of 2.5 times medium control value. Peptide pools are denoted by the first amino acid residue of each pool (see Figure 1).

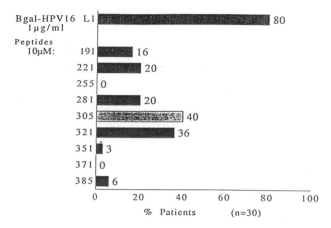

Percentage of patients responding to Bgal-HPV16 L1 antigen and peptide pools

Bgal-HPV16 L1 1 µg/ml — 80

Peptides 10µM:
191 — 16
221 — 20
255 — 0
281 — 20
305 — 40
321 — 36
351 — 3
371 — 0
385 — 6

% Patients (n=30)

Figure 3. Peptide pools are denoted by the first amino acid residue of each pool (see Figure 1).

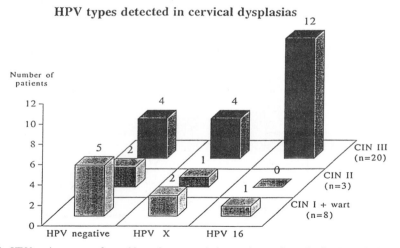

HPV types detected in cervical dysplasias

Number of patients

CIN III (n=20)
CIN II (n=3)
CIN I + wart (n=8)

HPV negative   HPV X   HPV 16

Figure 4. HPV typing was performed by polymerase chain reaction on formalin fixed cervical biopsies from patients.

CIN = cervical intraepithelial neoplasia.

HPV X = Samples positive using general purpose primers for HPV but not identified by type specific primers to HPVs 6,11,16, 18.

238

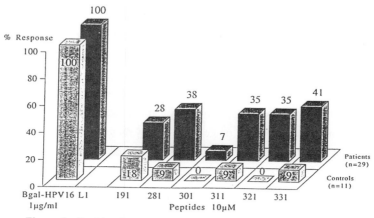

Proliferative T-cell responses to Bgal-HPV16 L1 antigen and peptides in patients and controls

Figure 5. Peptides denoted by first amino acid residue (see Figure 1).

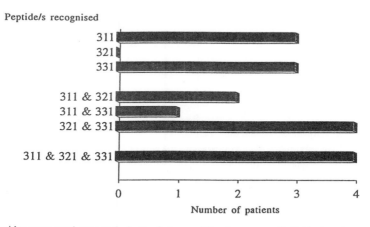

Number of patients responding to individual peptides spanning HPV16 L1 aa311-345

Figure 6. Peptides were used separately in the 3 day proliferation assays. Individual patient responses to them have been grouped as shown. Peptides denoted by first amino acid residue (see Figure 1).

responses to any of the peptide pools, we required that at least two of the 20 cell lines should recognise a pool of peptides and β gal-HPV16.L1. Applying these criteria to this patient only pools 305 and 385 gave specific responses.

A summary of the patients responses to the fusion protein and peptide pools is shown in Figure 3. Eighty percent (n=30) of the patients with all grades of cervical dysplasias responded to the fusion protein which could have been directed to either the HPV16.L1 molecule or the much larger β-galactosidase fusion partner, or both. The responses to the peptides revealed only the HPV16.L1 component of this response. It can be seen that 40% of the patients recognised pool 305-329 and the stimulation indices (SI) ranged from 2.5-17.9 (data not shown). A second pool, 321 (peptides 321-335, 325-339 and 331-345) was recognised by 36% of the patients. Other peptide pools (191-225, 221-265, 281-305 and 385-415) were recognised by patients but at lower levels ($\leq$20%).

HPV typing was performed on cervical biopsy material (n=31) and showed a 60% detection level of HPV16 in high grade cervical dysplasias (figure 4) of which two thirds gave proliferative T-cell responses to one or more peptide pools (data not shown).

In analysing the data it was evident that 76% of patients responded to the region 311-345 showing this to be a highly immunogenic part of the molecule. It was therefore decided to map this region using single peptides (15 mers overlapping by 5amino acids) instead of peptide pools. This part of the study was performed on a further 29 patients and 11 control subjects. The findings confirmed the original observations on pooled peptides (figure 5) with an overall response of 59% (18% in controls) to region 311-345 (35% to 311-325; 35% to 321-335 and 41% to 331-345), 38% and 28% to peptides 281-295 and 191-205 respectively. Individual responses to the three peptides within the 311-345 region where variable (figure 6). Some patients reacted to a single peptide (21%) while others responded to two of the three (24%) or all three (14%) peptides suggesting that overlapping T cell epitopes exist within this immunodominant region.

DISCUSSION

Patients with dysplasias and to a lesser extent disease free controls have the capability to mount proliferative T cell responses to HPV16.L1 (aa 199-409). These have been demonstrated by the generation of short term T-cell lines derived from their peripheral blood after two weeks amplification in the presence of an HPV16.L1 fusion protein followed by 3 day specificity assays using synthetic peptides of HPV16.L1. All the patients had active disease, as shown by histology on their cervical biopsies, at a mucosal site and in the majority of cases could demonstrate a T cell response to HPV16.L1 in their peripheral blood. It is clear from this study that secondary immune responses to HPV antigens are detectable in the systemic immune system following mucosal sensitisation. Whether these T cell responses provide adequate protection against HPV in individuals with different grades of cervical dysplasias is not known and awaits longitudinal studies on patients and should also include measurements of specific cytotoxic responses as well as serology to complete the picture. We have been unable to show that proliferation T cell responses to a particular region of HPV16.L1 can be positively linked to histological grading or disease activity (data not shown). What has been shown by epitope mapping is that there are immunodominant regions (aa 191-225, aa 281-295 and aa 311-345) on HPV16.L1 (aa 199-409) and the most readily detectable one is in the region 311-345. Within this region individual responses to it are highly variable which suggests that different modes of antigen processing and presentation via MHC class II occurs with individuals of different HLA type. Also, the T cell repertoire of an individual will further influence how this region is seen immunologically. Interestingly the 321-335 peptide was never seen on its own but was seen in association with the other two peptides. Taken together these findings would indicate that to induce an effective T helper response to HPV16.L1 aa311-345 in man it would require the whole region to be presented. Short peptides ($\pm$ 15 mers) or combinations of peptides are poor immunogens on their own and normally require a carrier molecule to make them more immunogenic. To circumvent the problems of using peptides as immunogens an alternative approach would be to use different types of HPV capsids containing L1 only to protect against genital warts and perhaps more importantly in the longer term the development of cervical dysplasias associated with high risk HPV types.

ACKNOWLEDGEMENTS

Imperial Cancer Reasearch Fund for the synthesis of the synthetic peptides to HPV16.L1; Guy's Special Trustees and UMDS for funding the project.

REFERENCES

Doorbar, J., Campbell, D., Grand, R. J. and Gallimore, P. H., 1986, Identification of the human papillomavirus 1a E4 gene products, *EMBO J.* 5: 355.

Stanley, K. K. and Luzio, J. P., 1984, Construction of a new family of high efficiency bacterial expression vectors: identification of cDNA clones coding for human liver proteins, *EMBO J.* 3: 1429.

van den Brule, A. J., Snijders, P. J., Raaphorst, P. M., Schrijnemakers, H. F., Delius, H., Gissmann, L., Meijer, C. J. and Walboomers, J.M., 1992, General primer polymerase chain reaction in combination with sequence analysis for identification of potentially novel human papillomavirus genotypes in cervical lesions, *J Clin Microbiol.* 30: 1716.

IMMUNOLOGICAL ASPECTS OF CERVICAL CARCINOMA

Carina G.J.M. Hilders, Jaap D.H. van Eendenburg, Yvonne Nooyen,
Gert Jan Fleuren

Department of Pathology
University of Leiden
P.O. Box 9603
2300 RC Leiden
The Netherlands

INTRODUCTION

The importance of Major Histocompatibility Complex antigens for the control of tumor growth by the host immune system has long been recognized. Especially in Human Papillomavirus related cervical carcinoma, in which the cellular immune system plays an important role[1-3], the efficacy of this immune response is strongly dependent on the presentation of tumor associated antigens by the HLA molecules. In this study we have investigated the relationship between expression of HLA class I and II molecules and immune cells in human cervical carcinomas with the objective to define aspects of immune responsiveness which might affect tumor progression.

MATERIAL AND METHODS

Tissue samples and preparation

Samples of normal cervical tissue (n=10), cervical intraepithelial neoplasia (n=25) and squamous cell carcinomas of the cervix (n=30) were kindly supplied by the Departments of Pathology and Gynecology of Leiden University Hospital and the

Immunology of Human Papillomaviruses
Edited by M.A. Stanley, Plenum Press, New York, 1994

Departments of Pathology and Gynecology of Leyenburg Hospital (The Hague). All the samples were obtained prior to treatment. The tissue was snap-frozen in liquid isopentane and stored at -70°C until sectioned for study.

Histopathological examination

The diagnosis of each lesion was made by using conventional histologic sections prepared from paraffin embedded tissue, stained with hematoxylin and eosin. Premalignant lesions of the cervix were classified as cervical intraepithelial neoplasia (CIN) grade 1,2 and 3. The twenty-five premalignant lesions composed of 11 CIN1, 5 CIN2 and 9 CIN3. The squamous cell carcinomas of the uterine cervix were classified as well-differentiated (grade 1), moderately differentiated (grade 2), and poorly differentiated (grade 3). The thirty squamous cell carcinomas were divided into 5 (17%) poorly -, 17 (57%) moderately -, and 8 (26%) well differentiated -, tumors.

Monoclonal antibodies

A panel of polyclonal antisera and monoclonal antibodies were used to identify different infiltrating immune cells, such as lymphocytes, NK-cells and macrophages and monomorphic as well as allele-specific HLA class I and II expression[4].

Immunohistochemistry

A three-step indirect immunoperoxidase technique was performed as described elsewhere[4].

Assessment

Slides were examined by two independent investigators. The proportion of tumor cells stained by each monoclonal antibody was assessed semi-quantatively and classified as: uniformly positive, heterogeneous, and uniformly negative. In each section the tumor stroma served as an internal positive control. The number of infiltrating immune cells was quantitatively asssessed by morphometry as infiltrating immune cells among the tumor cells (tumor infiltrating cells) or in stromal tissue (stromal infiltrating cells)[4].

Statistical analysis

The 'Chi-square test' and the '95% confidence interval for the percentage of agreement' statistics were applied to correlate different staining patterns.
To correlate the number of infiltrating immune cells in HLA +/+-,- tissue, we used the 'unpaired t-test'.

RESULTS

HLA class I expression

Normal cervical epithelium showed uniform staining of HLA class I antigens in the basal layers of the epithelium where the immature basal cells are situated. In cervical intraepithelial neoplasia (CIN), class I expression was also observed on the cells of the superficial layers of the epithelium, in concordance with the disturbed maturation of the basal cells and the degree of CIN. In cervical carcinoma there was a heterogeneous reduction of the expression of monomorphic class I antigens in 20% of the cases. Allele-specific loss was observed in 50% of HLA-A2 positive patients, in 66% of HLA-A3, in 56% of HLA-Bw4 and in 37% of HLA-Bw6 respectively[5].

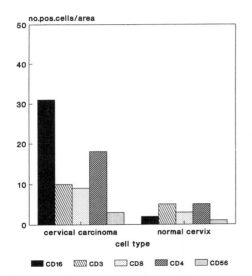

Figure 1. Infiltrating immune cells in cervical tissue.

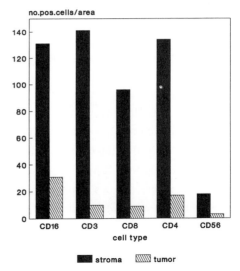

Figure 2. Stromal and tumor infiltrating cells in cervical carcinoma

HLA class II expression

In normal cervical tissue the class II antigens appeared to be restricted to the few immunocompetent cells present in the lower half of the epithelium. The HLA class II expression increased in advanced stages of CIN, although class II antigens were not seen on the epithelial cells, but was restricted to the increased number of immune cells, occurring throughout the dysplastic epithelium. *De novo* expression of monomorphic HLA class II antigens was observed in 80% of the cervical carcinomas. The different HLA class II loci were expressed in 80% for HLA-DR, 57% for HLA-DQ and 27% for HLA-DP on the tumor cells[4].

Infiltrating immune cells

Compared to normal cervical epithelium there was an increase in infiltrating immune cells present in cervical carcinoma (Figure 1). The majority of these tumor infiltrating cells were situated in the stromal bands surrounding the tumor cell foci. However, infiltrating cells were also situated in between the tumor cells. The infiltration of immune cells was not related to tumor necrosis. In all tumors, CD16 reactive monocytes/macrophages accounted for the majority of the infiltrating cells (stroma: 131 cells/area, tumor 32 cells/area). Next in frequency were T lymphocytes (stroma: 141 cells/area, tumor: 10 cells/area). Only few cells with an NK phenotype (CD3-, CD56+) were present (stroma: 18 cells/area, tumor 3 cells/area) and the CD22+ B cells were clustered in the stromal bands (stroma 94 cells/area) (Figure 2).

Infiltrating cells and HLA expression

By comparing the alterations of HLA class I expression on the tumor cells with the presence of infiltrating immune cells, we revealed a significant correlation between the downregulation of monomorphic HLA class I antigens on the tumor cells and a decrease in the tumor infiltrating CD8+ T lymphocytes. No such correlation was found between the stromal infiltrating CD8+ T lymphocytes and the HLA expression on the tumor cells. In addition, no correlations were found between allel-specific HLA class I expression and the presence of infiltrating immune cells.

Highly significant correlations were found between the abberant expression of HLA class II antigens on the tumor cells and an increase in tumor infiltrating CD3+/CD4+/CD8+ T cells, CD56+ NK cells and CD16+ macrophages. Locus-specific expression of the HLA clas II antigens on the tumor cells, revealed a significant correlation between *de novo* expression and an increase in tumor infiltrating immune cells[4].

DISCUSSION

The present study has shown that specific changes in HLA expression on cervical carcinoma may occur more often than previously accepted on the basis of W6/32 staining alone. By using an extensive panel of monoclonal antibodies directed against monomorphic- and polymorphic determinants of HLA class I and II antigens in a series of normal, premalignant and malignant cervical tissue, we could distinguish the selective changes of HLA expression in progression to cervical carcinoma. In normal cervical tissue and cervical intra-epithelial neoplasia, even though maturation and/or keratinization of epithelium is accompanied by a loss of class I expression, not a single sample of normal cervix or CIN from any patient lacked HLA class I expression, nor was there any change in locus/allele-specific expression. This means that the reduction or absence of class I expression is related to malignancy. Also the abberant HLA class II expression was confined to the tumor cells.

We also demonstrated, like several other immunohistological studies on cervical carcinoma[1-3], that high levels of mononuclear cell infiltrates are present in cervical tumor tissue, consisting predominantly of CD8+ T lymphocytes. Changes in monomorphic- as well as allele-speicif HLA class I and II expression can have direct effects on the immunogenicity of the tumor cells by interfering with immunosurveillance[6]. Also in cervical carcinoma, as shown in this study, correlations between tumor infiltrating immune cells and alterations in HLA class I or II expression on cervical carcinoma cells could be found. The alterations in HLA class I as well as HLA class II expression were demonstrated to have their effects only on the tumor infiltrating cells. *De novo* expression of HLA class II on the tumor cells resulted in a marked tumor induced infiltrate of immune cells, whereas in monomorphic HLA class I downregulated cervical tumors a significant decrease in tumor infiltrating CD8+ T lymphocytes was observed. By comparing these two phenomena it has become evident that the downregulation of HLA class I antigens dominates over the effect of *de novo* expression of HLA class II in regard to infiltration of CD8+ cells in cervical carcinoma. From these findings we deduce that the HLA class I expression on cervical carcinoma is of importance for triggering an *in situ* immune response. In addition, it becomes clear that in cervical carcinoma a correlation exists between HLA class I expression and tumor infiltrating CD8+ T lymphocytes. So probably these lymphocytes present *in situ* in cervical carinoma are thought to reflect a specific tumor-directed interaction rather than an inflammatory response, because their presence is associated with HLA class I expression on the tumor cells. These findings are indicative for the presence of HLA-restricted tumor-specific lymphocytes, thus promoting further characterization and assessment of the functional properties of these TIL in cervical carcinoma. In the presence of 1,000 U/ml of rIL-2, TIL from most solid tumors proliferate successfully. The majority of these lymphokine-activated TIL lyse a broad range of fresh and cultured tumor targets, exhibiting autologous tumor cytotoxicity as well as non-specific cytotoxic activity. In contrast, some human melanomas[7], breast cancers[8], sarcomas[9], renal cell carcinomas[10] and ovarian cancers[11] have yielded TIL that manifest more specific interactions with autologous tumor cells. Earlier studies on the isolation of TIL from cervical carcinoma[12], reported a minor TIL cell yield with a rather low and a-specific lysis. Therefore we are now developing methods to expand the initial TIL population from cervical carcinoma by the use of established autologous tumor cell lines as feeder cells in specialized culturing conditions. Preliminary results have shown that, by using the autologous cervical tumor cell lines as a homogeneous source of target cells, we are able to study the effectiveness and the mechanisms involved in antitumor reactivity.

Future clinical studies on immunotherapy, using tumor infiltrating lymphocytes in cervical carcinoma, have to take the alterations in HLA expression, as described in this study, into account, thus assisting a more precise delivery of treatment.

REFERENCES

1. T. Hachisuga, K. Fukuda, Y. Hayashi, T. Iwasaka and H. Sugimori, Immunohistochemical demonstration of histiocytes in normal ectocervical epithelium and epithelial lesions of the uterine cervix, *Gynecol Oncol.* 33:273 (1989).

2. M. Väyrynen, K. Syrjänen, R. Mäntyjärvi, O. Castr'n and S. Saarikoski, Immunophenotypes of lymphocytes in prospectively followed up human papillomavirus lesions of the cervix, *Genitourin Med.* 61:190 (1985).

3. A. Ferguson, M. Moore and H. Fox, Expression of MHC products and leucocyte differentiation antigens in gynaecological neoplasms: An immunohistological analysis of the tumour cells and infiltrating leucocytes, *Br J Obstet Gynaecol.* 52:551 (1985).

4. C.G.J.M. Hilders, J.G.A. Houbiers, H.H. Ravenswaay Claasen van, R.W. Velhuizen and G.J. Fleuren, The association between HLA-expression and infiltration of immune cells in cervical carcinoma, *Lab Invest.* in press:(1993).

5. C.G.J.M. Hilders, J.G.A. Houbiers, E.J.T. Krul and G.J. Fleuren, The expression of histocompatibility leukocyte antigens in the pathway to cervical carcinoma, *Am J Clin Pathol.* in press:(1993).

6. P.C. Doherty, B. Knowles and P.J. Wettstein, Immunological surveillance of tumors in the context of major histocompatibility complex restriction of T cell function, *Adv. Cancer Res.* 42:1 (1984).

7. L.M. Muul, P.J. Spiess, E.P. Director and S.A. Rosenberg, Identification of specific cytolytic immune responses against autologous tumor in humans bearing malignant melanoma, *J Immunol.* 138:(1987).

8. T. Sato, S. Takahashi, H. Koshiba and K. Kikuchi, Specific cytotoxicity of a long-term cultured T-cell clone on human autologous mammary cancer cells, *Cancer Res..* 46:4384 (1986).

9. S.F. Slovin, R.D. Lackman, S. Ferrone, P.E. Kiely and M.J. Mastrangelo, Cellular immune response to human sarcomas: cytotoxic T cell clones reactive with autologous sarcomas, *J Immunol.* 137:3042 (1986).

10. A.S. Koo, C.L. Tso, T. Shimabukuro, C. Peyret, J.B. Kernion de and A. Belldegrun, Autologous tumor-specific cytotoxicity of tumor-infiltrating lymphocytes derived from human renal cell carcinoma, *J Immunother.* 10:347 (1991).

11. C.G. Ioannides, R.S. Freedman, C.D. Platsoucas, S. Rashed and Y.P. Kim, Cytotoxic T cell clones isolated from ovarian tumor-infiltrating lymphocytes recognize multiple antigenic epitopes on autologous tumor cells, *J Immunol.* 146(5):1700 (1991).

12. A.K. Ghosh and M. Moore, Tumour-infiltrating lymphocytes in cervical carcinoma, *Eur J Cancer.* 28A(11):1910 (1992).

ANALYSIS OF TUMOUR-INFILTRATING LYMPHOCYTES IN CERVICAL CARCINOMA

Anna K. Ghosh, Suzanne Glenville, Jenny Bartholomew and Peter L. Stern

CRC Immunology Department
Paterson Institute for Cancer Research
Christie Hospital NHS Trust
Manchester M20 9BX
U.K.

INTRODUCTION

Infiltrating lymphocytes are readily seen in cervical tumours but little information is available regarding their functional properties. Methods have recently been developed that allow the isolation and propagation of tumour-infiltrating lymphocytes (TIL) in the presence of interleukin-2 (IL-2) which allows their functional characterisation. TIL from many solid human tumours eg. breast, ovary, lung and colon have been shown to proliferate in bulk culture under the influence of IL-2 and exhibit predominantly non-MHC restricted cytotoxicity with varying degrees of cytotoxicity against autologous and allogeneic targets. In contrast, TIL isolated from some malignant melanomas exhibit specific autologous tumour cytotoxicity. Evidence that cell-mediated immunity plays a role in the control of virus-induced tumours prompted a study to determine whether HPV related cervical tumours elicit a specific T cell response.

An initial study was undertaken to ascertain whether; A) TIL can be established in long-term culture in the presence of IL-2 from cervical tumour biopsies and B) Examine their phenotypic and functional characteristics. The outcome of this initial study demonstrated low auto-tumour cytotoxicity at the clonal level (Ghosh and Moore, 1992).

The present study is continuing this work and aims to; A) Develop cell lines from the primary biopsy; B) Expand TIL in the presence of autologous tumour in order to elicit a specific anti-tumour response; C) To ascertain whether TIL recognise HPV antigens on tumour cells.

MATERIALS AND METHODS

Initial Study. Fresh tumour tissues were obtained from 27 patients with cervical carcinoma prior to radiotherapy treatment at the Christie Hospital and Holt Radium Institute, Manchester. A piece of tissue was designated for immunohistology and the remaining tissue was disaggregated,digested with enzymes and set up in culture with rIL-2 (200 U/ml). In cases with sufficient material, a two-step density gradient consisting of 100% and 75% Lymphoprep was used to separate tumour cells and lymphocytes. These tumour cells were cryopreserved for use as target cells in cytotoxicity assays.

TIL cultures were expanded and analysed for cytotoxicity to NK, LAK, allogeneic and autologous tumour cell targets by standard ^{51} Cr cytotoxicity assays. In 6 cases TIL were cloned by limiting dilution in the presence of IL-2 and irradiated allogeneic PBLs and BSM (EBV-transformed B cell line). Immunophenotyping was performed by an alkaline phosphatase method (APAAP).

Present Study: Methods are being developed to improve the conditions for expanding tumour specific CTL . In order for sufficient tumour cells to be available for generating and characterising the cytotoxic profile of TIL, cervical carcinoma cell lines are being established from primary tumours. Enzyme digested tumour cell suspensions are plated onto irradiated 3T3 feeders and/or tumour tissue is minced finely and plated onto feeders. Cell lines are passaged onto fresh 3T3 cells every 7-10 days as necessary.

When tumour cell lines are established, TIL cultures are being set up at a lymphocyte to tumour cell ratio of 4:1 with irradiated autologous tumour and 20 U IL-2/ml. TIL are being cloned in the presence of IL-2, irradiated autologous tumour and BSM.

RESULTS

Initial Study: The main features of the initial study are summarised here. Immunohistochemical analysis of infiltrating cells in tumour biopsy sections demonstrated that the mean T4/T8 ratio in the tumour was 0.9 (range 0.3-2.6) and in the stroma 1.1 (range 0.5-1.9). Few CD25+ cells were observed. TIL were successively expanded in 16/27 cases. The outgrowth of TIL did not correlate with stage of disease or phenotype of infiltrating cells.

Bulk TIL cultures showed non-MHC restricted cytotoxicity in the majority of cases. CD8+ cells were the predominant subset in over 50% of cultures, with varying numbers of CD56+ and CD25+ cells. T cell clones isolated from two cases showed low autotumour cytotoxicity and in one of these cases cytotoxicity to Caski, an allogeneic cervical tumour (Table 1). These clones were CD3+CD4+CD56-or CD3+CD8+CD56-/CD56+. Clones isolated from four other cases exhibited non MHC-restricted cytotoxicity and the majority were of CD3+ CD4+ (or CD8+) CD56+ phenotype.

Table 1. Cytotoxicity and phenotype of bulk cultured tumour-infiltrating lymphocytes and representative clones from pt.16

	% Specific cytotoxicity				Phenotype			
	Auto-tu	Caski	K562	Mel 1	CD3	CD4	CD8	CD56
Bulk(day 14)	ND	4	24	6	76	40	32	10
Clone 1	6	3	0	0	+	+	–	-
Clone 2	2	9	0	0	+	-	+	-
Clone 8	7	19	0	0	+	-	+	-
Clone 10	0	14	0	0	+	+	-	-
Clone 11	13	25	0	0	+	+	-	-
Clone 12	2	27	0	0	+	+	-	-
Clone 13	19	36	0	6	+	-	+	+
Clone 14	11	29	2	9	+	-	+	+

Present Study: Immunohistochemical analysis of TIL in freshly disaggregated tumour cell suspensions show low numbers of infiltrating CD4+ and CD8+ lymphocytes. Tumour samples have been obtained from 23 cervical cancer patients. The conditions for *in vitro* culture of samples were investigated and optimised for the development of cell lines. One cell line, 778BG, has been established from a cervical tumour biopsy and one is in early passage at present. Characterisation of cell line 778BG is in progress. A TIL culture has been initiated from patient 778BG with irradiated autologous tumour cells as stimulators. A cytoassay performed at 21 days showed the bulk culture exhibits predominantly non-MHC restricted cytotoxicity, however a second cytoassay performed at 45 days showed a slight reduction in cytotoxicity against NK and LAK sensitive target cells with an increase in cytotoxicity to the autologous tumour (Figure 1). The TIL culture is being cloned by limiting dilution in the presence of autologous tumour cells. Clones obtained will be assayed against a panel of target cells to determine their specificity and MHC restriction.

SUMMARY AND FUTURE WORK

Initial studies demonstrated that TIL can be amplified and cloned from cervical carcinoma biopsies by expansion in IL-2. Low autotumour cytotoxicity was observed at the clonal level although the predominant cytolytic function is non MHC-restricted. The method of stimulation of TIL may affect the phenotype and specificity of effector cell generated. The presence of tumour cells may act as a further *in vitro* stimulus for propagation of tumour

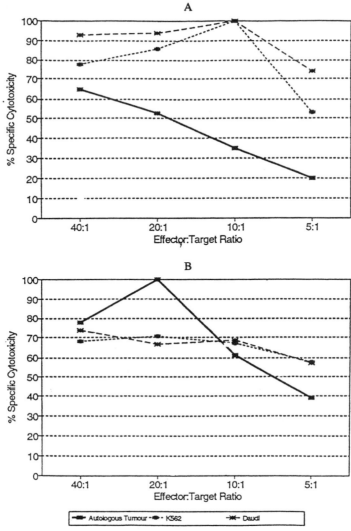

Figure 1. Cytotoxicity assay of bulk co-culture of TIL and autologous tumour (778BG).
A) 21 days in culture; B) 45 days in culture

specific CTL. This is exemplified by studies on melanoma where specific anti-tumour effector cells have been detected after coculture of lymphocytes derived from peripheral blood, tumour or draining lymph nodes in the presence of autologous tumour and IL-2. The genomic sequence coding for a series of CTL epitopes (MAGE) have now been identified providing firm evidence for the existence of tumour specific antigens (Van der Bruggen et al.,1991; Traversari et al.,1992). Methods are being developed to improve the conditions for generating and expanding tumour specific CTL dervived from cervical carcinomas. This involves the establishment of autologous tumour cell lines and co-culture of TIL in the presence of autologous tumour. The nature of the antigen(s) recognised by T cells on autologous cervical carcinoma cells is unknown; the candidacy of HPV-related products requires investigation.

The focus of future work will be to develop and characterise cell lines derived from cervical biopsies and generate specific tumour CTL. A major aim will be to determine whether HPV antigens are recognised by tumour specific CTL. This will be acheived by the use of target cells pulsed with HPV 16 derived peptides or recombinant vaccinia virus encoding HPV 16 E6 or E7.

REFERENCES

1. Ghosh A.K. and Moore M., 1992, Tumour-infiltrating lymphocytes in cervical carcinoma, *Eur J Cancer* 28A:1910.
2. Van der Bruggen P., Traversari C., Chomez P., Lurquin C., DePlaen E., Van Den Eynde B., Knuth A. and Boon T., 1991, A gene encoding an antigen recognised by cytolytic T lymphocytes on a human melanoma, *Science* 254: 1643.
3. Traversari C., Vander Bruggen P., Luescher I.F., De Plaen E., Amar-Costesec A. and Boon T., 1992 A nonapeptide encoded by human gene MAGE-1 is recognised on HLA-A1 by cytolytic T lymphocytes directed against tumor antigen MZ2-E, *J Exp Med.* 176:1453.

LYMPHOCYTE-MEDIATED NATURAL CYTOTOXICITY TO HPV16 INFECTED CERVICAL KERATINOCYTES

Rong Wu, Nicholas Coleman, Geoffrey Higgins,
Esther Choolun, Margaret A. Stanley

Department of Pathology
University of Cambridge
Tennis Court Road
Cambridge CB2 1QP
U K

Natural Killer (NK) cells are capable of mediating spontaneous antibody-independent and non-MHC restricted cytotoxicity against many human neoplastic and virally infected cells without prior sensitization[1]. The activity of NK cells can be augmented by several cytokines. Purified IL-2 (Interleukin-2) alone is able to cause direct activation of nonlytic PBLs (Peripheral blood lymphocytes) into LAK (Lymphokine Activated Killer) cells without known antigen stimuli in vitro[2]. LAK are capable of binding to and killing a broad range of neoplastic and normal tissues (both NK-sensitive and NK-resistant)[3,4]. IFNγ can also influence the immune response by modulating susceptibilility of targets [5].

In this paper, we have studied the susceptibility of HPV16-infected cervical keratinocytes to non-specific lysis by resting and IL-2-activated PBLs and the modulatory effect of IFNγ pretreatment of keratinocytes. Lysis was quantified using a non-isotopic method, based upon the colorimetric detection of LDH (lactate dehydrogenase) released from the lysed cells in a four hour cytotoxicity assay.

Immunology of Human Papillomaviruses
Edited by M.A. Stanley, Plenum Press, New York, 1994

MATERIALS AND METHODS

Preparation of Lymphocytes

Buffy coats of normal human volunteers were obtained from the East Anglian Blood Transfusion Centre (Cambridge, U.K.). Lymphocytes were isolated by density gradient centrifugation on Histopaque (density 1.083)(Sigma). Activation was achieved by culturing at 1×10^6/ml in RPMI$_{1640}$ with glutamine medium (Gibco) containing 100 units/ml of IL-2 (British Biotechnology Limited) and 20% Fetal Calf Serum(FCS) for four days at 37^{0}C in a 5% CO_2 -95% air atmosphere.

Target Cells

The cell lines were maintained in continuous culture in GMEM (Glasgow's modification of Eagle's medium) containing 10% FCS at 37^{0}C in a 5% CO_2 incubator. They are (i) cervical carcinoma derived keratinocytes: CaSki , SiHa (HPV16+); (ii) non malignant cervical keratinocytes, immortalised but non-transformed by HPV16 : W12 and (iii) normal ectocervical keratinocytes (HPV16 negative). IFNγ (Genzyme Ltd) was added in the concentration of 300 units/ml 48 hours before the cytotoxicity assays. K562 cells (derived from a patient with chronic myelogenous leukemia in blast phase) were used as a known NK sensitive cell line and were cultured in RPMI$_{1640}$ /10%FCS medium.

Cytotoxicity Assay

Keratinocytes were trypsinized, washed and resuspended in RPMI$_{1640}$ /2%BSA(Bovine Serum Albumin). Target cells were added to lymphocytes in different effector:target (E:T) ratios in triplicate. After incubating at 37^{0}C in 5% CO_2 -95% air incubator for four hours, reagents in CytoTox 96^{Tm} Non-Radioactive Cytotoxicity Assay Kit (Promega) were used according to the manufacturer's instruction. Absorbance at a wavelength of 490nm was recorded on a Elisa Reader (Dynatech MR500). The percentage of cytotoxicity was calculated using the formula given by Promega.

RESULTS AND DISCUSSION

NK cells are involved in cytolytic activity against a wide range of virus-infected cells and neoplasms. NK activity is independent of prior antigen sensitisation but can be increased by various stimuli. It has been reported that HPV-16 transformed vulvar keratinocytes (Sk-v) are

Table 1. Cytotoxicity of freshly isolated PBL's against Caski, SiHa and K562 cells

E:T	% cytotoxicity					
	Caski		SiHa		K562	
	+	-	+	-		
50:1	0	0	8	5	42	
20:1	0	0	8	4	25	
10:1	0	0	4	4	18	
5:1	0	0	4	2	9	
2:1	0	0	0	3	3	

+   300 IU. IFN-γ 48 hours before use

-     no IFN-γ pretreatment

E:T   Effector : Target ratio

Table 2. Effects of pretreatment with IL-2 on the cytotoxicity of freshly isolated PBL's against HPV-16 containing and normal cervical keratinocytes

	% cytotoxicity							
	Caski		SiHa		W12		N.Cx	
- IL-2								
E:T	+	-	+	-	+	-	+	-
50:1	26	4	16	5	4	2	5	4
20:1	25	2	11	5	3	2	4	0
10:1	25	0	5	1	2	1	0	0
5:1	12	0	3	0	2	0	0	0
2:1	10	0	0	0	0	0	0	0
+IL-2								
50:1	64	5	48	5	15	3	28	4
20:1	52	2	30	5	10	2	22	1
10:1	40	0	20	2	4	1	14	0
5:1	11	0	14	0	3	0	8	1
2:1	5	0	6	0	3	0	8	0

+   300 IU IFN-γ 48 hours before assay

-     No IFN-γ pretreatment

E:T   Effector to Target ratio

susceptible to lysis by NK cells, while normal human keratinocytes are resistant to the natural killing of NK cells[6].

To determine whether NK cells were functionally effective to lyse HPV-16 infected cervical keratinocytes, freshly isolated PBLs were used to kill CaSki and SiHa in vitro and K562 used as a positive control. Consistent with other findings, freshly isolated PBLs were effective to lyse K562[3] but minimally responsive to Caski and SiHa both with or without IFNγ pretreatment , suggesting that CaSki and SiHa were NK resistant, similar to other neoplastic epithelial cell lines (e.g. COLO, a colon carcinoma cell line; ZR, a breast carcinoma cell line)[3].

LAK cells show a broader range of target cell destruction, which includes both NK-sensitive and NK-resistant tumour cells as well as fresh noncultured, surgically obtained solid tumour cells[2]. The lytic activity expressed by LAK is not MHC-restricted. Some target cells have greater sensitivity than others.

In our report, LAK activity was shown to be E:T ratio dependent and cell line-dependent. Satisfactory cytotoxicity was produced at an E:T ratio of 10:1 or more . LAK showed the best killing on IFNγ pre-treated target cells in all cases. The cytolytic effect on CaSki and SiHa was better than that on W12 and normal cervix. Although LAK cells were effective at killing IFNγ pretreated W12 and normal cervix, they showed little killing of untreated cells. However, NK cells showed little increase in killing of IFNγ pre-treated target cells.Our results also suggest that the effects of IFNγ on cytotoxicity depend on the effects of IL-2. In this study, IL-2 and IFNγ played critical roles in the killing of cervical keratinocytes. The mechanisms responsible for the effects are under investigation.

ACKNOWLEGEMENTS

Wu Rong was supported as a visiting worker by the British Council. Geoffrey Higgins was supported by an ICRF Fellowship .

REFERENCES

1. D.Santoli, G. Trinchieri, and F.S. Lief: Cell-mediated cytotoxicity against virus-infected target cells in human. *J Immunol* 121:526 (1978)

2. E.A Grimm, R.J. Robb, J. A. Roth, L. M. Neckers, L.B Lachman, D.J. Wilson, and S.A. Rosenberg:Lymphokine-activated killer cell phenomenon. *J Exp Med.* 158:1356 (1983)

3. J. H. Phillips and L. L. Lanier: Dissection of the lymphokine-activated killer phenomenon. *J Exp Med.* 164:814 (1986)

4. E. A. Grimm, A. Mazumder, H. Z. Zhang, and S. A. Rosenberg: Lymphokine- activated killer cell Phenomenon.*J Exp Med* 155:1823 (1982)

5. R.Kurzrock : Interferon-gamma. In'Cytokine Therapy'. ed D.W Galvani and J.C.Cawley. University of Cambridge. Cambridge (1992)

6. J.Malejczyk, S.Majewski, S.Jablonska, T.T.Rogozinski and G. Orth: Abrogated Nk-cell lysis of human papillomavirus(HPV)-16-Bearing keratinocytes in patients with pre- cancerous and cancerous HPV-induced anogenital lesions. *Int J Cancer* 43, 209 (1989)

SKIN TEST REACTIVITY TO PAPILLOMA CELLS IS LONG LASTING IN DOMESTIC RABBITS AFTER REGRESSION OF COTTONTAIL RABBIT PAPILLOMAVIRUS INDUCED PAPILLOMAS

Reinhard M. Höpfl,[1] Neil D. Christensen,[2] Kurt Heim[3] and John W. Kreider[4]

Departments of [1]Dermatology and [3]Gynecology
University of Innsbruck
Austria
[2-4]Department of Pathology
The Pennsylvania State University
Hershey, PA

INTRODUCTION

Human papillomaviruses (HPVs) are strictly epithelial pathogens and there is increasing evidence that infection by high risk HPV types has to be regarded as a major risk factor in the development of certain cancers such as the carcinoma of the cervix. Increased incidence of HPV induced lesions and cancer is a complication in immunosuppressed individuals, particularly in those patients with disturbed cell mediated immunity[1,2]. Conversely, prophylactic and therapeutic vaccination may represent a promising strategy to deal with the HPV associated health threat[3]. If successful, vaccines would have a profound effect on HPV associated morbidity and mortality with major benefits in both developed and in underdeveloped countries. However, our understanding of the role of the immune system in controlling HPV infection is still fragmentary.

Immunology of Human Papillomaviruses
Edited by M.A. Stanley, Plenum Press, New York, 1994

Evidence for a role of T-cells in regression is suggested by mononuclear cell infiltrates in warts during regression[4,5], but reported lymphoproliferative responses to PV antigens measured *in vitro* are low[6,7]. Application of skin tests to study immune responses to HPV *in vivo* was first published in 1977[8] and the reintroduction of this test for PV research in 1991 demonstrated delayed type hypersensitivity (DTH) to the major capsid protein L1 of HPV 16 in patients with cervical intraepithelial neoplasia (CIN)[9].

Advantages of *in vivo* analyses of complex immune responses by skin tests are obvious. Skin tests are extremely sensitive and injection of antigens intracutaneously mimics natural infection, since PV antigens are presented to the immune system via an epithelial surface. However, ethical considerations restrict application of skin tests in patients and demand exploitation of suitable animal models such as a newly developed mouse model[10] and the "Shope papilloma carcinoma complex" of rabbits[11]. We have recently demonstrated strong DTH skin test reactivity in cottontail rabbit papillomavirus (CRPV) infected domestic regressor rabbits with infectious CRPV particles but not with denatured virions or capsid proteins[12]. Early post infection events may have taken place[13], and virally derived early antigens or undefined cellular antigens of infected keratinocytes may have been additional targets presented to the immune system.

If a specific cellular immune response to papilloma cells is detectable by skin tests and plays a role in regression of CRPV papillomas in rabbits, then this response should be strongest in regressor rabbits. Generation of fresh autologous papilloma cells for rabbits whose papillomas had already regressed is possible only in the athymic *(nu/nu)* mouse xenograft system[14]. Production of these papilloma cells allowed us to test the above hypothesis in the "Shope" model system.

METHODS

Animals

Rabbits were inoculated with CRPV prepared from wild cottontail papilloma extracts[15]. Regressor rabbits consisted of nine animals with spontaneous and complete disappearance of papillomas. Regressor status was confirmed by resistance to reinfection with CRPV-DNA[16]. Progressors consisted of ten animals with persisting papillomas. Five uninfected animals served as naive controls.

Papilloma cells

Laboratory production *in vivo* of autologous papilloma cells was achieved for all animal groups alike with the athymic *(nu/nu)* mouse xenograft system modified as previously described[14]. Briefly, split-thickness chips of rabbit ear skin were washed in 70%

ethanol, cut into pieces with a sterile scalpel and incubated for 1 h at 37°C with phosphate-buffered saline (PBS) extracts from wild cottontail papillomas. Skin grafts were inserted subcutaneously into anaesthetized mice. Cysts (after 6 to 8 weeks of growth) were excised, and the keratin cores plus attached surrounding mouse tissues were removed. Conventional paraffin sections were prepared from papillomatous cyst walls and stained with hematoxylin and eosin (H&E) and by immunoperoxidase method for detection of PV group-specific antigen (Dako, Carpenteria CA, USA). These sections showed papillomatous changes, consisting of koilocytosis, hyperplasia and hyperkeratosis. Nuclei positive for group-specific antigen were seen. A crude suspension of tissue fragments was prepared mechanically by mincing with sharp scissors without further enzymatic treatment as described previously[17]. Large tissue fragments were removed by passage through a 15-gauge needle. A final concentration of approximately 10^6 tissue fragments per ml PBS was prepared and used within one hour for skin tests. Mouse tissue, removed from the surface of the cysts, and uninfected rabbit ear skin chips were used to prepare suspensions for control antigen preparations.

Skin tests

The procedure consisted of the intracutaneous injection of 0.03 ml test solution containing autologous papilloma cells into the shaved ear skin of rabbits through a 15-gauge needle as described recently[12]. Control preparations were injected into the contralateral ear. In addition, every papilloma cell containing solution was injected into 2 or 3 randomly chosen allogeneic -rabbits from the two other animal groups. Ear swelling was monitored over 5 days and measured to the nearest 0.01 mm with a constant tension thickness gauge. Biopsies for routine H&E staining were taken from additional skin tests at days 1, 2 and 3.

Statistics

Significance levels were determined at the upper 95% confidence limit of the average ear swelling at the same time point after injection of the corresponding autologous or allogeneic papilloma cells into the control animals. Swellings thicker than the mean swelling in naive rabbits + 2x standard deviations (SD) were considered positive. Statistical analyses were performed using the Fisher's exact probability test and the Mann-Whitney U test.

RESULTS

Swelling and histopathology had a biphasic course. After intense swelling within hours after papilloma cell inoculation, ear thickness decreased constantly. Later a more persistent skin induration was seen. Swelling increased between 48 and 72 hours in some cases and was measurable up to 7 days. Histopathology in early stages showed infiltrates with predominantly polymorphonuclear cells. Later biopsy specimens contained more mononuclear lymphocytes (data not shown).

Response to autologous papilloma cells

Skin test reactivity was more pronounced in regressors when compared to progressors (Figure 1). This was most obvious in the later phase of the reaction. After 72 hours, 8 of 9 regressors, but only 2 of 10 progressors had skin tests that were judged positive (p = 0.0044).

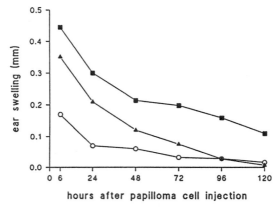

Figure 1 Time course of swelling to autologous papilloma cells: Average ear swelling in 9 regressor rabbits (■),in 10 progressors (▲ and in 5 naive control rabbits (o). Particularly in regressor rabbits an early response was followed by long lasting induration suggestive for DTH.

Response to allogeneic papilloma cells and control preparations

Data obtained with allogeneic papilloma cells injected in a crossover fashion into the different two animal groups were essentially identical as seen with autologous papilloma cells (Figure 2). Regressors reacted more strongly (mean swelling: 0.256 mm; SD = 0.24) than progressors (mean swelling: 0.121 mm; SD = 0.08) to allogeneic papilloma cells. When results obtained with allogeneic injections were compared to autologous tests, the only statistically significant difference was increased response of naive rabbits to allogeneic cells. The mean swelling was 0.137 mm (SD = 0 0.098). At injection sites of autologous papilloma cells a mean swelling of only 0.06 mm (SD = 0.0228) was measured. No significant skin test reactivity was observed with mouse tissue or rabbit keratinocytes containing control solutions.

DISCUSSION

The kinetics of the skin test reaction to papilloma cells appeared to be similar to the response following injection of viral antigens into CRPV infected rabbits[12]. In both experiments, time course and histopathology of the reaction were suggestive of a DTH response. This is in line with demonstrated DTH response to PV antigens in patients[8,9], and in a recently developed mouse model[10]. There is evidence for antigen specificity of the reaction, since there was no significant reactivity to control preparations and naive rabbits did not have a strong primary response even to allogeneic papilloma cells. In addition, injections of papilloma cells in a crossover fashion excluded the possibility that confounding factors such as preparation variables contributed to the strong response in regressor rabbits.

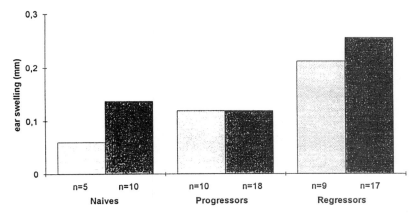

Figure 2 Average ear skin swelling to autologous (light) versus allogeneic (dark) papilloma cells 48 hours after injection of cell suspensions. Strongest response in regressors in both tests.

It is important to note that a positive skin test in regressors was detectable up to 2 years after complete regression of papillomas. Since our model system mimics natural infection of CRPV very closely, it is intriguing to hypothesize that the strong DTH reaction found in regressors may reflect a natural immune response that occurs during spontaneous regression. Indeed, vaccination with papilloma cells did increase the frequency of regression of "Shope" papillomas of rabbits[17]. However, this vaccination study did not provide direct evidence for a specific PV-reactive immunological response. Our studies further support a possible role of DTH as a mechanism for regression, since the most significant difference between progressor and regressor reactivity was seen in the late phase of the skin test reaction. DTH involved in defence against skin pathogens seems to be plausible from a clinical standpoint. Induction of non-PV-specific DTH has been used successfully as a therapeutic regimen for recalcitrant common warts[18].

We conclude that DTH reactivity to papilloma cells exists in CRPV infected rabbits. This reactivity seems to be long lasting in rabbits that have undergone complete regression of papillomas. However, the target antigens of the T-cells in these positive skin test reactions still remains to be determined. Since responses in regressing flat warts are directed to basal keratinocytes[19], it is most likely that the antigens involved are early viral proteins expressed by infected cells. Further application of skin tests may be a powerful tool to address this question and to identify regression antigens, which may be successfully used for adjuvant immunotherapy.

ACKNOWLEDGEMENTS

This study was supported by NIH grants Ca-47622, NOI-AI-82687 and the Jack Gittlen Memorial Golf Tournament. Prof. Peter Fritsch was instrumental in obtaining funds for R.M.H. who was supported by the grant JO-577 MED of the Erwin Schrddinger Foundation.

REFERENCES

1. R. Hoover and J.F. Fraumeni, Risk of cancer in renal transplant patients, *Lancet* ii. 55 (1973).
2. M. Laga, J.P. Icenogle, R. Marsella, A.T. Manoka, N. Nzila, R.W. Ryder, S.H. Vermund, W.L. Heyward, A. Nelson and W.C. Reeves, Genital papillomavirus infection and cervical dysplasia - Opportunistic complication of HPV infection, *Int J Cancer* 50:45 (1992).
3. M.S. Campo, Vaccination against papillomavirus, *Cancer Cells* 3:421 (1991).
4. M. Okabayashi, M.G. Angell, N.D. Christensen and J.W. Kreider, Morphometric analysis and identification of infiltrating leucocytes in regressing and progressing Shope rabbit papillomas, *Int I Cancer* 49:919 (1991).
5. H. Tagami, A. Ogino, M. Takigawa, S. Imamura and S. Ofugi, Regression of plane warts following spontaneous inflammation: a histopathological study, *Br J Dermatol* 90:147 (1974).
6. H.A. Cubie, M. Norval, L. Crawford, L. Banks and T. Crook, Lymphoproliferative response to fusion proteins of human papillomaviruses in patients with cervical intraepithelial neoplasia, *Epidemiol Infect.* 103:625 (1990).
7. F.C. Charleson, M. Norval, E.C. Benton and J.A. Hunter, Lymphoproliferative response to human papillomaviruses in patients with cutaneous warts, *Br J Dermatol.* 127:551 (1992).
8. J. Viac, J. Thivolet and Y. Chardonnet. Specific immunity in patients suffering from recurring warts before and after repetitive intradermal tests with human papillomavirus, *Br J Dermatol.* 97:365 (1977).
9. R. Höpfl, M. Sandbichler, N. Sepp, K. Heim, E. Miiller-Holzner, B. Wartusch, O. Dapunt, I. Jochmus-Kudielka, J. Ter Meulen, L. Gissmann and P. Fritsch, Skin test for HPV type 16 proteins in cervical intraepithelial neoplasia, *Lancet* 337:373 (1991).

10. C. S. McLean, J. S. Sterling, J. Mowat, A.A. Nash and M. A. Stanley, Delayed-type hypersensitivity response to human papillomavirus type 16 E7 protein in a mouse model, *J General Virol.* 74:239 (1993).

11. J.W. Kreider and G.L. Barlett: The Shope papilloma-carcinoma complex of rabbits: A model system of neoplastic progression and spontaneous regression, *Adv Cancer Res.* 35:81 (1981).

12. R. M. Höpfl, N. D. Christensen, M.G. Angell and J. W. Kreider, Skin test to assess immunity against Cottontail Rabbit Papillomavirus Antigens in Rabbits with Progressing Papillomas or after Regression, *J Invest Dermatol.* 101:127 (1993).

13. M.G. Angell, N.D. Christensen and J.W. Kreider, An in vitro system for studying the initial stages of cottontail rabbit papillomavirus (CRPV) infection, *J Virol Methods* 39:207 (1992).

14. J. W. Kreider, M.K. Howett, A. E. Leure-Dupree, R.J. Zaino and J. A. Weber, Laboratory production in vivo of infectious human papillomavirus type 11, *J Virol.* 61:590 (1987).

15. J.W. Kreider. "Viruses in Naturally Occurring Cancers. Book A," Cold Spring Harbor Press, Cold Spring Harbor(1980).

16. J.L. Brandsma and W. Xiao, Infectious Virus Replication in Papillomas Induced by Molecular Cloned Cottontail Rabbit Papillomavirus DNA, *J Virol.* 67: 567 (1993).

17. C.A. Evans, L.R. Gorman, Y.Ito and R.S. Weiser, A vaccination procedure which increases the frequency of regressions of Shope papillomas of rabbits, *Nature* 193:288 (1962).

18. M.F. Naylor, K.H. Neldner, G.K. Yarbrough, T.J. Rosio, M. Iriondo and J. Yeary, Contact immunotherapy of resistant warts, *J Am Acad Dermatol.* 19:679 (1988).

19. S. Aiba, M. Rokego and H. Tagami, Immunohistological analysis of the phenomenon of spontaneous regression of numerous flat warts, *Cancer* 58.1246 (1986).

MODULATION OF THE DTH RESPONSE TO HPV 16 E7

Mark Chambers, Zhang Wei, Nicholas Coleman, Anthony Nash and
Margaret Stanley

Department of Pathology
Tennis Court Road
Cambridge CB2 1QP
UK

INTRODUCTION

We have developed an animal model which mimics a number of aspects of clinical
infection with HPV. In this system 10^7 keratinocytes expressing HPV 16 E7 protein are
grafted onto syngeneic mice using a transplantation technique which permits the
reformation of a differentiated epithelium. By this route viral antigens may be presented
to the immune system in a manner comparable to the natural infection. Subsequent
intradermal challenge of the recipients at a site distant from the graft with an HPV-16 E7
recombinant vaccinia virus (vacc-E7) results in a delayed type hypersensitivity (DTH)
response[1].

We have evidence that there is a threshold cell inoculum below which immune
sensitisation does not occur and a DTH response cannot be induced by challenge with
vacc-E7[2]. This phenomenon suggests a lack of priming by low levels of antigen and has
interesting parallels with the natural infection where in the early phase low levels of E6/E7
are expressed[3,4]. We decided to test the hypothesis that priming with subthreshold cell
numbers would result in the induction of non-responsiveness on subsequent challenge with
high levels of HPV-16 antigen and to investigate whether such unresponsiveness would
be maintained on multiple challenge with the protein. The murine model previously

described[1], was modified to permit the formation of two grafts on opposite flanks of the mouse with the grafting procedures separated by one week.

MATERIALS AND METHODS

DTH assay protocol

Balb/c mice at 6-8 weeks of age were used. In the single grafting protocol a sterile glass coverslip was inserted subcutaneously into the left flank. On day 7 this was

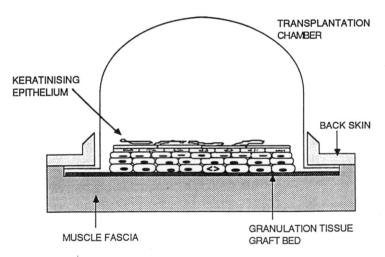

Figure 1. Diagram of the grafting chamber.

removed, a silicone transplantation chamber (Figure 1) inserted into the skin pocket which has been produced and the appropriate inoculum of cells injected through the dome of the grafting chamber. In the double grafting protocol, a glass coverslip was subcutaneously on both the right and left flank, the coverslip in the left flank was removed at day 7, the silicone grafting chamber was inserted over the granulation bed and the appropriate inoculum of keratinocytes injected through the lid of the grafting chamber. At day 14 the coverslip is removed from the right flank, the transplantation chamber inserted and the keratinocyte graft injected into the chamber.

Mice were challenged with recombinant HPV-16 antigen by intr-dermal injection into the left or right ear. The response to antigen was assayed by measuring the ear thickness in the challenged and unchallenged ears with a micrometer.

Cell lines

The NEK 16 cell line was used in these experiments. This line is an immortalised but non-tumorigenic mouse keratinocyte cell line derived after transfection of primary adult mouse epidermal cells with the plasmid pJ4Ω.16, the properties of this line have been described previously[1].

Recombinant HPV-16 E7 protein

A bacterial fusion protein of the maltose binding protein and HPV-16 E7 was produced using the pMAL vector system (New England Biolabs). The fusion protein was cleaved with thrombin and the E7 component purified by loading onto DEAE sephadex A50 resin. A suspension of this was used for ear injections (SE7): a 20μl inoculation representing 440ng of E7 protein. A suspension of Sephadex resin alone was included as a control.

A baculovirus generated HPV16 E7 protein was prepared and isolated using polyacrylamide gel electrophoresis (PAGE). After Coomassie blue staining the gel slice containing E7 was excised, placed in a minimal volume of saline and forced through syringe needles of ever decreasing size. A 20μl inoculum of this reagent known as PACE7 was injected into the ear of animals, a similarly treated gel slice containing no protein (PAC) was used as a control.

Recombinant vaccinia viruses expressing HPV-16 E7 or HPV-16 L1 have been described previously[1].

RESULTS AND DISCUSSION

The specificity of the DTH response to E7 after priming with 10^7 NEK 16 cells and intra-dermal challenge in the ear with vacc-E7 is shown in Figure 2, confirming the previous data[1].

To determine whether a DTH response could be induced to E7 protein alone when injected intra-dermally, mice were grafted with 10^7 16 and then challenged after 7 days with PACE7 or E7 generated as a bacterial fusion protein. As can be seen from the data in Figure 3 there was no significant response to PACE7 at 24 or 48 hours following ear challenge. We speculated that the ability of vacc-E7 to induce a response might be related to the ability of vaccinia to induce a non-specific inflammation at the site of inoculation. To test this, 48 hours after the initial ear challenge we inoculated the same sites with 2×10^7pfu of vacc L1; the subsequent ear swelling response was measured over 4 days and as can be seen from Figure 3 became significantly greater than controls only in the PACE7 challenged group. This is a significant observation for two reasons. First it demonstrates that a specific DTH response can be elicited with E7 protein alone and secondly that local inflammation plays an important part, at least in this model system, in the induction of the response, possibly by recruiting macrophages to the site of the sequestered allergen. These observations were confirmed using SE7 protein (data not shown) and the results in Figure 4 show that the phorbol ester TPA, an agent known to induce non-specific inflammation in skin could effect the same response as vaccinia although repeated applications of TPA were required.

In view of our observations that for the NEK line there was a threshold inoculum (10^6 cells) below which a DTH response could not be induced[2] although an epithelium was reformed (Appleby and Stanley unpublished results) we speculated the sub-optimal levels of priming with antighen might induce immunological non-responsiveness in this system. To address this question we used the

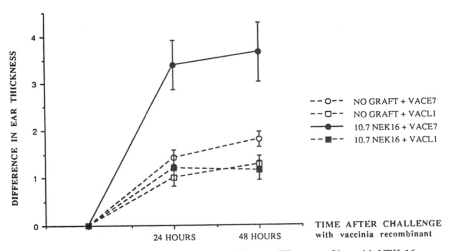

Figure 2. The DTH response to challenge with vacc-E7 post grafting with NEK 16.

immunological non-responsiveness in this system. To address this question we used the double graft protocol and the results of this experiment are shown in Figure 5. DTH reactivity was significantly diminished in mice initially grafted on the left flank with 5×10^5 NEK 16, followed 7 days later with a right flank graft of 10^7 cells and then challenged intradermally with the bacterial recombinant protein SE7 (combined with TPA). No DTH

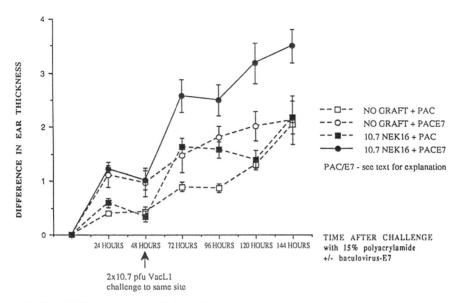

Figure 3. The DTH response to challenge with baculovirus derived HPV-16 E7 protein after NEK 16 grafting.

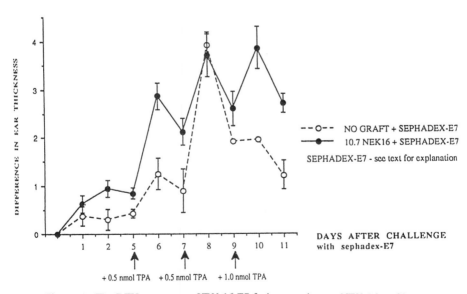

Figure 4. The DTH response to HPV-16 E7 fusion protein post NEK 16 grafting.

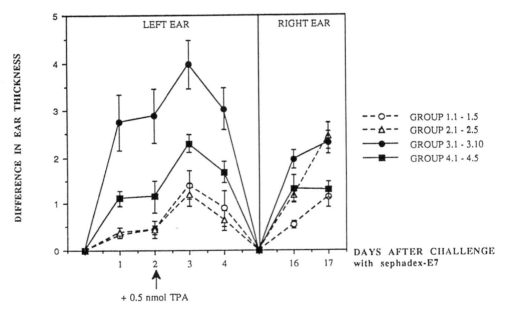

	DAY 7	DAY 14	DAY 21	DAY 36
GROUP	LEFT FLANK	RIGHT FLANK	LEFT EAR	RIGHT EAR
1.1 - 1.5	NO GRAFT	NO GRAFT	SEPHADEX	VacE7
2.1 - 2.5	NO GRAFT	NO GRAFT	SEPHADEX-E7	VacE7
3.1 - 3.10	NO GRAFT	10^7 NEK16	SEPHADEX-E7	VacE7
4.1 - 4.5	$5x10^5$ NEK16	10^7 NEK16	SEPHADEX-E7	VacE7

Figure 5. The establishment and maintenance of DTH attenuation in mice sub-optimally primed with NEK 16. Ear swelling was measured at days 22-25 with a micrometer and expressed as left ear thickness minus right ear thickness. 0.5nM TPA was applied to the left ear on day 23. Right ear thickness was measured on day 36 before injection with vacc-E7. The increase in right ear thickness was measured on days 37 and 38.

was observed in non-grafted animals but a strong DTH response was evident in mice grafted only with 10^7 NEK 16. Mice were then re-challenged 14 days after the SE7 inoculation by intra-dermal injection in the right ear with 2×10^7 pfu of vacc-E7. Mice sham grafted and challenged with SE7 displayed DTH reactivity on the second challenge with vacc-E7 indicating the priming effect of E7. Mice initially grafted with 10^7 NEK 16 as expected retained their response to E7 but in contrast the mice initially grafted with 5×10^5 NEK 16 remained unresponsive. We conclude that in these mice priming with low numbers of HPV-16 expressing cells resulted in immunological unresponsiveness to 3 challenges of E7 spanning a period of 31 days.

DISCUSSION

The observations reported here have important implications for human infection with HPV and for vaccination strategy. Cell mediated immunity has been implicated in the eradication of HSV[5,6], HPV[1,7] and recently HIV[8]. Some years ago it was suggested that HIV may evade elimination by the immune system by inducing "low zone" tolerance[9]. Our results support the concept that HPV evades immune eradication in sites such as the uterine cervix by inducing quiescence of the DTH effector response. HPV 6 E7 mRNA has been detected in the basal layer of low-grade squamous intra-epithelial lesions of the cervix[4], and since E7 has been shown to act as a tumour rejection antigen in a mouse model[10] the induction of immunological unresponsiveness to it would enable HPV-16 to persist and exert its oncogenic effects. Our evidence suggests that this unresponsiveness may be induced by presentation to the immune system of viral antigen in low concentrations. Higher concentrations of E7 do successfully induce DTH, a response consistent with observations in regressing warts[7], which reflect an effective host response to HPV infection. In some systems however excessive amounts of antigen may favour B-cell stimulation rather than DTH responses[11]. In designing strategies for immuno - intervention against HPV therefore, the amount of antigen presented to the immune system may be a critical factor in determining the overall clinical outcome.

ACKNOWLEDGEMENTS

Mark Chambers was supported by the Nita King studentship, the Harnett Fund (University of Cambridge) and the T'siao T'siao Fund, Downing College, Cambridge. Zhang Wei and Nicholas Coleman were supported by ICRF.

REFERENCES

1. C.S. McLean, J.C Sterling, J. Mowat, A.A. Nash and M.A. Stanley, Delayed hypersensitivity response to the human papillomavirus type 16 E7 protein in a mouse model, *J Gen Virol*. 74:239 (1993).

2. M.A. Chambers, W. Zhang, N. Coleman, A.A. Nash and M.A. Stanley, "Natural" presentation of human papillomavirus type 16 E7 protein to immunocompetent mice results in antigen-specific sensitisation or sustained unresponsiveness, *submitted for publication*.

3. M.H. Stoler, C.R. Rhodes, A. Whitbeck, S.M. Wolinsky, L.T. Chow and T.R. Broker, Human papillomavirus type 16 and 18 expression in cervical neoplasias, *Human Pathol.* 23:117 (1992).

4. G.D. Higgins, D.M. Uzelin, G.E. Phillips and C.J. Burrell, Presence and distribution of human papillomavirus sense and antisense transcripts in genital cancers, *J Gen Virol.* 72:885 (1991).

5. W.A. Anderson and E.D. Kilbourne, A herpes simplex skin test diagnostic of low protein antigen content from cell culture fluid, *J Invest Dermatol.* 37:25 (1961).

6. A.A. Nash, H.J. Field, P.G. Gell and P. Wildy, Cell mediated immunity in herpes simplex infected mice: induction, characterisation and anti-viral effects of delayed type hypersensitivity, *J Gen Virol.* 48:351 (1980).

7. S. Aiba, M. Rokugo and H. Tagami, Immunohistologic analysis of the phenomenon of spontaneous regression of numerous flat warts, *Cancer* 6:1246 (1986).

8. M. Clerici, F.T. Hakim, D.J. Venzon, C.W. Hendrix, T.A. Wynn and G.M. Shearer, Changes in interleukin-2 and interleukin-4 production in asymptomatic, human immunodeficiency virus-seropositive individuals, *J Clin Invest.* 91:759 (1993).

9. R.J. Sharpe and R.T. Schweitzer, The LAV/HTLV-III virus may evade elimination by the immune system by inducing low zone tolerance to itself, *Med Hypotheses* 20:421 (1986).

10. L.P. Chen, E.K. Thomas, S.L. Hu, I. Hellstrom and K.E. Hellstrom, Human papillomavirus type 16 nucleoprotein E7 is a tumour rejection antigen, *Proc Natl Acad Sci USA.* 88:110 (1991).

11. P.A. Bretscher, A strategy to improve the efficacy of vaccination against tuberculosis and leprosy, *Immunol Today* 13:342 (1992).

FINE CHARACTERIZATION OF THE HPV16 E7 49-57 TUMOR PROTECTIVE CYTOTOXIC T CELL EPITOPE "RAHYNIVTF"

Mariet C.W. Feltkamp[1,2], Michel P.M. Vierboom[1], Jan ter Schegget[2], Cornelis J.M. Melief[1], and W. Martin Kast[1]

[1]Department of Immunohematology & Blood Bank
University Hospital
Leiden PO Box 9600
2300 RC Leiden
The Netherlands
[2]Department of Virology
Academic Medical Centre
Meibergdreef 15
1100 AZ Amsterdam
The Netherlands

INTRODUCTION

Human papillomavirus (HPV) DNA, predominantly of the HPV16 genotype, can he detected in more than 90% of the human cervical carcinomas[1]. The "high risk" HPV types, including HPV16, are believed to play an important role in the pathogenesis of human cervical cancer. The ability of HPV16 to *in vitro* immortalize human keratinocytes[2] and the dependence on HPV16 expression for preservation of the transformed phenotype of cervical cancer-derived cell lines[3] suggests direct involvement of HPV 16 in the multi-step process of cervical carcinogenesis. Cervical cancer and other HPV-related cancers are more commonly seen in immunosuppressed individuals[4,5]. This suggests that proper immunosurveillance interferes with HPV-associated tumor development and that T cell immunity, in particular mediated by cytotoxic T lymphocytes (CTL), is important in the defense against virus induced tumors.

CTL recognize antigenic peptides (CTL epitopes) which are presented at the cell surface in the antigen-presenting cleft of an MHC class 1 molecule. This is the result of intracellular protein processing in which peptides, after degradation and stable complex formation with major histocompatibility complex (MHC) class 1 heavy and light chain (β_2-microglobulin), are transported to the cell surface[6]. A prerequisite for every peptide serving as a CTL epitope is therefore binding to an MHC class I molecule, which can be tested. With this knowledge proteins of interest can be screened for possessing potential CTL epitopes.

In a recent study[7] we generated all possible 9-mer peptides (n=240) overlapping by 8 amino acids (aa) from the HPV16 E6 and E7 protein sequences and tested those for their ability to bind to the murine MHC class 1 H-2K^b and D^b molecules making use of the antigen-processing defective cell line RMA-S[8]. Via this method we identified 5 "high" affinity K^b and/or D^b binders, among which the D^b binder E$_7$ 47-57 (RAHYNIVTF). We demonstrated that RAHYNIVTF is not only a class I binder but also a CTL epitope, since it induces CTL through peptide immunization of C57BL/6 (B6) mice (H-2^b haplotype) which lyse RAHYNIVTF-loaded syngeneic cells and, importantly, also lyse HPV16 transformed tumor cells. Moreover, RAHYNIVTF-immunized mice were resistant to a challenge with the same HPV16 tumor cells suggesting a CTL-mediated protective immune response against an HPV16 tumor[7].

For further knowledge and application it is important to know whether RAHYNIVTF is the precise CTL epitope. In general D^b molecules present naturally processed peptides of 9 aa in length[9]. However, since several exceptions to this rule have been described, one can not assume that the 9-mer RAHYNIVTF is the precise epitope on the basis of its length. Length requirements for a CTL epitope dictated by the antigen-presenting groove of an MHC class I molecule are very strict[10]. Only epitopes of the right length will bind optimally in the class I groove and effective use of peptides of sub-optimal length requires logs excess of peptide compared to the optimal length epitope[10]. We synthesized length-variants of the RAHYNIVTF peptide and tested those for their ability to bind to D^b. We demonstrate that, among these length-variants, RAHYNIVTF is the best D^b binder. Its sequence is compared with the described D^b specific peptide motif[11].

Furthermore, we addressed the question whether RAHYNIVTF, apart from a CTL response, also induces a T cell proliferative response because of a partial overlap with a previously identified epitope for T helper cells (T$_h$ epitope), HPV16 E$_7$ 48-54 (DRAHYNI)[12]. We did not observe proliferation *in vitro* against the 9-mer peptide - RAHYNIVTF indicating that RAHYNIVTF does not contain a T$_h$ epitope.

MATERIALS AND METHODS

Peptides and Immunization

Peptides were generated by solid phase strategies on a multiple peptide synthesizer (Abimed AMS 422) by repeated cycles in which addition of Fmoc protected amino acids to a resin of polystyrene was alternated with a Fmoc deprotection procedure. Peptides were cleaved from the resin and side chain protective groups were removed by treatment with aqueous TFA. Peptides were analyzed by reversed phase HPLC, lyophilized and dissolved in 0.5% DMSO in PBS before use. Once dissolved the peptides were stored at -70⁰C. When used for immunization, 100 μg (50 μl of 2 mg/ml peptide solution) peptide was extensively mixed with 50 μl complete Freund's adjuvant (CFA, Difco, Detroit Mi, USA). The 100 μl mixture was s.c. injected in the base of the tail in B6 mice which were held under specific pathogen free conditions.

The "RMA-S MHC Class I-Peptide-Binding Assay"

RMA-S cells were cultured for 36 hours at 26⁰C in culture medium in the presence of 2% human pool serum. Cells were washed twice in serum-free medium and filled out in 96 well U-bottom microtiter plates, 2.5×10^5 cells/well in serum-free medium. Peptides were added at the given concentrations. After a 4 hour incubation in a total volume of 50μl at 26⁰C, cells were washed in PBS supplemented with 0.5% BSA and 0.2% azide (further referred to as PBA) and incubated with mAb 28.14.8S (anti D^b)[13] for 30 minutes on ice. Cells were washed and incubated with FITC-labelled goat anti mouse F(ab')₂-fragments for 30 minutes on ice. Subsequently, cells were washed twice in PBA, suspended in PBA and transferred to tubes. Cell samples were analyzed in a FACscan^R flow cytometer (Becton Dickenson, Mountain View CA, USA) and the fluorescence index (mean channel number (MCN) in the presence of peptide minus MCN in the absence of peptide divided by the MCN in the absence of peptide) was calculated for each peptide.

T Cell Proliferation Assay

Ten days after immunization the inguinal lymph nodes were collected and made into a single cell suspension. The responder cells were filled out in a 96 well flat-bottom plates, 10^5/well. To each well was added 5×10^4 stimulator cells, the MHC class II⁺ B cell line of C57BL/10 origin (H-2^b) "771" [14], which were pre-incubated for 1 hour at room temperature with 2 times the given end concentration of peptide. After 4 days at 37⁰C, the cells were pulsed with 1μCi/well of ³H-labelled thymidine for 4 hours. Thymidine incorporation was measured on a Beta-plate® liquid scintillation counter (Wallac, Turku, Finland). The proliferation index (Pi) was calculated as follows: (cpm in the presence of peptide)-(cpm in the absence of peptide) divided by (cpm in the absence of peptide).

RESULTS

Recently we demonstrated that the 9-mer CTL epitope RAHYNIVTF is a "high" affinity D^b-binding peptide[7]. To establish whether RAHYNIVTF is the optimal length peptide for Db~binding we generated peptides around the RAHYNIVTF aa sequence varying in length between 20 and 8 aa. They were tested for binding to the "empty" Db molecules on RNA-S cells[8]. RMA-S cells were incubated with the peptides in titrated amounts from 100 µg to 0.1 ng/ml (10x dilution steps), and the level of D^b expression on the cell surface, a measure for D^b-binding[7], was analyzed by FACS. The results of a representative experiment are shown in Table 1, displayed as peptide concentrations resulting in a half maximum level of D^b expression ([1/2 max]). From this table we conclude that RAHYNIVTF has the relatively highest affinity for H-2D^b.

Table 1. Overview of the D^b-binding capacity of RAHYNIVTF length-variants.

HPV16 E7	aa sequence	[1/2 max], µg/ml [1]
43 – 62	GQAEPDRAHYNIVTFCCKCD	> 100
48 – 58	DRAHYNIVTFC	66
48 – 57	DRAHYNIVTF	3
49 – 58	RAHYNIVTFC	7
48 – 56	DRAHYNIVT	> 100
49 – 57	RAHYNIVTF	1
50 – 58	AHYNIVTFC	21
48 – 55	DRAHYNIV	> 100
49 – 56	RAHYNIVT	7
50 – 57	AHYNIVTF	> 100
51 – 58	HYNIVTFC	> 100

[1] Peptide concentration which results in half maximum D^b expression on RMA-S cells following peptide incubation.

Since the optimal length D^b-binder and CTL epitope RAHYNIVTF[7] partially overlaps with the T_h epitope DRAHYNI[12], we investigated whether RAHYNIVTF is capable of inducing a proliferative T cell response. We immunized B6 mice with 100 µg of the 20-mer peptide GQAEPDRAHYNIVTFCCKCD, a peptide against which a strong proliferative response can be measured *in vitro* when it is used for immunization *in vivo* [12]. After 10 days the inguinal lymph node cells were isolated and brought into culture in the presence of MHC class II$^+$ syngeneic stimulator cells pre-incubated with peptide. After a culture period of 4 days in the presence of peptide, T cell proliferation was assessed by measuring the incorporation of ^{3}H-labelled thymidine. The results are shown in Table 2.

Table 2. Peptide-specific proliferation of inguinal lymph node cells isolated from GQAEPDRAHYNIVTFCCKCD-immunized B6 mice.

Stim. cells[1] (+/-)	Peptides aa sequence	Peptide concentration, μg/ml				
		100	50	25	12.5	0
−	−					0,0
+	−					2,0
+	GQAEPDRAHYNIVTFCCKCD	22.1[2]	11.6	6.3	4.0	
+	DRAHYNIVTFC	3.4	2.7	2.8	2.8	
+	DRAHYNIVTF	1.6	3.0	3.3	2.8	
+	RAHYNIVTFC	2.9	3.3	3.0	3.2	
+	DRAHYNIVT	1.6	2.3	2.7	2.5	
+	RAHYNIVTF	3.1	3.1	3.7	2.9	
+	AHYNIVTFC	1.8	2.4	2.6	2.4	

[1] "771", a C57BL/10 (H-2^b) B cell line[14]. [2] Proliferation index (PI)

The inguinal lymph node cells from GQAEPDRAHYNIVTFCCKCD-immunized B6 mouse clearly proliferate *in vitro* in the presence of this 20-mer peptide in a concentration- dependent manner. However, the same responder cells do not proliferate against any of the other shorter peptides, including RAHYNIVTF. In conclusion, inguinal lymph node cells isolated from a GQAEPDRAHYNiVTFCCKCD-immunized B6 mouse do not proliferate against RAHYNIVTF whereas the same cells exhibit good proliferation against the control 20-mer GQAEPDRAHYNIVTFCCKCD.

DISCUSSION

Recently we have identified a 9-mer peptide from HPVI6, E7 49-57 RAHYNIVTF, which is a "high" affinity MHC class I D^{b}binder and acts as a CTL epitope when loaded on syngeneic target cells for CTL obtained from RAHYNIVTF-immunized B6 mice[7]. Additionally, RAHYNIVTF seems to be present as a naturally processed CTL epitope on HPVI6-transformed tumor cells, since these cells are lysed by RAHYNIVTF-directed CTL[7]. Finally, B6 mice immunized with RAHYNIVTF are protected against a tumor challenge with HPV 16-transformed cells[7]. The fine characterization of this CTL epitope is now carried out in this study with respect to peptide length required for optimal D^b binding and induction of T cell proliferation.

We tested length-variant peptides around RAHYNIVTF for binding to D^b. From Table 1 it is clear that from all the peptides tested RAHYNIVTF displays the lowest [1/2 max] and is therefore the best D^{b}binder among them. Since, in general, it is observed that the best MHC class I-binding peptide within a sequence harboring a CTL epitope is indeed the CTL epitope[10], it is very likely that the optimal D^b-binder RAHYNIVTF is also the optimal length CTL epitope. If RAHYNIVTF is therefore the naturally processed CTL epitope present on HPV16-expressing cells, as is suggested by *in vitro* lysis of HPV16 transformed cells by RAHYNIVTF-directed CTL[7], the F needs to be included as a C terminal anchor in the D^b allele-specific peptide motif[11].

Because of the partial overlap of CTL epitope E_7 49-57 RAHYNIVTF with the Th epitope E_7 48-54 DRAHYNI[12], we investigated whether RAHYNIVTF induced a proliferative response. Inguinal lymph node cells from B6 mice immunized with the 20-mer peptide GQAEPDRAHYNIVTFCCKCD were *in vitro* stimulated with RAHYNVTF length variants (Table 2). The three T_h sequence-containing peptides DRAHYNIVTFC, DRAHYNIVTF and DRAHYNIV did not induce T cell proliferation which, at first sight, seems to contradict with the data described by Tindle et al[12]. However, in that particular study proliferative responses were measured against the 19-mer peptide QAEPDRAHYNIVTFCCKCD and N- or C-terminal aa deletion-variants thereof. Using that strategy a "minimal T cell-proliferative epitope" was determined, E_7 48-54 DRAHYNi. In fact the DRAHYNI peptide itself was not used for proliferation induction.

On the basis of our study it is most unlikely that the 7-mer DRAHYNI itself will induce T cell proliferation, which is in concordance with the recently emerged principles for MHC class II-binding peptides. These peptides are found to be 12-24 aa long[15,16], supporting our observation that only the DRAHYNI-containing 20-mer peptide GQAEPDRAHYNIVTFCCKCD induced proliferation, in contrast to the shorter DRAHYNI containing peptides (Table 2).

Like the other short peptides, RAHYNIVTF did not induce a proliferative T cell response. it is therefore unlikely that RAHYNIVTF, apart from a CTL epitope, also harbors a T_h epitope. A reflection thereof could be the fact that we never observed peptide (including - GQAEPDRAHYNIVTFCCKCD)-specific T cell proliferation following immunization with RAHYNIVTF itself (data not shown). Taken these data together, we assume that upon vaccination with RAHYNIVTF only a CTL response is induced and that the observed *in vivo* protection against a tumor induced by HPV16-transformed cells following RAHYNIVTF immunization is at the account of the RAHYNIVTF-directed anti-tumor CTL response.

ACKNOWLEDGEMENTS

This study was supported by the Dutch Cancer Society (NKB) grant RUL 93-588. W. Martin Kast is a senior fellow of the Royal Netherlands Academy of Arts and Sciences.

REFERENCES

1. A.J.C. Van den Brule, J.M.M. Walhoomers, M. du Maine, P. Kenemans, and C.J.L.M. Meijer, Difference

in prevalence of human papillomavirus genotypes in cytomorphologically normal cervical smears is associated with a history of cervical intraepithelial neoplasia. *Int J Cancer* 48:404 (1991)

2. G. Pecoraro, D. Morgan, and V. Defendi, Differential effects of human papillomavirus type 6, 16, and 18 DNAs on immortalization and transformation of human cervical epithelial cells. *Proc Natl Acad Sci USA* 86: 563 (1989)

3. M. Von Knehel Doeberitz, T. Bauknecht, D. Bartsch, and H. zur Hausen, Influence of chromosomal integration on glucocorticoid-regulated transcription of growth-stimulating Papillomavirus genes E6 and E7 in cervical carcinoma cells. *Proc Natl Acad Sci USA* 88:1411 (1991)

4. M.1. Alloub, B.B.B. Barr, K.M. McLaren, I.W. Smith, M.ll. Bunney, and G.E. Smart, Human papillomavirus infection and cervical intraepithelial neoplasia in women with renal allografts. *Br Med J.* 298:153 (1989)

5. M. Laga, J.P. Icenogle, R. Marsella, A.T. Manoka, N. Nzila, R.W. Ryder, S.H. Vermund, W.L. Heyward, A. Nelson, and W.C. Reeves, Genital papillomavirus infection and cervical dysplasia - opportunistic complications of HIV infection. *Int J Cancer* 50: 45 (1992)

6. J.J. Monaco, A molecular model of MHC class-I-restricted antigen processing. *Immunol Today* 13:173-179 (1992)

7. M.C.W. Feltkamp, H.L. Smits, M.P.M. Vierboom, R.P. Minnaar, B.M. de Jongh, J.W. Drijfhout, J. ter Schegget, C.J.M. Melief, and W.M. Kast. Vaccination with cytotoxic T lymphocyte epitope containing peptide protects against a tumor induced by human papillomavirns type 16-transformed cells. *Eur J Immunol.* 23:2242 (1993).

8. H.-G. Ljunggren, C. Ohlen, P.Hoglund, L.Franksson, and K. Karre, The RMA-S lymphoma mutant; consequences of a peptide loading defect on immunological recognition and graft rejection. *Int J Cancer* Supplement 6: 38 (1991)

9. K. Falk, O. Rotschke, S. Stevanovic, G. Jung, and H.-G. Rammensee, Allele-specific motifs revealed by sequencing of self-peptides eluted from MHC molecules. *Nature* 351: 290 (1991)

10. T.N.M. Schumacher, M.L.H. De Bruijn, L.N. Vernie, W.M. Kast, C.J.M. Melief, J.J. Neefjes, and H.L. Ploegh, Peptide selection by MHC class I molecules. *Nature* 350: 703 (1991)

11. O. Rotschke, and K. Falk, Naturally-occurring peptide antigens derived from the MHC class-I-restricted processing pathway. *Immunol. Today* 12: 447 (1991)

12. R.W. Tindle, G.J.P. Fernando, J.C. Sterling, and I.H. Frazer, A "public" T-helper epitope of the E7 transforming protein of human papillomavirus 16 provides cognate help for several E7 B-cell epitopes from cervical cancer-associated human papillomavirus genotypes. *Proc Natl Acad Sci USA* 88: 5887 (1991)

13. K.Ozato, and D.H. Sachs, Monoclonal antibodies to Mouse MHC. 111. Hybridoma antibodies reacting to antigens of the H-2^b haplotype reveal genetic control of isotype expression. *J Immunol.* 126: 317 (1981)

14. E.J.A.M. Sijts, F. Ossendorp, E.A.M. Mengede, P.J. Van den Elsen, and C.J.M. Melief, An immunodominant MCF Murine Leukemia Virus-encoded CTL epitope, identified by its MHC class I binding motif, explains MuLV type specificity of MCF-directed CTL. *J Immunol.* in press.

15. A.Y. Rudensky, P. Freston-Huriburt, S.-C. Hong, A. Barlow, and C.A. Janeway, Sequence analysis of peptides bound to MHC class ll molecules. *Nature* 353: 622 (1991)

16. J.H.Brown, T.S Jardetski, J.C. Gorga, L.J. Stern, R.G. Urban, J.L. Strominger, and D.C. Wiley, Three dimensional study of the human class II histocompatibility antigen HLA-DR1. *Nature* 364: 33 (1993)

VACCINATION OF CATTLE WITH L2 PROTEIN PREVENTS BPV-4 INFECTION

G.M. McGarvie,[1] L.M. Chandrachud,[2] J.M. Gaukroger,[2] G.J. Grindlay,[1] B.W. O'Neil,[2] J.W. Baird,[2] E.R. Wagner,[1] W.F.H. Jarrett[2] and M.S. Campo[1]

[1]Beatson Institute for Cancer Research
CRC Beatson Laboratories
[2]Dept. of Veterinary Pathology, University of Glasgow
Garscube Estate
Glasgow, G61 1BD
UK

INTRODUCTION

Papillomaviruses can infect and cause tumours in both cutaneous and mucousal epithelia. The virus induced tumours can progress to squamous cell carcinoma, as in the case of HPV-16 associated cervical carcinoma (zur Hausen, 1991) and BPV-4 associated alimentary cancer in cattle (Campo & Jarrett, 1986). There is a requirement for prophylactic and therapeutic vaccines which would protect against infection and accelerate rejection of established tumours. Potential vaccines are now possible with the use of recombinant proteins. Vaccination studies are difficult in humans for several reasons and in addition little is known about the immune response to papillomavirus. We have used BPV-4 infection in cattle as a model system allowing the opportunity for vaccination studies using the early and late proteins of BPV-4 and analyses of the immune response. We have previously shown that vaccination with the E7 protein inhibits the development of papillomas and causes early rejection of papillomas (Campo et al, 1993). This is accompanied by an increase in E7 specific antibodies and T cells. We have now shown that immunisation with the late protein, L2, of BPV-4 gives virtually complete protection against BPV-4 infection (Campo et al, 1993). In this report we investigate the immune response to the L2 protein in vaccinated and unvaccinated cattle in order to understand the reason for the protective effect of L2.

METHODS

Production of Fusion Proteins

The early (E) E7 and late (L) L2 open reading frames (ORFs) were cloned in pGEX (Smith & Johnson, 1988) and in the pUR plasmid series (Ruther & Muller-Hill, 1983) to produce Glutathione-S-Transferase (GST) and β-galactosidase (βGal) fusion products respectively as described previously (Campo et al, 1993) (Figure 1a). Briefly the E7 recombinant [nucleotides (nt)652 to 1249] represents the E7 protein from amino acids (aa) -21 to 98. The L2 ORF (nt3987 to 5585) was cloned in its entirety representing aa -8 to 524 (L2w) and as three fragments, nt 4042 to 4610, nt 4610 to 4989 and nt 4989 to 5629 representing peptides from aa 11 to 200 (L2a), 201 to 326 (L2b) and 327 to 524 (L2c). The fusion peptides were partially purified by the preparation of inclusion bodies. βGal fusions were further purified by SDS-PAGE to be used as antigens in ELISA.

Vaccination

Vaccination with GST-E7 and GST-L2. The cattle were divided into two groups of 15 (groups 1 and 2) and one group (group 3) of 17 animals. Each animal in group 1 was given 1mg GST-E7 and 1mg total GST-L2 (L2w,a,b,c ratio 1:5:5:5) and each animal in group 2 was given 1mg GST-L2 in Freund's incomplete adjuvant (FIA). The vaccination was repeated 4 weeks later. Two weeks after boost all the animals were challenged with 10^{11} BPV-4 particles in the palate. The animals were examined every 3 to 4 weeks and the number and size of papillomas was determined. Blood was taken from each animal before vaccination, 4 weeks after the first vaccination, at challenge and 4, 7 and 11 weeks after challenge for immunological analysis.

Long Term Studies

Twelve vaccinated animals from group 1 and 2 above were kept for 1 year and then rechallenged with BPV-4

Vaccination with GST-L2 in Aluminium Gel

Cattle were divided into three groups of 12. Groups 1 and 2 were vaccinated with 1mg and 0.1mg GST-L2 (L2w,a,b,c) respectively in aluminium gel using a similar vaccination strategy and challenge as above.

ELISA

Microtitre plates were coated with 0.1 g βGal-L2w or 1 g L2a, b or c as indicated in coupling buffer (100mM $NaHCO_3$, 10mM EDTA, pH 9.6) at 4°C overnight. Plates were blocked with 10% goat serum, 5% non fat milk, 0.5% Tween in PBS for 1 hour at 37°C. Doubling dilutions of sera were added and incubated overnight at 37°C. Goat anti bovine IgG alkaline phosphatase (1:500) followed by an alkaline phosphatase substrate kit (Biorad) was used for detection and the plates were read at 405nm.

Neutralisation Assay

3×10^{11} particles of BPV-4 were incubated with sera from cattle at 4°C overnight then used to infect bovine foetal palatine tissue for 1 hour at 37°C. The tissue was implanted subcutaneously in the left flank of athymic nude mice. After 24 weeks the mice were sacrificed and implants were scored for the presence or absence of papillomas. Foetal calf serum (FCS) was used as a control.

RESULTS

Immunisation With The L2 Protein Prevents Papilloma Development

We have previously shown that the L2 protein of BPV-2 induced early rejection of fibropapillomas of the skin in cattle (Jarrett *et al*, 1991). We speculated that the L2 of BPV-4 may potentiate the effect of E7 if administered in combination. Fifteen animals were vaccinated with GST-E7 and GST-L2 and fifteen with GST-L2 alone then all animals including the control group were challenged with virus and examined for papillomas at 4, 7 and 11 weeks after challenge (Figure 1). In the control group most of the cattle progressed through the normal stages of papilloma development having several stage 2 and 3 lesions by 11 weeks after challenge. Five animals had few or no lesions but it is not unusual to find resistance in some animals as this is a common disease in Britain (Jarrett, 1985). Only 4 animals from the two vaccinated groups developed any lesions and two of them were clear by 7 weeks after challenge. The vaccinated animals were still papilloma free 44 weeks after challenge compared to controls which still had papillomas. Twelve of the vaccinated cattle were kept for one year and then rechallenged with BPV-4. Two of the animals had small papillomas 5 weeks after rechallenge but all were papilloma free by 7 weeks after challenge (data not shown). Vaccination with L2 alone or in combination with E7 gave almost complete protection from BPV-4 infection and this was almost certainly due to L2.

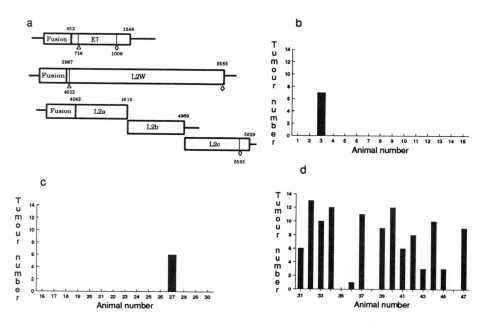

Figure 1. Development of papillomas. (a) fragments cloned in pUR and pGex, the triangle and diamond represent initiation and termination codons respectively. (b, c & d) Number of tumours in calves 11 weeks after challenge (b) group 1, E7 + L2 vaccine (c) group 2, L2 vaccine (d) group 3, controls.

In a second vaccination trial using L2 peptides only at 1mg and 0.1mg with aluminium gel as an adjuvant only one vaccinated animal developed any papillomas compared to 11 out of 12 in the control group (data not shown). L2 is therefore effective as a protective vaccine at lower doses and when administered in aluminium gel. This is relevant for human vaccine development as aluminium gel is an accepted adjuvant for human use.

L2 Specific Antibodies Are Present In The Sera Of Vaccinated Animals

Blood was taken from all the cattle before vaccination, 4 weeks after the first vaccination, 2 weeks after the second vaccination (challenge) and 4, 7 and 11 weeks after

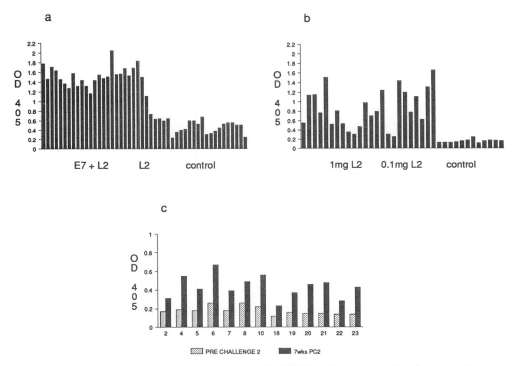

Figure 2. IgG response to L2w (a) Vaccination trial with GST-E7 & L2, sera from 7 weeks post challenge. (b) Vaccination trial with 1 & 0.1mg GST-L2 in aluminium gel, sera from 4 weeks post challenge. (c) Long term studies, sera from 7 weeks post 2nd challenge.

challenge and the sera was tested by ELISA for the presence of antibodies to the whole L2 protein (L2w). All the vaccinated animals had a high titre of antibodies to L2w (Figure 2). L2 specific antibodies were present before challenge increasing after challenge and decreased again by 11 weeks after challenge. L2 specific antibodies were not detected in the sera of cattle in the control groups. Vaccinated cattle that were rechallenged after 1 year were analysed for the presence of L2 specific antibodies at 5 and 7 weeks after the second challenge (Figure 2c). The presence of L2 specific antibodies indicates activation of the memory arm of the immune system.

The Majority Of L2 Antibodies Are Directed Against The C-Terminal

L2 has been cloned in three fragments to produce three fusion peptides, L2a, L2b and L2c (Figure 1a). These peptides were used as antigen in ELISA to identify if the response was directed to one part of the L2 protein. Sera from 6 animals were analysed. Figure 3 indicates that the majority of the cattle recognise L2c, the C-terminal portion of L2 (aa 327-524) with a small response against L2a, the N-terminal portion. The response to L2a was only seen at challenge and no animal responded to L2b, the middle portion of L2. This indicates that the major antibody epitope is contained within L2c.

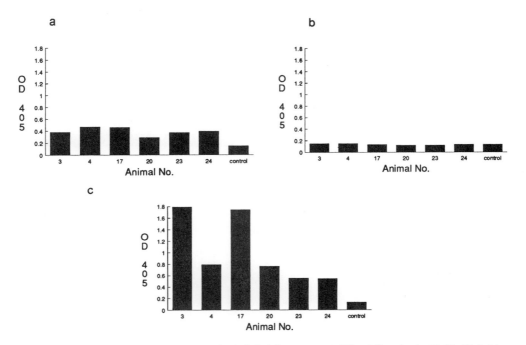

Figure 3. IgG response to L2 fragments, animals 3 & 4 from group 1 (E7 + L2), animals 17, 20, 23 & 24 from group 2 (L2). (a) L2a. (b) L2b. (c) L2c.

Vaccinated Animals Have Virus Neutralising Antibodies

BPV-4 infected bovine foetal palatine tissue implanted subcutaneously in athymic nude mice results in the development of papillomas at the site of implant. This system was used to determine the virus neutralising capability of sera from 4 vaccinated and 3 unvaccinated cattle at 7 weeks after challenge by incubating the virus with the sera prior to infection. Implants were scored for the presence or absence of a papilloma (Table 1). When foetal calf serum was used as a control, 4 out of 6 implants contained papillomas.

From 20 implants of tissue infected with BPV-4 after incubation with sera from vaccinated cattle none contained papillomas. This indicates that sera from the vaccinated cattle are capable of neutralising infectivity of BPV-4. Four out of twelve implants had papillomas using sera from 3 of the control cattle. Interestingly serum from a control animal (34) at 18 weeks after challenge, when the cow had several stage 3 papillomas, had virus neutralising activity. It has not been determined which viral protein the neutralising activity is directed against but these experiments show that vaccination with a recombinant protein can induce viral neutralisation.

Table 1. Neutralisation of BPV-4 in athymic mice

Vaccine	Bovine No.	Papillomas/ Implants	Total P/I
sera from 7 wks PC			
FCS		4/6	4/6
E7 + L2	1	0/4	
E7 + L2	3	0/4	
			0/20
L2	17	0/6	
L2	24	0/6	
control	36	1/3	
control	37	2/5	4/12
control	42	1/4	
serum from 18 wks PC			
control	34	0/6	0/6

DISCUSSION

We have demonstrated that vaccination of cattle with recombinant L2 protein of BPV-4 prior to challenge with BPV-4 is effective in preventing the development of papillomas in these animals. This can be achieved if the vaccine is administered using Freund's Incomplete Adjuvant or Aluminium gel as an adjuvant. Vaccination with two doses of 0.1mg GST-L2 is sufficient to protect the cattle and the cattle remain immune to viral infection for at least one year. The sera of vaccinated cattle all have a high titre of antibodies to L2 as determined by ELISA. Using the 3 fragments of L2, a,b and c, indicates the majority of this response is directed against the C-terminal portion of the protein with a small response against the N-terminal portion. Whether the C-terminal peptide (L2c) is sufficient to protect the cattle is currently being determined. Antibodies in the sera from vaccinated cattle are virus neutralising as demonstrated by the nude mouse xenograft system. L2 is the minor capsid protein and there is evidence that part of it is exposed on the surface of the virion and it is probable that the neutralising activity is directed against this portion of the protein. Other studies looking at CRPV infection in rabbits demonstrated that recombinant L2 protein of CRPV could protect rabbits from CRPV infection (Christensen *et al*, 1991; Lin *et al*, 1992). Virus neutralising antibodies could be generated by vaccinating rabbits with L2. The fact that two animal model systems both using natural host and virus can be protected against viral infection by recombinant L2 protein has strong implications for HPV L2 having a protective effect against HPV.

REFERENCES

Campo, M.S. and Jarrett, W.F.H.,1986, Papillomavirus infection in cattle: viral and chemical cofactors in naturally occurring and experimentally induced tumours,*in*: Papillomaviruses, Ciba foundation symposium. 120:117-135, ed. D. Evered and S. Clark, John Wiley, New York.

Campo, M.S., Grindlay,G.J., O'Neil, B.W., Chandrachud, L.M., McGarvie, G.M. and Jarrett, W.F.H., 1993, Prophylactic and therapeutic vaccination against a mucosal papillomavirus, *Journal of General Virology* 74:945-953.

Christensen, N.D., Kreider, J.W., Kan, N.C. and DiAngelo,S.L., 1991, The open reading frame L2 of cotton tail rabbit papillomavirus contains antibody-inducing neutralising epitopes, *Virology* 181:572-579.

Jarrett, W.F.H., 1985, The natural history of bovine papillomavirus infection, *in*:Advances in Viral Oncology, vol 5:83-102, ed. G.Klein, Raven Press, New York.

Jarrett, W.F.H., Smith, K.T., O'Neil, B.W., Gaukroger, J.M., Chandrachud, L.M., Grindlay, G.J., McGarvie, G.M. and Campo, M.S., 1991, Studies on vaccination against papillomaviruses: prophylactic and therapeutic vaccination with recombinant structural proteins, *Virology* 184:33-42.

Lin, Y-L., Borenstein, L.A., Selvakumar, R., Ahmed, R. and Wettstein, F.O., 1992, Effective vaccination against papilloma development by immunization with L1 or L2 structural proteins of cottontail rabbit papillomavirus, *Virology* 187:612-619.

Ruther, U. and Muller-Hill, B., 1983, Easy identification of cDNA clones, EMBO *Journal*, 2:1791-1794.

Smith, B.D. and Johnson, K.S., 1988, Single step purification of polypeptides expressed in *Escherichia coli* as fusions with glutathione-s-transferase, *Gene* 67:31-40.

zur Hausen, H., 1991, Human papillomaviruses in the pathogenisis of anogenital cancer, *Virology* 9-13.

IMMUNE RESPONSES TO HPV 16 E7

Merilyn H. Hibma, M. Tommasino, G. Van Nest[1], S.J. Ely, M. Contorni[2],
R. Rappuoli[2] and L.V. Crawford

ICRF Tumour Virus Group,
Department of Pathology,
University of Cambridge,
Cambridge CB2 1QP,
UK
[1]Chiron Corporation,
Emeryville,
USA
[2]IRIS,
via Fiorentina 1,
53100 Siena,
Italy

INTRODUCTION

There is a strong association between the presence of HPV DNA and the
transformation of cervical tissue to malignancy. This link provides a rare opportunity to
target a tumour immunologically through specific proteins of the causal agent. Proteins
involved in transformation are linked to the malignant phenotype and are therefore likely
to be maintained in tumours.

We chose to look at the immune response to the transforming protein E7 to
determine whether immunisation with this protein could elicit a protective response
against HPV16 expressing target cells.

Immunology of Human Papillomaviruses
Edited by M.A. Stanley, Plenum Press, New York, 1994

MATERIALS AND METHODS

The complete E7 protein encoding ORF of HPV16 was expressed in the fission yeast *Schizosaccharomyces pombe*[1]. This protein was previously shown to have a phosphorylation pattern identical to that of protein expressed in higher eukaryotes[2]. Urea solubilised E7 extracted from mechanically disrupted yeast cells was purified on hydroxyapatite. The urea was then removed by dialysis from E7 containing fractions.

Baby mouse kidney cells (BMK) derived from Balb/c mice were transformed with both myc and the entire HPV16 genome. Expression of the E7 ORF was confirmed in these cells by immunoprecipitation. The tumour forming dose was determined to be 5×10^4 cells injected subcutaneously (sc).

Groups of eight Balb/c mice were immunised with purified yeast E7. Animals received a single dose sc of either 0μg, 10μg or 50μg of E7, with Freund's Complete Adjuvant (FCA) or 0μg or 50μg of E7 with adjuvant MF59[3]. After 7 weeks, a second dose of an equal amount was administered by the same route. Animals immunised with FCA received the second immunisation with Freund's Incomplete adjuvant (FIA). Fourteen weeks following the primary immunisation, animals were challenged with 5×10^4 HPV16/myc BMK cells, sc on the flank. Mice were bled 6 weeks following the primary immunisation and three weeks following the secondary immunisation. Serum IgM and IgG antibody responses to E7 were measured by ELISA and tumour development was noted.

The effect of time between immunisations was determined in a second experiment. Mice were immunised at four or seven week intervals between primary and secondary immunisations and challenge. A further comparison was made between intraperitoneal (ip) and sc immunisations in the seven week group.

To characterise the effect of the route of immunisation on protection, groups of 8 mice were immunised at four weekly intervals with 0, 25 or 50μg E7 in MF59, either ip or sc. Four weeks following the second boost, mice were challenged with tumour cells.

RESULTS

The amount and class of antibody produced in response to E7 in mice was dependent on both protein dose and the adjuvant used. Animals immunised with FCA had weak IgM responses, in contrast to MF59 which stimulated primarily IgM (Fig. 1). The serum IgG response to E7 was poor in the presence of MF59, although good IgG responses were induced using FCA and E7 (Fig. 2). The larger protein dose in FCA immunised animals induced significantly greater levels of IgG late in the response.

Mice in the FCA immunised groups were equally susceptible to tumour challenge (Table 1). Animals immunised ip with the adjuvant MF59 and E7 showed a delay in the onset of tumour development.

Where mice had been immunised with MF59 and E7 sc at either four or seven weekly intervals, there was no difference total numbers of tumours developed (Table 2). There was however some indication of protection against challenge in mice that were immunised ip.

Table 1. Effect of immunisation with E7 on tumour development.
Groups of eight mice immunised with E7 in either MF59 or FCA/FIA were challenged with 5×10^4 HPV16/myc BMK cells, subcutaneously. Mice were killed when tumours reached 1cm in any dimension and the time following challenge was noted.

	Mean survival time (weeks)	Final no. of animals with tumours at 10 weeks
0μg E7+FCA/FIA	4.2±0	8
10μg E7+FCA/FIA	4.2±0	8
50μg E7+FCA/FIA	4.2±0	8
0μg E7+MF59	5.7±0.7	6
50μg E7+MF59	8.8±4.7	5

Table 2. The effect of immunisation with E7 in MF59 on protection against subsequent tumour challenge.
Groups of 8 mice were immunised subcutaneously with no protein or E7 and MF59 at either 7 week intervals or at 4 week intervals. Mice were challenged either 4 weeks or 7 weeks following the second immunisation and the number of mice with tumours was assessed 8 weeks following challenge.

	7 week intervals	4 week intervals	7 week intervals
	sc	sc	ip
0μg E7+MF59	6	6	NT
50μg E7+MF59	7	6	3

On repeating the comparison between routes of immunisation with MF59 and E7 with four weekly intervals between immunisations and challenge, mice immunised ip were better protected against subsequent challenge than those immunised sc (Table 3). Antibody responses in protected mice were characterised by low IgG (Fig. 3) and when IgG was detected it was predominantly of the IgG2a subclass (Table 4).

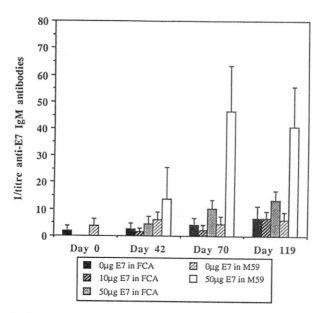

Figure 1. Serum antibody responses to immunisation with E7 in either FCA/FIA or MF59.
Peripheral blood was removed from mice one week prior to and 3 weeks following secondary immunisation and 3 weeks following challenge with tumour cells. Serum IgM was measured by ELISA at these times.

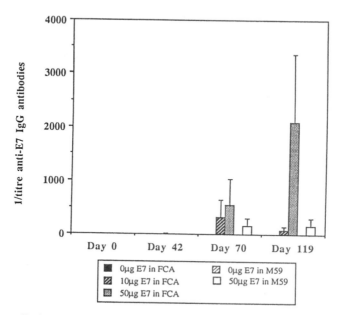

Figure 2. Serum antibody responses to immunisation with E7 in either FCA/FIA or MF59.
Peripheral blood was removed from mice one week prior to and 3 weeks following secondary immunisation and 3 weeks following challenge with tumour cells. Serum IgG was measured by ELISA at these times.

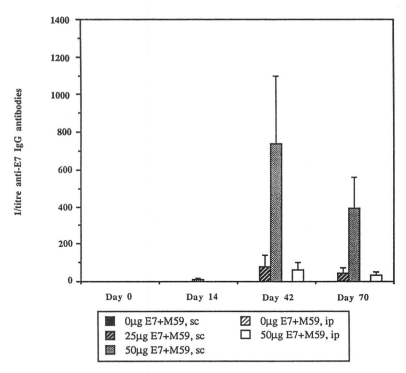

Figure 3. Serum antibody responses to immunisation with E7 and MF59 either subcutaneously or intraperitoneally.

Mice were sampled 2 weeks following primary immunisation, 2 weeks following secondary immunisation and 2 weeks following challenge. Serum IgG was measured by ELISA at these times.

Table 3. The effect of route of immunisation with E7 in MF59 on protection against subsequent tumour challenge.

Groups of eight mice were immunised either intraperitoneally or subcutaneously with no protein or E7 and MF59 at 4 week intervals. They were challenged 4 weeks following the second immunisation and the number of mice that had developed tumours 8 weeks following challenge was assessed.

	sc immunisation	ip immunisation
0μg E7+MF59	4	4
25μg E7+MF59	3	NT
50μg E7+MF59	4	0
0μg E7+no adjuvant	5	NT

Table 4. The Relationship between Ig Class and Tumour Development in mice immunised with E7 and MF59 sc.

Serum IgG, IgG1 and IgG2a antibodies against E7 were measured in mice immunised with E7 and MF59 either intraperitoneal or subcutaneously.

Animal No.	Route	IgG	IgG1	IgG2a	Tumour
21	sc	+(weak)	+	-	+
22	sc	-	-	-	+
23	sc	+	+/-	+	-
24	sc	+	+	+	-
25	sc	+	+	+	-
26	sc	+	NT	NT	+
27	sc	+	+	+	-
28	sc	-	-	-	+
53	ip	+(weak)	-	-	-
54	ip	-	-	-	-
55	ip	+	+	-	-
56	ip	+(weak)	+	-	-
57	ip	+	-	+	-
58	ip	+	-	-	-
59	ip	-	-	-	-
60	ip	+(weak)	+	-	-

DISCUSSION

Immunisation with yeast expressed E7 can generate both IgM and IgG antibodies specific for that protein. Although sc immunisation with protein and FCA generated good IgG titres, these animals were not protected against challenge with the tumorigenic cell line. In contrast, sc immunisation with MF59 and protein stimulated a stronger IgM response and these animals were partially protected against tumour challenge. The immunisation of animals with protein and MF59 ip conferred greater protection against challenge than the same dose and adjuvant sc.

An association has been established between the secretion of IgG1 antibodies by B cells activated by Th2 cells and IgG2a and Th1 cell activation[4]. Results presented here indicate that protection was high in groups where class switch was low. Further, IgG2a was measured in protected animals immunised sc, indicating involvement of the Th1 cell lineage. Although the possibility of involvement of other cell populations such as cytotoxic T lymphocytes mustn't be discounted, clones of the Th1 lineage can kill appropriate target cells[5] and may do so in this case. The absence of IgG2a in the majority of protected animals immunised ip may relate to the sensitivity of the assay, rather than an absence of activation of Th1 cells.

The selective activation of Th1 and Th2 cell populations may depend on the type of antigen presenting cell stimulated. There is some evidence to suggest that dendritic cells stimulate Th1 whereas B cells activate Th2 cells. Clearly this may be influenced by the route of immunisation and could account for the marked effect that route of immunisation has on protection.

We must now further this study by directly examining the effector cell population involved in this protective response.

ACKNOWLEDGEMENTS

The authors gratefully acknowledge the assistance of the ICRF Animal Unit in these experiments.

REFERENCES

1. Tommasino, M., Contorni, M., Scarlato, V., Bugnoli, M., Maundrell, K., and Cavalieri, F., Synthesis, phosphorylation, and nuclear localisation of human papillomavirus E7 protein in *Schizosaccharomyes pombe*, *Gene*, 93:265 (1990)

2. Tommasino, M., Corntorni, M., and Cavalieri, F., HPV16 E7 phosphorylation in fission yeast: characterisation and biological effects, *Gene*, 111:93 (1992)

3. Van Nest, G., K.S. Steimer, N.L. Haigwood, R.L. Burke and G. Ott., Advanced adjuvant formulations for use with recombinant subunit vaccines. In: Vaccines '92. Modern Approaches to New Vaccines. Eds. R.M. Chanock, R.A. Lerner, F. Brown and H. Ginsburg. Cold Spring Harbor Laboratories, Cold Spring Harbor, N.Y., pp. 57-62 (1992).

4. Sandor, M., Gajewski, T., Thorson, J., Kemp, J., Fitch, F., and Lynch, R., CD4+ Murine T cell clones that express high levels of immunoglobulin binding belong to the interleukin 4-producing T helper cell type 2 subset, *J Exp Med.*, 171:2171 (1990)

5. Bottomly, K., A functional dichotomy in CD4+ T lymphocytes, *Immunol Today* 9:268 (1988).

USE OF DOUBLE *ARO SALMONELLA* MUTANTS TO STABLY EXPRESS HPV16 E7 PROTEIN EPITOPES CARRIED BY HBV CORE ANTIGEN

Patricia Londoño,[1] Robert Tindle,[3] Ian Frazer,[3] Steve Chatfield,[2] and Gordon Dougan[1]

[1]Department of Biochemistry
Imperial College of Science, Technology and Medicine
London SW7 2AY
UK
[2]Vaccine Research Unit
Medeva Group Research
Imperial College of Science, Technology and Medicine
London SW7 2AY
UK
[3]Lions Immunology Laboratory
Princess Alexandra Hospital
Brisbane
Queensland
Australia

INTRODUCTION

Attenuated *Salmonella* strains have been used as vectors for delivering antigens from other pathogens via the oral route[1]. These organisms are particularly efficient in eliciting mucosal responses as well as cellular and humoral responses against the heterologous antigen. Among the characterised of these attenuated *Salmonella* strains are genetically engineered *aro* mutants which are defective in one more of the genes required for the synthesis of aromatic compounds, including para-aminobenzoic acid and aromatic

Immunology of Human Papillomaviruses
Edited by M.A. Stanley, Plenum Press, New York, 1994

amino acids[2]. *S.typhimurium aro*A, *aro*D double mutants have been used as carriers to deliver a variety of heterologous antigens to the mammalian immune system. Examples are the P.69 Pertactin antigen of *Bordetella pertussis*[3] and tetanus toxin fragment C. The nucleocapsid of the Hepatitis B Virus (HBV), also known as **core** antigen, is a complex polymer made up of approximately 180 copies of a single 21KDa polypeptide which spontaneously assemble together into 27 nm diameter particles[5]. In spite of being internal viral antigens, the particles are very powerful humoral and cellular immunogens[6]. An important feature of the core particles is their ability to provide T helper determinants for B lymphocytes directed against epitopes of other molecules physically linked to them[7,8]. This carrier ability has been exploited for eliciting immune responses against peptide sequences from different viruses. Chimeric core particles with inserted heterologous epitopes from human rhino virus, HBV, HIV and murine cytomegalovirus have been successfully used to elicit B and T cell responses in mice (for a review see 9). The strongest antibody responses were obtained when insertions were made in an immunodominant region of the protein known as the **e1 loop**. This region is thought to be an exposed loop structure accessible to the immune system in the surface of the core particle[10].

The E7 protein of Human Papilloma Virus has been considered a target for developing a vaccine against HPV-associated cervical cancer in women. This protein contains B and T cell epitopes which have been mapped by different research groups with very consistent results[11,12]. We have chosen an immunodominant region of the HPV16 E7 protein to express it in a double *aro Salmonella* mutant as an insertion within the e1 loop of HBV core particles. This construct will allow us to test the feasibility of immunising animals against papilloma virus using an E7 protein peptide. The initial results towards this aim are summarised in this paper.

RESULTS

Cloning of the HPV16 E7 Peptide into the HBV Core Antigen Gene using a *Salmonella* Vector

Plasmid pGA was constructed to express the full length HVB core antigen gene in *Salmonella*. It is a pAT153 derivative which carries a copy of the core antigen gene under the control of a modified ***nir*B** promoter. The wild type *nir*B promoter, belongs to a family of promoters associated with the regulation of nitrite metabolism. *Nir*B is activated by nitrites in the environment as well as by anaerobic conditions. This promoter has been successfully used in *Salmonella* to drive the expression of heterologous antigens *in vivo*[4]. Presumably it can be switched on by signals such as the low oxygen tension found intracellular environments within host tissues. The use of inducible promoters such as *nir*B results in a more stable expression of the antigen.

The sequence of the HPV16 E7 peptide chosen for this study comprised 21 amino acid residues, which corresponded to residues number 35 to 54 of the protein sequence: EDEIDGPAGQAEPDRAHYNI (single letter aminoacid code). To insert this peptide into the core antigen gene, a pair of 72 nucleotide-long sense and antisense oligonucleotides, encoding these amino acid residues, were synthesised. NheI compatible sequences were engineered at both ends of the oligonucleotides so that they could be inserted into the unique Nhe I site of pGA. This restriction site is located in a region which encodes the e1 loop. The resulting plasmid, depicted in Figure 1, was named pGAE716.

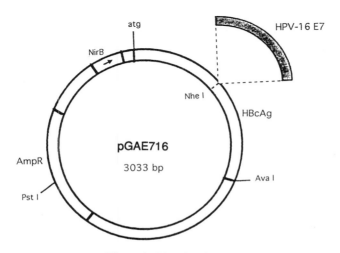

Figure 1. Plasmid pGAE716.

Expression of Core Antigen Recombinant Molecules Containing Epitopes from the HPV E7 Protein

Plasmids pGA and pGAE716 were electroporated into **S.typhimurium** BRD 509, an *aro*A *aro*D double mutant[3], to produce strains BRD969 and BRD974 respectively. Expression of both core antigen and the chimeric E7/core antigen occurred when the transformed *Salmonella* was growing under low oxygen tension in a liquid media. Bacteria transformed with pGAE716 produced a distinct polypeptide of the expected molecular weight which reacted with two murine monoclonal antibodies produced against HPV16 E7, namely 4F and 6D. These antibodies recognised two different determinants within the cloned peptide sequence[12] (Data not shown).

Plasmid Stability and Persistence of *Salmonella* Strains BRD969 and BRD974 in BALB/c Mice

Groups of female BALB/c mice (6 week old) were immunised with a single dose of either BRD509, BRD969 or BRD974. Each animal received an inoculum of 10^{10} *Salmonella* by the oral route. On days 7 and 14, four mice from each group were sacrificed to evaluate the ability of the *Salmonella* to invade the host reticuloendothelial system. The numbers of viable bacteria present in Peyer's patches, mesenteric lymph nodes, livers and spleens were enumerated. Table 1 shows the estimated results of the total number of *Salmonella* found on each organ, based on viable counts carried out in LB plates with and without ampicillin.

These results show that both BRD969 and BRD974 were able to colonise all organs examined with similar efficiency as BRD509, the parental strain. On the other hand, they indicate that on average 100% of the *Salmonella* recovered from organs of animals inoculated with bacteria harbouring either of the two plasmids was resistant to ampicillin. Therefore neither pGA nor pGAE716 seem to be significantly segregated from the transformed bacteria during the host invasion process.

Table 1. Growth of *S.typhimurium* in the organs of mice following oral inoculation.

STRAIN	DAY/ MEDIA	LOG10 VIABLE ORGANISMS/ORGAN (2SE)			
		PEYER PATCHS.	MESENT LMPH NDS.	SPLEEN	LIVER
BRD509	7 LB	4.3(2.0)	2.8(0.8)	2.1(1.5)	2.8(2.0)
	14 LB	2.7(1.5)	2.5(1.5)	0.8(1.0)	0.1(0.2)
BRD969	7 LB	3.0(2.7)	2.0(0.9)	3.4(3.2)	3.1(0.9)
	7 AMP	3.0(2.4)	2.6(2.4)	2.9(3.4)	3.0(1.0)
	14 LB	2.0(0.9)	2.5(0.4)	1.1(1.7)	1.0(1.2)
	14 AMP	2.5(1.7)	2.0(0.6)	0.9(1.8)	0.8(1.1)
BRD974	7 LB	2.5(3.2)	1.5(1.7)	1.6(2.4)	1.2 2.8)
	7 AMP	2.5(3.2)	1.9(0.5)	1.4(2.5)	1.1(2.8)
	14 LB	1.4(1.8)	2.0(0.9)	1.2(0.7)	1.0(1.2)
	14 AMP	2.3(0.8)	2.0(0.7)	0.8(1.5)	0.9(1.2)

CONCLUSIONS

Epitopes of the E7 papilloma protein can be inserted in the e1 loop of the HBV core antigen and expressed in *Salmonella aro* mutants using the nirB promoter. The antigenicity of the epitopes is retained when expressed as part of the core polypeptide, as demonstrated by its reactivity with anti E7 monoclonal antibodies. When used to orally immunise mice, the *S.typhimurium aroA, aroD* mutant expressing the HPV16 E7/ HBV core construct can invade and persist in host tissues. This should facilitate the production of an immune response against the E7 peptide. The immune response against this construct is at present being investigated.

REFERENCES

1. S. Chatfield, R.A. Strugnell, and G. Dougan, Live *Salmonella* as vaccines and carriers of foreign antigenic determinants, *Vaccine* 7: 495 (1989).

2. S.K. Hoiseth, and B. Stocker, Aromatic-dependent *Salmonella typhimurium* are non-virulent and effective as live vaccines, *Nature* 291:238, (1981).

3. R. Strugnell, G. Dougan, S. Chatfield, I. Charles, N. Fairweather, J. Tite, J.L. Li, J. Beesley, and M. Roberts, Characterisation of a *Salmonella typhimurium aro* vaccine strain expressing the P.69 antigen of *Bordetella pertussis, Infect Immun.* 60:3994, (1992).

4. S. Chatfield, I. Charles, A. Makoff, M. Oxer, G. Dougan, D. Pickard, D. Slater, and N. Fairweather, Use of the *nir*B promoter to direct the stable expression of heterologous antigens in *Salmonella* oral vaccine strains: Development of a single-dose oral tetanus vaccine, *Bio-Technology* 10: 888, (1992).

5. A. Budkowska, S.J. Wai-kuo, J.L. Gerin, Immunochemistry and polypeptide composition of hepatitis B core antigen (HBcAg), *J Immunol.* 118:1300, (1977).

6. K. Murray, S.A. Bruce, A. Hinne, Hepatitis B virus antigen made in microbial cells immunises against viral infection, *EMBO J.* 3:645, (1984).

7. D.R. Millich, A. McLachlan, A. Moriarty, Immune response to hepatitis B virus core antigen (HBcAg): Localisation of T-cell recognition sites within HBcAg/HBeAg, *Immunology* 139:1223, (1987).

8. B.E. Clarke, A.R. Carroll, M.J. Francis, Chimeric proteins based on hepatitis B core antigen form highly immunogenic particles, in:"Vaccines 89," H. Ginsberg, F. Brown, R.A. Lerner, R.M. Chanock (eds), Cold Spring Harbor Laboratory, New York, (1988).

9. M.J. Francis, Use of hepatitis B core as a vehicle for presenting viral antigens, *Rev Human Biol.* 1:62, (1992).

10. P. Arogs, and S. Fuller, A model for the hepatitis B core protein: prediction of antigenic sites and relationship to RNA virus capsid proteins, *EMBO J.* 7:819, (1988).

11. S. Comerford, D.J. McCance, G. Dougan, and J. Tite, Identification of B anti-cell epitopes of the E7 protein of human papillomavirus type 16, *J Virol.* 65:4681, (1991).

12. R.W. Tindle, J. Smith, H.Geysen, L. Selvey, and I. Fraser, Identification of B epitopes in human papillomavirus type 16 E7 open reading frame protein, *J Gen Virol.* 71:1347, (1990).

AN EXPERIMENTAL TETRACYCLIN AND VITAMIN A THERAPY OF HPV INFECTIONS OF THE LOWER FEMALE GENITAL TRACT

J. Madej, A. Basta, J. G. Madej Jr. and M. Strama

Department of Gynecology and Oncology
Collegium Medicum
Jagiellonian University
23 Kopernika Street
Cracow
Poland

Papilloma lesions of the lower female genital tract (LFGT) belong to the group of sexually transmitted diseases. Four stages of papilloma lesions are distinguished, i.e. papilloma lesions non-suspected of CIN or cancer, papilloma lesions suspected of CIN or cancer; they both are visible as proliferative forms. There are also subclinical lesions, usually suspected of CIN in colposcopic evaluation, and the so-called latent lesions with no colposcopic pattern and only with positive virological tests and/or koilocytosis[1,2,3]. The purpose of this paper is the introduction of our results of experimental oral tetracyclin and vitamin A treatment of these lesions.

A stimulus for this clinical trial was the suggestion that chlortetracyclin hydrochloride is effective against the so-called "large" viruses, and vitamin A plays a leading role in the processes of differentiation and maturation of squamous epithelium [4,5,6].

Initially we used only chlortetracyclin hydrochloride, and subsequently tetracyclin hydrochloride with the addition of vitamin A. The combination was employed only in clinical forms of papilloma, usually called condyloma, after colposcopy, cytology and when necessary after a histological evaluation.

Table 1. Type of HPV infection and localisation within LFGT - treatment with Teracycline and vitamin A after 1988 (N=206)

LOCALIZATION	OVERT	TYPE OF INFECTION		
		Subclinical forms	Latent	HPV infection and intraepithelial neoplasia
Cervix	12	38	24*	46
Vagina	18	4		2
Vulva	24	2		6
Multifocal	24	3		3
Total	78	47	24	57

*In cervical/vaginal smears there were noted koilocytes. IPR and/or hybridization tests were positive.

After 1988, the diagnostic procedure was complemented by virological tests, immunoperoxidase reaction and/or HPV DNA typing test. Auroemycine was used for the first time with a positive reaction in papilloma vulvae of a girl [7]. This result stimulated us to continue the clinical trial with the additional use of Vitamin A. It appeared that good results were obtained only when the drugs were administered orally. In this way we further treated 72 women with clinical lesions, and 5 men - sexual partners of infected women, with penile and/or anal region papilloma lesions [2,8,9]. Satisfactory results were obtained in 62 women and in all the men. As it followed from our observations, the best results were achieved after 1-3 series of treatment applied with a monthly interval after each one. One series consisted of 6.0-8.0 Tetracyclin and fifty 12,000 I.U. capsules of vitamin A, administered twice a day. The lesions disappeared as early as 2 weeks, and the latest 3-4 months after treatment.

After 1988, this therapy was employed in all the cases of typical papilloma (condyloma) lesions, papilloma subclinical lesions, latent lesions, and exceptionally in cases with coexistence of CIN 1-2 (Table 1). All other cases, i.e. with histologically confirmed CIN 3 and typical papilloma lesions containing HPV type 16/18 especially within the cervix, were treated by conisation and in exceptional cases by cryosation. The presented material did not include cases on concomitant *Chlamydia trachomatis* infections. Completed regression of lesions after tetracyclin and vitamin A treatment was noted in 53 (67.9%) of patients belonging to our stages I and II, i.e. with over papillomas; in 34 (72%) cases of subclinical forms, and in 18 (75%) cases of latent lesions. In comparison with the group of untreated cases, only the results in stage IV were statistically insignificant.

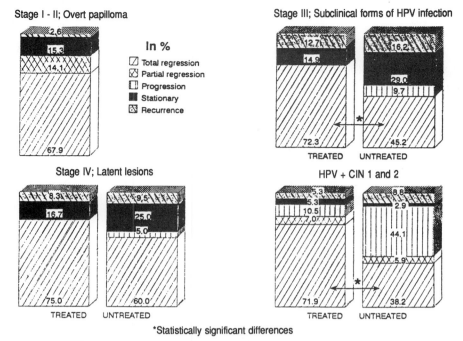

Figure 1. Tetracycline and Vitamin A Treatment After 1988.

Finally we determined also the statistically significant regression of CIN 1-2 concomitant with HPV infections in cervical lesions. Our results confirm the opinion of Grub[5] and Basta[6] that vitamin A deficiency is a possible factor in the development of CIN in cases of HPV infections.

Summing up, it can be concluded that tetracyclin and vitamin A therapy is successful in selected cases of clinical papilloma and in subclinical stages of HPV Infections within LFGT, especially of the cervix. This therapy brings about the regression of CIN, VAIN and VIN of lower grades in cases of their coexistence with HPV infections. Therefore, this treatment of papillomas may be also recognized as prophylaxis of CIN of LFGT.

REFERENCES

1. J. Madej, Das Problem der Papillomavirus-Entstehung und der Veränderung an der Portio, in: "Beller=Graef-Seitzer Gegensätzliche Auffasungen in der Geb. u. Gynäk", HUF-V, Mühlheim (1988).

2. J. Madej, A. Basta, J.G. Madej Jr. and M. Strama, Colposcopy staging and treatment of papillomavirus infection of the cervix, Clin Exp Obst Gyn., 19:34 (1992).

3. J. Madej, A. Basta, J.G. Madej Jr. and M. Strama, Colposcopy findings of HPV infection of lower genital tract, in:: "XVI Int. Ain Shams Med. Congress, Infection and Diseases, Cairo, p. 175 (1993).

4. J. K. Podlewski and A. Chwalibogowska-Podlewska, Medicaments of contemporary therapy, (in Polish), PZWL, Warszawa, (1990).

5. G. S. Grubb, Human papillomavirus and cervical neoplasia, Int J Epidem., 1:15 (1986).

6. A. Basta, The association of human papilloma virus infections, blood serum vitamin A level and cervical intraepithelial neoplasia, *in:* 7th World Congress of Cervical Pathology and Colposcopy, Inter. Publ. *in: Med Scien Tech.*, Parthenon Publishing Group Ltd., Lancs, UK (1992).

7. J. Madej et al., Papilloma vulvae with a colposcopy picture similar to squamous-cells carcinoma in a child, (in Polish), *Przegl Lek.*, 25:374 (1969).

8. J. Madej, Successful trial treatment of condyloma acuminatum with chlortetracyclin, *Przegl Lek.*, 25:758, (1969).

9. J. Madej and A. Loster, Spitze Kondylome - Tetracyclin und Vitamin A haben auch Erfolg, *Med Trib.*, 42:23 (1984).

RETINOIDS AND IFNα SYNERGISTICALLY DECREASE TUMOR CELL-INDUCED ANGIOGENESIS AND STIMULATE LYMPHOCYTE INDUCED ANGIOGENESIS

Slawomir Majewski[1], Andrzej Szmurlo[1], Maria Marczak[1], Magdalena Malejczyk[1], Maria Noszczyk[1], Werner Bollag[2] and Stefania Jablonska[1]

[1]Department of Dermatology
Warsaw School of Medicine
Koszykowa 82a
02-008 Warsaw
Poland
[2]Pharmaceutical Research
F. Hoffmann-La-Roche Ltd.
CH-4002 Basle
Switzerland

INTRODUCTION

The growth of solid tumors requires a vascular supply, formed in the process of tumor-induced angiogenesis (TIA) (Folkman, 1990). TIA is an active sprouting of capillaries and new blood vessel formation due to some tumor cell-derived angiogenic factors capable of stimulating endothelial cell proliferation and migration (Folkman and Klagsburn, 1987). TIA was shown to precede or accompany malignancy not only in various experimental systems (Bouck, 1990) but also in natural human tumors of the cervix, skin, breast and bladder (Folkman, 1990). The presence of newly formed blood vessels on the surface of the cervix can indicate an underlying but invisible tumor (Sillman, et al., 1981). Quantitation, either by routine histology or immunohistochemistry, of the number of blood vessels on tissue sections of breast carcinoma was shown to be useful for estimation of relapse-free survival rate (Weidner et al., 1992) and probability of the metastatic disease (Horak et al., 1992).

Various experimental strategies that limit tumor angiogenesis were also shown to slow or abrogate tumor growth (Maione and Sharpe, 1990). Since most of the known inhibitors of angiogenesis exhibit also severe host toxicity, new less toxic antiangiogenic agents might be useful in the clinical practice. One group of such candidate compounds could be retinoids, shown in our previous studies to be strong angiogenic inhibitors (Majewski et al., 1986; Majewski et al., 1989; Rudnicka et al., 1991). Another group of compounds of special interest are interferons, which are capable of inhibiting TIA without major toxic effects (Sidky and Borden 1987).

The aim of the present study was to compare antiangiogenic and antiproliferative activity of various retinoids, interferon α-2a and their combinations in an in vivo model of cutaneous angiogenesis in the mouse. We also studied an immunomodulatory properties of these compounds by means of lymphocyte-induced angiogenesis assay in the same mouse system.

MATERIAL AND METHODS

Cells

Skv keratinocytes were established from vulvar intraepithelial neoplasia and were found to harbor integrated HPVI6 DNA sequences (Schneider-Maunoury et al., 1987; 1990). In vivo (in nude mice) and in vitro propagation of Skv cells led to selection of weakly tumorigenic Skv-el and Skv-11 parental lines and their tumorigenic Skv-e2 and Skv-12 counterparts. In addition we used HeLa cells harboring HPVI8 DNA. The cells were grown in vitro in a standard MEM with 10% FCS. The cell proliferation was studied by direct cell counting after trypsin/EDTA detachment.

Tumor cell-induced angiogenesis (TIA) and lymphocyte-induced angiogenesis (LIA)

We used previously described method (Sidky and Auerbach 1975) with some modifications (Majewski et al., 1984). In brief, Balb/c female mice were X-ray immunosuppressed and injected intradermally with human cell lines or with freshly isolated human peripheral blood mononuclear cells (PBMC). Three days after cell injection the mice were killed, their skin was prepared from the underlying muscles and the angiogenic reaction was evaluated at the inner surface of the skin by counting newly formed blood vessels at the site of cell injection (Sidky and Auerbach 1975). In order to study anti-angiogenic potential of retinoids (all-trans RA, 9-cis RA, 13-cis RA) and

IFNα-2a, these compounds were administered i.p. at the doses 2.5mg/kg and 5,000 U/kg, respectively, for 5 consecutive days before angiogenesis induction.

RESULTS

We found that IFNα-2a and all retinoids tested markedly inhibited angiogenesis induced by tumorigenic human cells (in Table 1 it is shown for tumorigenic HeLa cells, but similar results were obtained with other tumorigenic cells, i.e. Skv-e2 and Skv-12 lines). Combined administration of retinoids and IFNα-2a led to a synergistic inhibition of TIA. None of the retinoids significantly inhibited angiogenesis induced by nontumorigenic cells (data not shown).

Table 1. The effects of retinoids, IFNα-2a and their combinations on angiogenic capability of HPV18 harboring cell line.

Treatment of the mice with:	Angiogenesis (mean number ± SD of newly formed blood vessels)
Vehiculum	27.8 ± 2.3 (46)
IFNα-2a	21.5 ± 3.3 (41)
Trans RA	22.7 ± 5.1 (20)
9-cis RA	24.1 ± 3.2 (15)
13-cis RA	19.7 ± 2.3 (13)
IFNα-2a + Trans RA	14.9 ± 3.0 (8)
IFNα-2a + 9-cis RA	16.0 ± 2.0 (20)
IFNα-2a + 13-cis RA	15.1 ± 2.3 (14)

All group different from the control at p<0.01. In parentheses numbers of i.d. injections of HeLa cells.

The retinoids given systemically into the mice slightly stimulated (p<0.05) angiogenesis induced by i.d. injection of PBMC from 15 healthy individuals (not shown). Studies on the effect of retinoids (10^{-7}M) and IFNα-2a on cell growth in vitro also revealed differences in relation to tumorigenicity of the cells. The nontumorigenic Skv cells were more sensitive to the inhibitory effect of retinoids as compared to the tumorigenic counterpart cells. IFNα-2a in combination with retinoids had an synergistic inhibitory effect on proliferation of nontumorigenic Skv cells (Table 2).

Table 2.The effects of retinoids, IFNα-2a and their combination on the proliferation of HPV16-harboring keratinocytes.

Cell treatment	Proliferation inhibition (%) of:	
	Skv-11 (nontu)	Skv-12 (tu)
IFNα-2a	27*	43*
Trans RA	4	2
9-cis RA	23*	0
13-cis RA	31*	16
IFNα-2a + Trans RA	37*	36*
IFNα-2a + 9-cis RA	40*	36*
IFNα-2a + 13-cis RA	44*	44*

* Significantly different form the control at least at $p<0.05$

DISCUSSION

The exact mechanism of the synergistic anti-TIA effect of retinoids and IFNα-2a is not known, but it could be due to a decrease of angiokine production by tumor cells or to inhibition of endothelial cell proliferation. The synergistic effects of retinoids and IFNα-2a on TIA and on tumor cell proliferation, as well as immunostimulatory activity of these compounds (as manifested by increased LIA) could explain, in part, the high efficacy of combined therapy of advanced cutaneous and cervical HPV-associated carcinomas (Lippman et al., 1992a; 1992b).

REFERENCES

Bouck, N., 1990, Tumor angiogenesis: the role of oncogenes and tumor suppressor genes, *Cancer Cells* 2:179.

Folkman, J., 1990, What is the evidence that tumors are angiogenesis dependent? J. *Natl. Cancer Inst.* 82:4.

Folkman, J., Klagsburn, M., 1987, Angiogenic factors, *Science* 235:442.

Horak, E.R., Leek, R., Klenk N., 1992, Angiogenesis, assessed by platelet/endothelial cell adhesion molecules, as indicator of node metastases and survival in breast cancer, *Lancet* 340:1120.

Lippman, S.M., Parkinson, D.R., Itri, L.M., Weber, R.S., Schantz, S.P., Ota, D.M., Schusterman, M.A., Krakoff, I.H., Gutterman, J.U., Hong, W.K., 1992, 13-cis retinoic acid and interferon α-2a: effective combination therapy for advanced squamous cell carcinoma of the skin, *J Natl Cancer Inst.* 84:235.

Lippman, S.M., Kavanagh, J.J., Paredes-Espinoza, M., Delgadillo-Madrueno, F., Paredes-Casillas, P., Hong, W.K., Holdener, E.E., Krakoff, I.H., 1992. 13-cis retinoic acid plus interferon α-2a: highly active systemic therapy for squamous cell carcinoma of the cervix, *J Natl Cancer Inst.* 84:241.

Maione, T.E., Sharpe, R.J., 1990, Development of angiogenesis inhibitors for clinical applications, *TIPS* 11:457.

Majewski, S., Kaminski, M., Szmurlo, A., Kaminska, G., Malejczyk, J., 1984, Inhibition of tumour-induced angiogenesis by systemically administered protamine sulphate, *Int J Cancer* 33:831.

Majewski, S., Polakowski,I, Marczak, M., Jablonska, S., 1986, The effects of retinoids on lymphocyte- and transformed cell line-induced angiogenesis, *Clin Exp Dermatol.* 2:317.

Majewski, S., Marczak, M., Jablonska S., Rudnicka, L., 1989, Effects of retinoids on angiogenesis and on the proliferation of endothelial cells in vitro, *in:* "Pharmacology of Retinoids in the Skin", U. Reichert, B. Shroot, ed., Karger, Basle, pp.94.

Rudnicka, L., Marczak, M., Szmurlo, A., Makiela, B., Skiendzielewska, A., Majewski, S., Jablonska, S., 1991, Acitretin decreases tumor cell-induced angiogenesis, *Skin Pharmacol.* 4:150.

Schneider-Maunoury, S., Croissant, O., Orth, G., 1987, Integration of human papillomavirus type 16 DNA sequences: a possible early event in the progression of genital tumors, *J Virol.* 61:3295.

Schneider-Maunoury, S., Pehau-Arnaudet, G., Breitburd, F., Orth, G., 1990, Expression of the human papillomavirus type 16 genome in SK-v cells, a line derived from a vulvar intraepithelial neoplasia, *J Gen Virol.* 71: 809.

Sidky, Y.A., Borden, E.C., 1987, Inhibition of angiogenesis by interferons: effects on tumor- and lymphocyte-induced vascular responses, *Cancer Res.* 47:5155.

Sidky, Y.A., Auerbach, R., 1975, Lymphocyte-induced angiogenesis: A quantitative and sensitive assay of the graft- vs-host reaction, *J Exp Med.* 141:1084.

Sillman, F., Boyce, J.,and Fruchter, R., 1981, The significance of atypical vessels and neovascularization in cervical neoplasia, *Am J Obstet Gynecol.* 139:154.

Weidner, N., Folkman, J., Pozza, F., Bevilacqua, P., Allred, E.N., Moore, D.H., Meli, S., Gasparini, G., 1992, Tumor angiogenesis: a new significant and independent prognostic indicator in early-stage breast carcinoma, *J Natl Cancer Inst.* 84:1875.

RELEASE OF SOLUBLE TUMOR NECROSIS FACTOR-α (TNF-α) RECEPTOR BY HPV-ASSOCIATED NEOPLASTIC CELLS

Jacek Malejczyk,[1] Magdalena Malejczyk,[2] Slawomir Majewski,[2] Anna Hyc,[1] Françoise Breitburd,[3] Gerard Orth,[3] and Stefania Jablonska[2]

[1]Department of Histology and Embryology, Warsaw Medical School
Chalubinskiego 5, PL-02004 Warsaw, Poland
[2]Department of Dermatology, Warsaw Medical School
Koszykowa 82a, PL-02008 Warsaw, Poland
[3]Unité des Papillomavirus, Institut Pasteur
25 rue du Dr. Roux, F-75724 Paris-Cédex 15, France

INTRODUCTION

There is a growing evidence that immunological system is involved in surveillance against HPV-associated neoplasia.[1] The immune mechanisms responsible for eradication of HPV-induced tumors may include direct participation of natural killer (NK) cells,[2] activated macrophages,[3] and cytotoxic T lymphocytes.[4] Furthermore, growth and dissemination of potentially malignant lesions may be under control of locally released immunoregulatory anti-tumor cytokines including interferons,[5] interieukin-6,[6] transforming growth factor-ß,[7] as well as tumor necrosis factor-α (TNF-α).[8]

TNF-α is a pluripotent immunoregulatory cytokine displaying cytotoxic or cytostatic effect against a variety of tumor cell lines.[9] Recently, we have found that it is spontaneously expressed and released by a non-tumorigenic SKv keratinocyte cell line harboring and expressing integrated HPV16 DNA sequences.[8] TNF-α released by SKv cells exerted an autocrine growth limiting effect upon their growth[8] and upregulated in an autocrine manner expression of an intercellular adhesion molecule-1 (ICAM-1).[10] Expression of ICAM-1 has been found to be necessary for SKv cell lysis by NK cells (M. Malejczyk et al., unpublished observation), it is therefore possible that endogenous TNF-α may also play an important part in induction of susceptibility of HPV-transformed cells to cell-mediated cytotoxic responses.

Immunology of Human Papillomaviruses
Edited by M.A. Stanley, Plenum Press, New York, 1994

It is possible that tumorigenic progression of HPV-transformed neoplastic cells is, at least partially, associated with an escape from under local and systemic immune and cytokine surveillance. Accordingly, SKv cell lines displaying high tumorigenic potential in nude mice were found to be resistant to antiproliferative effect of endogenous TNF-α.[11] The mechanism of escape of SKv cells and possibly other HPV-transformed neoplastic cells from under endogenous TNF-α-mediated surveillance is unclear. It may be related to a decreased expression of TNF-α receptors (TNF-αR),[10,11] as well as to spontaneous release of soluble TNF-αR (sTNF-αR) displaying TNF-α neutralizing activity.[12] Therefore, the aim of the study was to evaluate shedding of sTNF-αR by different SKv cell lines and the levels of circulating sTNF-αR in sera of patients suffering from lesions induced by different types of HPV.

MATERIALS AND METHODS

Patients

The study included three groups of patients: (i) 25 patients with condylomata accuminata (CA) associated with HPV6 and 11; (ii) 17 patients with skin warts (SW) associated mostly with HPV1, 2, and 3 including 3 renal allograft recipient persons; and (iii) 7 patients with epidermodysplasia verruciformis (EV) associated with EV-specific HPVs, mainly HPV5 and 8. As control served 32 sex- and age-mached healthy persons displaying no detectable symptoms of HPV infection.

SKv cell lines

SKv keratinocytes were established from vulvar intraepithelial neoplasia and were found to harbor integrated HPV16 DNA sequences and to express HPV16 E6 and E7 oncoproteins.[13,14] In the present study we used two distinct SKv cell types, SKv-e and SKv-l cells, differing in an arrangement of HPV16 DNA integration.[13] Both groups of SKv cells were represented by weakly tumorigenic SKv-e1 and SKv-l1 parental lines as well as their respective highly tumorigenic SKv-e2 and SKv-l2 derivates. Tumorigenic potential of all tested SKv cell sublines was confirmed by their transplantation into the nude mice. The cells were propagated *in vitro* in MEM supplemented with 10% FCS, 2 mM L-glutamine, 10 mM HEPES, and antibiotics as described elsewhere.[8] For generation of SKv cell-conditioned media (CM), the cells were cultured for 48 h and then the cell-free supernatants were harvested and stored frozen until used.

Evaluation of cell-associated TNF-αR expression by SKv cells

Expression of cell-associated TNF-αR by different SKv cell sublines was estimated by ^{125}I-TNF-α binding assay as described.[8] Briefly, the cells were incubated with different concentrations of ^{125}I-TNF-α (Amersham International, Buckinghamshire, UK) and the radioactivity bound to the cells was evaluated in a gamma-counter. Nonspecific binding was determined in the presence of 100 fold molar excess of unlabeled TNF-α and was substracted. The number of TNF-αR per cell was then calculated by Scatchard analysis.

Evaluation of sTNF-αR

Evaluations of type I sTNF-αR in SKv CM and patients' sera were performed by means of specific enzyme-linked immunobiological assay (ELIBA) ready-to-use kits (kindly offered by Drs. N. Drees and H. Gallati of the Hoffmann-La Roche, Basel, Switzerland), according to the attached protocols.

SKv cell proliferation assay

To evaluate effect of sTNF-R on growth of SKv keratinocyte sublines, the cells were cultured in replicate wells of 24-well tissue culture plates with or without human recombinant (r) type I and II sTNF-αR (kindly supplied by Drs. N. Drees and H. Gallati, Hoffman-La Roche, Basel, Switzerland). The cell number increase was then evaluated by cell counting in Bürker's chamber after 48 h of culture.

Table 1. Expression of cell-associated TNF-αR and spontaneous release of type I sTNF-αR by different SKv cell lines.

	Number of TNF-αR/cell[1]	Amount of sTNF-αRI in CM (ng/10^7 cells)[2]	sTNF-αRI/membrane TNF-αR ratio
SKv-e cells			
SKv-e1	11,000	3.72 ± 0.24	3.38
SKv-e2	3,000	3.34 ± 0.32	11.13
SKv-1 cells			
SKv-l1	18,000	5.69 ± 0.35	3.16
SKv-l2	9,000	11.81 ± 0.27[3]	13.12

[1]Approximated number calculated from 3 independent experiments.
[2]Results are mean ± SE obtained from evaluation of 3 different CM preparations.
[3]Significantly higher ($P < 0.05$) by Student-t test as compared to SKv-l1 cells.

RESULTS

Accordingly to our recent observations,[10,11] TNF-α binding assay has revealed that highly tumorigenic SKv cells expressed significantly lower number of TNF-αR than their weakly tumorigenic parental lines (Table 1). Analysis of spontaneous shedding of TNF-αR by different SKv cell lines showed that CM from all tested sublines contained sTNF-αRI. No type II sTNF-αR were detected. Relative sTNF-αRI release rate was similar in weakly tumorigenic parental SKv-e1 and SKv-l1 lines and was considerably higher in highly tumorigenic SKv-e2 and SKv-l2 cells (Table 1).

To evaluate whether sTNF-αR may influence growth of SKv cells they were cultured in the presence of an excess of rsTNF-αRI or rsTNF-αRII. As seen in Figure 1, both types of sTNF-αR significantly stimulated growth of weakly tumorigenic SKv-e1 and SKv-l1 cells while having little or no effect on highly tumorigenic SKv-e2 and SKv-l2 cells. Furthermore, both sTNF-αR stimulated growth of weakly tumorigenic cells up to the level of highly tumorigenic ones.

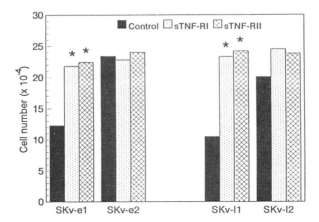

Figure 1. Effect of human rsTNF-αRI and rsTNF-αRII on proliferation of SKv cells. SKv cells were cultured in the presence of 1 ng/ml of each type of sTNF-αR and their number was evaluated after 48 h. The cells in medium alone served as control. * - Stimulation statistically significant at least at $P < 0.05$ by Student-t test.

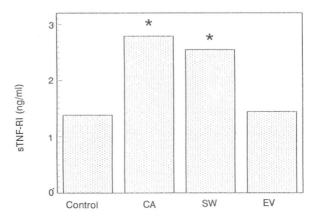

Figure 2. Detection of type I sTNF-αR in sera of patients suffering from different HPV-associated lesions. * - The amount of sTNF-αR significantly higher ($P < 0.05$) as compared to control healthy persons by Student-t test.

Evaluation of sera from patients with CA showed the significantly increased levels of circulating sTNF-αRI (Figure 2). In this group, the highest amounts of sTNF-αRI were detected in patients with long lasting reccurrent lesions. An elevated levels of sTNF-αRI were also detected in SW patients, this, however, could be due to the very high amounts of circulating receptors in renal transplant recipients. On the contrary, the levels of circulating sTNF-αRI in patients with EV were in normal range.

DISCUSSION

Results of the present work show that HPV16-harboring SKv keratinocytes spontaneously release type I but not typeII sTNF-αR and this is consistent with an observation that keratinocytes express exclusively TNF-αRI.[8,15] Spontaneous shedding of sTNF-αR was also observed in case of other tumor cell lines[16] suggesting that this phenomenon may be a common feature of some neoplastic cells. A relative rate of shedding of sTNF-αRI by SKv cells was increased in highly tumorigenic lines. Inasmuch as sTNF-αR display TNF-α neutralizing ability, their increased shedding may contribute to tumorigenic progression of HPV-transformed cells. Accordingly, rsTNF-αR significantly stimulated growth of weakly tumorigenic SKv cell lines suggesting that these molecules may enable HPV-harboring cell escape from under autocrine TNF-α growth limitation.

It has been reported that sera of patients suffering from different types of cancer contained the increased levels of both types of sTNF-αR, and the amounts of circulating receptors correlated with the severity of the disease.[16] In the present study, we demonstrated elevated amounts of sTNF-αRI in sera of patients with benign CA and patients with SW. The reason of increased levels of sTNF-αRI in sera of these patients is unknown, however, it cannot be excluded that they may be, at least partially, a result of shedding from HPV-harboring cells. Inasmuch as the highest levels of circulating receptors were found in heavily immunosuppressed patients, it is possible, that the presence of circulating sTNF-R may be a factor that promote persistance and dissemination of the lesions. The prognostic value of the circulating sTNF-αR in some HPV-associated disorders remains, however, to be elucidated.

Surprisingly, in EV patients in spite of immunosuppression sTNF-αRI levels were in normal range. These people are heavily infected with EV-specific HPVs, and the lesions were found to produce large amonts of TNF-α[17] and displayed high level of TNF-αR expression (S. Majewski, unpublished observation). It is conceivable that local interactions of TNF-α with its cellular and soluble receptors are responsible for not increased levels of sTNR-αRI in the circulation.

Acknowledgments

This study was supported by the Warsaw Medical School Grants D14 and VId/2.

REFERENCES

1. S. Jablonska, S. Majewski, and J. Malejczyk, Die Immunologie von HPV-Infektionen und der Mechanismus einer latenten Infektion, *Hautarzt* 43:305 (1992).
2. J. Malejczyk, S. Majewski, S. Jablonska, T.T. Rogozinski, and G. Orth, Abrogated NK-cell lysis of human papillomavirus (HPV)-16-bearing keratinocytes in patients with pre-cancerous and cancerous HPV-induced anogenital lesions, *Int. J. Cancer* 43:209 (1989).

3. L. Banks, F. Moreau, K. Voudsen, D. Pim, and G. Matlashewski, Expression of the human papillomavirus E7 oncogene during cell transformation is sufficient to induce susceptibility to lysis by activated macrophages. *J. Immunol.* 146:2037 (1991).

4. L. Chen, M.T. Mizuno, M.C. Singhal, S.-L. Hu, D.A. Galloway, I. Hellström, and K.E. Hellström, Induction of cytotoxic T lymphocytes specific for a syngeneic tumor expressing E6 oncoprotein of human papillomavirus type 16, *J. Immunol.* 148:2617 (1992).

5. K.F. Trofatter, Interferon treatment of anogenital human papillomavirus-related diseases. *Dermatol Clin.* 9:343 (1991).

6. J. Malejczyk, M. Malejczyk, A. Urbanski, A. Köck, S. Jablonska, G. Orth, and T.A. Luger, Constitutive release of IL-6 by human papillomavirus type 16 (HPV16)-harboring keratinocytes: a mechanism augmenting the NK-cell-mediated lysis of HPV-bearing cells. *Cell. Immunol.* 136:155 (1991).

7. C.D. Woodworth, V. Notario, and J.A. DiPaolo, Transforming growth factors beta 1 and 2 transcriptionally regulate human papillomavirus (HPV) type 16 early gene expression in HPV-immortalized human genital epithelial cells. *J. Virol.* 64:4767 (1990).

8. J. Malejczyk, M. Malejczyk, A. Köck, A. Urbanski, S. Majewski, N. Hunzelmann, S. Jablonska, G. Orth, and T.A. Luger, Autocrine growth limitation of human papillomavirus type 16-harboring keratinocytes by constitutively released tumor necrosis factor-α. *J. Immunol.* 149:2702 (1992).

9. B. Beutler and A. Cerami, The biology of cachectin/TNF - a primary mediator of the host response, *Ann. Rev. Immunol.* 7:625 (1989).

10. S. Majewski, M. Skopinska, M. Malejczyk, F. Breitburd, G. Orth, S. Jablonska, and J. Malejczyk, Spontaneous expression of intercellular adhesion molecule 1 and tumorigenic progression of human papillomavirus type 16-harboring keratinocytes: a relationship to autocrine regulation by tumor necrosis factor α, Submitted for publication.

11. J. Malejczyk, M. Malejczyk, S. Majewski, F. Breitburd, T.A. Luger, S. Jablonska, and G. Orth, Increased tumorigenicity of human papillomavirus type 16-harboring keratinocytes is associated with resistance to endogenous tumor necrosis factor-α-mediated growth limitation, *Int. J. Cancer*, in press.

12. J. Malejczyk, M. Malejczyk, F. Breitburd, S. Majewski, A. Urbanski, N. Expert-Besançon, S. Jablonska, G. Orth, and T.A. Luger, Progressive growth of human papillomavirus type 16-harboring keratinocytes is associated with spontaneous release of soluble TNF-α receptor/TNF-α inhibitor. Submitted for publication.

13. S. Schneider-Maunoury, O. Croissant, and G. Orth, Integration of human papillomavirus type 16 DNA sequences: a possible early event in the progression of genital tumors. *J. Virol.* 61:3295 (1987).

14. S. Schneider-Maunoury, G. Pehau-Arnaudet, F. Breitburd, and G. Orth, Expression of the human papillomavirus type 16 genome in SK-v cells, a line derived from vulvar intraepithelial neoplasia. *J. Gen. Virol.* 71:809 (1990).

15. U. Trefzer, M. Brockhaus, H. Loetscher, F. Parlow, A. Kapp, E. Schöpf, and J. Krutmann, 55-kd tumor necrosis factor receptor is expressed by human keratinocytes and plays a pivotal role in regulation of human keratinocyte ICAM-1 expression, *J. Invest. Dermatol.* 97:911 (1991).

16. D. Aderka, H. Engelmann, V. Wernik, Y. Skornick, Y. Levo, D. Wallach, and G. Kushtal, Increased serum levels of soluble receptors for tumor necrosis factor in cancer patients, *Cancer Res.* 51:5602 (1991).

17. S. Majewski, N. Hunzelmann, R. Nischt, B. Eckes, L. Rudnicka, G. Orth, T. Krieg, and S. Jablonska, TGFß-1 and TNFα expression in the epidermis of patients with epidermodysplasia verruciformis, *J. Invest. Dermatol.* 97:862 (1991).

CONTRIBUTORS INDEX

SUBJECT INDEX